The Desktop Guide to
Herbal Medicine

*The Ultimate Multidisciplinary Reference
to the Amazing Realm of Healing Plants,
in a Quick-Study, One-Stop Guide*

BRIGITTE MARS, A.H.G.

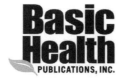

**Basic
Health**
PUBLICATIONS, INC.

The information contained in this book is intended to educate, delight, and expand your under-standing of the healthful and beautiful herbs that grace this planet and to empower you to take responsibility for your own health. In cases of serious health concerns, please see a qualified health-care professional.

The publisher does not advocate the use of any particular healthcare protocol but believes the information in this book should be available to the public. The publisher and author are not responsible for any adverse effects or consequences resulting from the use of the suggestions, preparations, or procedures discussed in this book. Should the reader have any questions con-cerning the appropriateness of any procedures or preparation mentioned, the author and the publisher strongly suggest consulting a professional healthcare advisor.

Basic Health Publications, Inc.
28812 Top of the World Drive
Laguna Beach, CA 92651
Phone: 949-715-7327 • www.basichealthpub.com

Library of Congress Cataloging-in-Publication Data

Mars, Brigitte.
    The desktop guide to herbal medicine : the ultimate multidisciplinary reference to the amazing realm of healing plants, in a quick-study, one-stop guide / Brigitte Mars.
        p. cm.
    Includes bibliographical references and index.
    ISBN 978-1-59120-193-9
    1. Herbs—Therapeutic use—Handbooks, manuals, etc. I. Title.

    RM666.H33M3666   2007
    615'.321—dc22

                                                                2007005889

Editor: Nancy Ringer
Typesetter/Book design: Gary A. Rosenberg
Cover design: Mike Stromberg

Printed in the United States of America

10   9   8   7   6   5   4   3   2   1

Contents

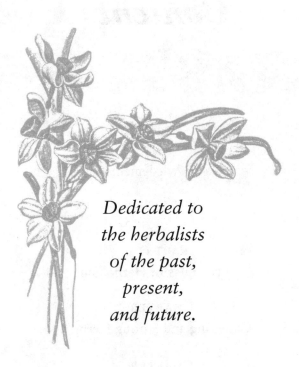

*Dedicated to
the herbalists
of the past,
present,
and future.*

Acknowledgments

My heartfelt thanks go out to my publisher, Norman Goldfind, who has always supported my work in bringing the message of good health to the people of our planet.

Nancy Ringer, editor extraordinaire, you have so many amazing skills for which I am always grateful. Many thanks to Carol and Gary Rosenberg for their editing, typesetting, and artistic skills.

Thanks always to Rosita Arvigo, Beth Baugh, Matthew Becker, Mark Blumenthal, Jane Bothwell, Mary Bove, Chanchal Cabrerra, Diana Diluca, Ann Drucker, Cascade Anderson Geller, Rosemary Gladstar, Mindy Green, Christopher Hobbs, David Hoffman, Juliano, Sara Katz, Kathi Keville, Henriette Kress, Laura Lamun, Alicia Bay Laurel, Rob McCaleb, Pamela Montgomery, Cynthia Pileggi, Jermey Safron, Debra St. Claire, Rick Scalzo, Farida Sharan, "Herbal Ed" Smith, Jill Stansbury, Lesley Tierra, Michael Tierra, Roy Upton, Susun Weed, Dr. Roger Wicke, David Winston, David Wolfe, and my herbally oriented sons-in-law, Mitch Stegall and Dr. Christopher Daugherty (daymaker); you are all beautiful and beloved! Thanks to Sam Fuqua, Ned McCrumb, Kaylene Proctor, and the gang at Pharmaca for their special help. Much honor to the late greats Terrence Mckenna, William Lesassier, Dr. John Christopher, Dr. Alfred Vogel, and Jeanine Parvati Baker.

Tom Pfeiffer, you have helped me in a thousand and one ways for more than thirty years. Rainbeau Harmony Mars and Sunflower Sparkle Mars, you make my life amazing! Much love.

Introduction

reetings and radiant blessings,
Herbal medicine has been with us since the beginning, one of the many aspects of humankind's symbiotic relationship with the natural world. It is the most time-tested healing tradition in the world, having evolved over hundreds of thousands of years in disparate regions and diverse cultures. Research into the amazing health benefits of the plant world will certainly continue, but herbal medicine has already benefited millions of people over the centuries. That's a lot more than prescription drugs can claim!

As a practitioner of herbal healing for more than thirty-five years, having witnessed how herbs improve the health of our planet's population every day, I feel a deep enthusiasm and appreciation for the plant world. When we begin to work with plants as healing allies, we improve our health, and we also empower ourselves to take charge of our health. In a time when treatment is still valued over prevention, when the technology of medicine can outstrip our ethical understanding of it, and when treatment options can be decided by insurance administrators, taking control of our own health is vital.

Herbal medicine is not a "diagnose and treat" program. It is a holistic approach to maintaining a vibrant, energetic, balanced state of being that is best practiced every day. When illness or injury occur, the goal is to treat the source of the problem, rather than the symptoms, by helping the body call up its own healing mechanisms. Most plant medicines work gently in this manner, but some are strong and sometimes harsh. Ailment is matched to therapy: when gentle measures will do, gentle measures can be taken, but when aggressive therapy is needed, the plant world stands at the ready. And when herbal medicine is woven together with the scientific wonders of Western medicine, treatment possibilities are unparalleled.

Practicing herbal medicine on a daily basis encourages us to focus on not only the maintenance of our own health but also that of our planet. When we bring herbs into our lives, we tend to become glad custodians of the earth, eager to protect and nurture the vast potential of the natural world around us. We learn that existence in all forms is about balance: In order to benefit from the natural world, we must also benefit it. When we nurture the plants, they are able to nurture us.

This book is intended to be a companion in the pursuit of a natural balance: the study, prescription, and use of herbs to achieve vibrant health, mitigate illness, and correct physiological imbalances, in ourselves and in the world at large. May it fill you with knowledge that is practical, helpful, and healthful. And may your countenance blossom with radiance and health.

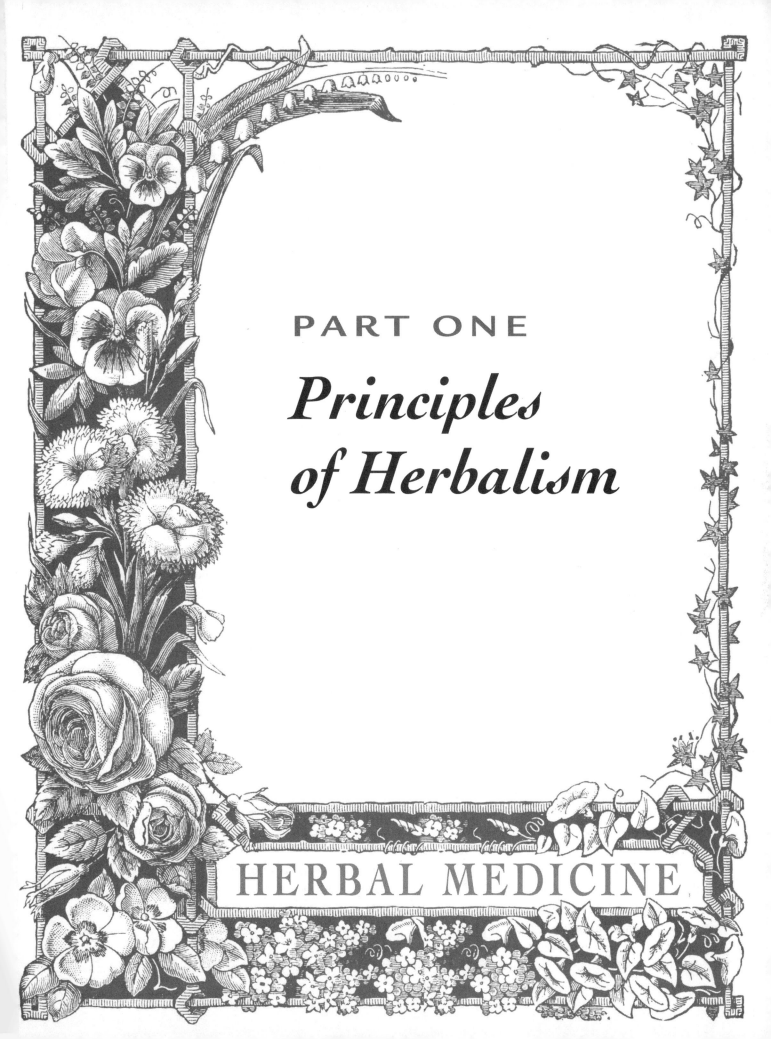

PART ONE

Principles of Herbalism

HERBAL MEDICINE

1. *Gathering and Storing Herbs*

athering herbs is a great adventure, whether you purchase herbs from a retail outlet or head out into the wilds to collect them yourself. The following guidelines will help guide you along the way. With good humor at the ready and good study under your belt, finding the herbs you need, and storing them so that they last, can be an aromatic, textural, and visual treat!

SHOPPING FOR HERBS

Herb shops are fun places. If you don't have one near you, many offer their wares online (see the resources at the end of this book). The staff are usually quite friendly, enjoying the company of both people and plants. When asked for assistance they can instruct you on how to bag up the herbs you want, whether the price code needs to be marked on the bag, and any other procedures that are not clearly posted in the area. Sometimes the shops offer workshops on using herbs, which can be tremendously helpful in the study of herbal medicine. The more experience you can get, the better!

Do your best to seek out organically cultivated herbs. Not only do they have the most healing properties (pesticides are designed to destroy, not heal), but organic cultivation is healthier for the planet and creatures that live upon it. Sometimes you may find supplies of *wildcrafted* herbs; these are herbs that have been collected from the wild. If you use wildcrafted plants, be sure they were harvested in a sustainable method that respects the environment and ensures the continuation of that species. Avoid using plants that are endangered or at risk.

Dried herbs should look and smell almost like the fresh product. Look for good color. An herb that was originally green when fresh should not look like yellow straw when dried. Bright golden calendula flowers should still show their hue. Nettles should still be bright green.

WILDCRAFTING

Learning to wildcraft, or collect wild plants, in your own neck of the woods will greatly enhance your pleasure in practicing herbal medicine, as well as your sense of connection to the earth.

The most important rule of wildcrafting is to make sure you collect the proper species. Some plants have poisonous lookalikes. Be especially careful with mushrooms, as a mistake can easily be fatal. Also be sure to collect the correct plant part—for example, blue elderberries are wonderful, but the leaves are toxic. And know that animals have different physiologies; just because an animal eats a plant doesn't mean it is safe for humans to ingest.

Avoid collecting plants within 50 feet of a busy road, in areas that are sprayed with herbicides or pesticides, or in areas known to be polluted or contaminated. Ask permission before gathering on private land.

Any known endangered species must be left alone; do not harvest it from the wild. With any species, identify the grandfather/mother plant in a stand of plants—it's usually the largest or the first to flower—and leave it to ensure the continuation of the strongest of the species. Never take more than 10 percent of what's there. Vary the places you collect from.

Collect plants in a way to ensure the continued

survival of the species. If all you need are the leaves and flowers, take only some tops from the plants; cutting back plants in this manner can actually help promote new growth. You might also thin plants growing together, as you would thin plants in your garden, to give the other plants more room. If you're collecting roots, which will destroy the plants, plant ripe seeds in the hole you've dug and fill the holes with soil.

If possible, spray or water plants the day before you harvest them to clean any extra dirt or debris off them. Gather leaves and flowers in the morning, after the dew has risen and before the sun is too hot.

The part of the plant you want to harvest usually determines the time of the year when you should collect it:

- **Leaves** are best taken just as the plant begins to flower, when its energy is still in the leaves.

- **Flowers** are best taken when they are just starting to open.

- **Fruit** (such as rose hips) is best when it is fully ripe, and seeds are best when they are fully ripe and dry.

- **Bark** is best collected in the spring or fall. If taken after a spell of damp weather, bark will separate more easily. Never girdle (remove the bark from all the way around) a tree, as this will impair the sap's ability to rise.

- **Roots** generally are ideal in the fall, after the plant has completed its cycle and the life force of the plant goes back into its roots and inner bark. Biennial or perennial roots can also be collected in the spring of the second year. There are exceptions, of course. Echinacea is harvested only after three years and ginseng after seven years. Scrub roots well after collecting them.

- **Gums** and **resins** are best collected in hot, dry weather.

Leaves and flowers are usually collected during the time of the full moon. Roots are said to be best when collected during the time of the new moon.

Ask permission from and give thanks to the herbs you gather. My friend Debra St. Clare likes to remind people, "Bless it before you pick it." Sing while collecting! Be joyful!

DRYING HERBS

Drying herbs makes them available all year round. When herbs are dried, their cell walls break down, which enables the properties of the plants to be easily released when the herbs are rehydrated.

Dry herbs in the shade in a warm, well-ventilated area. They may be dried on a nylon or stainless-steel screen, in a shallow box, or loosely in a paper bag. (If you're drying the herbs in a paper bag, punch many holes in the bag for ventilation.) Some have found drying herbs in a paper bag in the backseat of the car very effective. You also can tie herbs in small bunches and string them up in an attic or warm room to dry. For herbs that contain a lot of moisture, I sometimes spread a clean sheet on the top floor (the hottest area of our home) and spread the herbs out on the sheets until they are dry. Cut large roots in half lengthwise to ensure quicker drying.

Most herbs dry in four to seven days. When leaves and flowers crumble between your fingers, that is a good indication they are dry enough; if they bend and remain flexible, they probably still contain moisture that needs to evaporate. To test a root for dryness, slice into it in a couple of places; if the root is dry to the touch in its center, it's ready to be stored. Storing undried herbs in a glass jar is likely to result in mold. A method to test for dryness is to seal a sample of herb in a small, dry, glass jar. If droplets of moisture appear on the lid, the herb's moisture content is still too high and the drying process must be resumed.

Store herbs as soon as they are fully dried. They don't need to become a collecting area for dust and cobwebs.

STORING HERBS

Whether your dried herbs were bought at the store or collected from your garden and dried in your attic, they must be stored properly. Clean, dry glass jars make the best herb storage containers. (Plastic does not make a good storage container, because it's permeable and does not protect the flavor of the herbs.) Be sure that the jars are completely dry—check for moisture especially under the rims—and remove any cardboard inner lid. Amber-colored glass bottles (I've used recycled bottles that some types of vitamins are sold in), which protect their contents from light, are great.

Light and heat deteriorate the quality of dried herbs. Many people make the mistake of storing their herbs out on a sunny windowsill or on top of the stove, where they degrade in quality quickly. Instead, keep teas in a cupboard, where they will be protected from light and heat, to better conserve their flavors and therapeutic properties.

Be sure to label your storage containers. Six months from now, it might be difficult to recognize catnip from oregano! I also like to write the Latin name of the plant on the storage label. After you've written and said them a few times, these beautiful, poetic names become part of your memories. It is also a good idea to write the date of when you purchased or dried the plant material.

Many herb books will tell you that dried leaves and flowers keep for one year and roots and barks for two to three years. However, taste, color, and smell are the most reliable indicators of potency. You may find that some herbs, when stored properly, keep for much longer. Nature provides more herbs every year, so ideally you should purchase or harvest no more than you are likely to use within the year.

2. *Making Herbal Medicines*

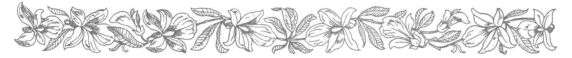

Hydrotherapy, as healing with water is known, has been around for as long as humankind. And why not? Water is an adaptable conductor of many types of energies, from electricity to magnetism to heat. It is also a solvent, capable of leaching constituents away from other compounds and carrying them in itself. In this way water, and its cousins alcohol and vegetable oils, are able to be infused with the properties of healing herbs.

It's simple to imagine how those properties can be transferred to the human body when we ingest the liquid formulation, such as with a tea or tincture. But those infused liquids are no less powerful when applied topically. The human skin not only is a barrier encasing and protecting the bones, organs, and tissues but also is a large organ of elimination and absorption. The pores of the skin release wastes through perspiration; they also take in constituents they come into contact with. Herb-infused liquids, therefore, when applied topically, give over to us the nutrients and healing elements they carry. Better yet, topical applications allow us to bring those constituents to the specific site where they are needed—to a wound via a compress, for example, or to an infection in the eye via an eyewash.

Following is some advice on making original herbal formulations, and after that brief descriptions of how to use such formulations in whatever form is necessary, from herb baths to teas, poultices, steam inhalations, and more.

MAKING YOUR OWN HERBAL FORMULAS

Years before the age of herbalists, people who lived close to the earth and used herbs for healing were called simplers. The lovely art of simpling is the use of a local mild herb over an extended period. Simpling is a great way to deeply connect with all the aspects of a plant's power and to learn more about the unique flavor and properties of that individual plant. One of my favorite simples is nettles.

But herbal medicines need not be limited to using a single plant at a time. Many wonderful medicines with great flavor and therapeutic potential can be made by blending herbs. When you are creating your own formulas by mixing herbs together, it is helpful to know as much as possible about their effects, and of course about any possible side effects, in order to evaluate their potential synergy. However, don't be afraid to play around with combinations of herbs that are generally regarded as safe. Contemplate the flavor, feeling, or healing property you want to create, and then get to work trying to create it.

It's fine to combine fresh and dried herbs in a formula. For example, dried store-bought cinnamon can be paired with fresh spearmint from the garden. You also can mix tea-bagged herbs with loose herbs, allowing them to steep together.

Formulation is not a rigid science—there are many different ways to create a formula, and a certain formula may have a different effect in different people. Skill comes with study and experience. The following points should help beginners get started:

- In general, a standard herbal formula consists of one part roots, two parts leaves, and three parts flowers and/or seeds.

- Ten percent of any herbal formula usually consists of a stimulating herb that will help transport the benefit of the other herbs to where it is needed. Some examples of stimulating carriers are angelica, cinnamon, cloves, and ginger.

• It may help to determine the main organ that needs help (for example, the skin) and then add herbs to support three systems that affect that organ (for example, the lungs, liver, and large intestine).

• Study the physiology of the health concern you want to address. Understand its energy, and understand the energy of the person experiencing the health concern. For example, a person who feels cold all the time may benefit from warming herbs like cinnamon and ginger, and an overly warm person might appreciate cooling herbs like peppermint and spearmint.

• See the whole being, not the health concern. A healthier lifestyle, in terms of emotional health, diet, and exercise, can do as much to encourage healing as an herbal therapeutic.

• Try to create formulas using a few herbs that cover several purposes. For example, ginger can warm a person who feels cold all the time, and it also will relieve his or her indigestion or rheumatism.

• When you're developing formulas, make small batches the first time around. Label each batch with its ingredients, its intended use, and the date of its creation. You don't want to serve up something fantastic and not be able to recreate such a pleasure! I love to purchase colorful label books from Dover Publications. They feature stick-on labels with angels, fairies, seasonal themes, antique themes, and more. When you have a blend you like, make up a fun or catchy name for it and add it to your recipe file.

BATHS

To prepare a bath with herbs, brew a strong batch of herb tea, using about $\frac{1}{2}$ cup of herbs in half a gallon of water and simmer for twenty minutes. Then strain the tea into the tub. You also can simply tie a handful of herbs in a dark-colored washcloth and throw it, or a few ready-made tea bags, into very hot running water as you fill the tub. When the water has reached the right level, turn it off and allow the herbs to steep in the bath while you floss or check your e-mail. When the bathwater has cooled to a comfortable temperature, get down into it. If you prepared the bath with the herb-filled cloth, use it to scrub your body as you deeply inhale the aromatherapeutic benefits. Close a curtain around the bath to hold in the scented steam.

COMPRESSES

Compresses are a way to use herbs topically to help heal wounds, inflammation, rashes, and skin infections; relieve pain, soreness, and spasms; improve circulation; and stimulate sweat glands and the lymphatic system.

To make a compress, soak a clean towel in hot or cold herb tea, then wring it out and apply the cloth to the area needing treatment. Cover the damp cloth with a dry towel to help it stay hot or cold. When the compress temperature changes (the hot cools down or the cold warms up), resoak the cloth in the tea and reapply. Repeat several times.

A hot compress increases circulation and is especially beneficial in cases of backache, arthritic pain, and sore throat. After the final hot compress cools down, apply a cool compress to the area briefly. Making the compress of hot ginger tea increases its potency.

A cold compress constricts blood flow and is best for hot, inflamed conditions such as swellings. When a cold-compress treatment is done, keep the treated area warm afterward to avoid chilling the person receiving treatment. Peppermint tea makes an extremely potent cold compress.

The best indicator of whether a hot or cold compress is needed is the opinion of the patient; he or she should be asked whether hot or cold would give the best relief. In some cases, both hot and cold are needed. For example, a headache is best resolved by a hot compress on the back of the neck and a cold compress on the forehead.

EYEWASHES

Eyewashes can be used to soothe tired, inflamed, and/or infected eyes. Some even claim they can improve vision. The washes causes the blood vessels of the eyes to contract and then relax. They are an excellent therapeutic practice for eyes that are getting lots of use from reading and sitting in front of a computer.

Herb teas used as eyewashes should be somewhat weaker than teas for ingestion. Use just 1 scant teaspoon of herb per cup of water, and simmer at a low boil for 10 minutes to assure sterility. Use a strainer with a very fine mesh to strain the tea to avoid getting particles of herbs in your eyes, and cool the tea to body temperature before administering.

To administer an eyewash, you'll need an eyecup, available at any pharmacy. Especially in cases of eye infections, it is important to sterilize the eyecup between uses either by running it through a dishwasher with a heated drying cycle or by bringing water to a boil, pouring it into the eyecup, and letting it sit for 1 minute.

Pour enough of the strained tea into the sterilized eyecup to fill it. Lean back and pour the mixture into one of your eyes, being sure to blink several times so the eye is well bathed. Repeat with the other eye.

Make eyewashes fresh for each day of use to avoid introducing bacteria into the eyes. If you're repeating treatment through the day, you can brew the tea in the morning and refrigerate any extra. Allow the refrigerated tea to reach room temperature before using it, and discard whatever is left over at the end of the day.

Use only those herbs that are recommended for eyewashes.

FACIAL STEAMS

A facial steam is an excellent way to deeply cleanse your skin, relax facial muscles, and improve circulation, all the while giving yourself an invigorating rosy glow. It's a lovely treatment to indulge in before a special party or when you want to look your best. At most, facial steams should be done once or twice a week.

Undergoing a facial steam is like absorbing an herbal tea through the pores of your skin. First, wash your face. Then pour 1 quart of boiling water over a handful of herbs in a glass bowl. Tie back your hair. Lean over the bowl and drape a towel over your head. Keep your face about 10 inches away from the water to avoid getting burned. Inhale the sensuous steam for 5 to 7 minutes, lifting the towel to vent steam as necessary.

FOOT AND HAND BATHS

Many of the body's nerve endings are in the hands and feet, so hand and footbaths can feel especially delicious. They can lessen the symptoms of many conditions, such as arthrtis, colds, flu, and poor circulation.

Footbaths, in particular, can help improve conditions of the lungs, bladder, prostate, and uterus. They also can be very therapeutic in treating odoriferous and aching feet, as well as in helping to reduce cellulite, swelling, calluses, leg cramps, and varicose veins. And they are an excellent preventive treatment at the first signs of a cold, sore throat, headache, or congestion in the eyes and ears, as the heat draws congestion away from the respiratory system. Footbaths can, depending on the health concern being addressed and the ambient temperature, be hot or cold, or they can alternate between hot and cold. They are a lovely precursor to a foot massage, or better yet, you can massage the feet while soaking them.

To prepare the bath, make a standard herbal tea using about 1 gallon of water for a footbath or $\frac{1}{2}$ gallon for a hand bath. Strain out the herbs and pour the tea into a wide basin. Place your bare feet or hands in the basin, and enjoy the relaxing sensation until the water cools down. If you have a warm condition—inflammation, such as from a sprain, or fever or headache—a cool washcloth on the forehead can be a nice addition; refresh it every two to three minutes. Afterward, pour cold water over the top and bottom of your feet and hands, then dry the skin thoroughly.

An especially potent treatment is to soak your hands for 8 minutes in the morning and to soak your feet for 8 minutes in the evening. For children, half that amount of time is sufficient.

HAIR RINSES

A hair rinse is a wonderful treatment both therapeutically and cosmetically. Bring 1 quart of water to a boil and add 4 heaping teaspoons of your choice of herbs. Stir, cover, and let sit 1 hour. Strain into a large plastic squeeze bottle. Add 1 tablespoon apple cider vinegar. Pour the strained tea slowly over your hair. Don't rinse it out; just let it dry and enjoy the subtle radiance.

INFUSED OILS

Infused oils can be applied directly to the skin as a treatment. They also can be used as massage oils or as the base for salves.

It's preferable to use dried herbs in making infused oils, as moisture can cause the oil to become rancid more quickly. If you're using fresh herbs, allow them to wilt first, which will get rid of some of their moisture. Make sure all of your equipment is dry before getting started.

The infusion is usually prepared in one of three ways:

- Place the herbs in the top part of a double boiler and cover with oil. Make sure there's water in the bottom part of the double boiler. Cook over very low heat for about three hours.
- Combine the herbs and oil in a jar with a tight-fitting lid. Place a pan of hot water in an oven set to the lowest heat setting. Place the jar in the pan. Let "cook" for several hours.
- Combine the herbs and oil in a slow cooker (such as a Crock Pot). Set the cooker to the low heat setting and cook for a couple of hours.

When the oil is ready, strain out the herbs by pouring the oil through a stainless-steel strainer or potato ricer lined with clean muslin. If you press the herbs that collect in the strainer, keep the oil you get from pressing separate from the rest, since it will contain more water and should be used soon.

Store the infused oil in a glass jar with a tight-fit-

ting lid. Fill the jar entirely; having an air space at the top can encourage bacterial growth. You can top off the jar with more carrier oil if necessary to fill it. You can also add more herbs to the oil to make it stronger, if you want; you'll simply have to strain them out before using the oil. (If you do add herbs to the oil, you may find that bubbles develop in the oil. These are from gases in the herbs and are not a sign of rancidity.)

Keep the jar in a cool, dark location, or even the refrigerator, where they will keep for several months to several years.

LINIMENTS

A liniment is made the same way as a tincture (see page 13), but the menstruum used is isopropyl (rubbing) alcohol or apple cider vinegar. Be sure to label the bottle you're storing the liniment in "For external use only"; you wouldn't want to mistake it for a tincture.

MASSAGE OILS

Find a clean, dry bottle; I like to use a plastic bottle with a squeeze top, so that if it falls to the floor during a massage, you don't have to deal with a disaster. Pour into this bottle 4 ounces of a carrier oil, such as almond, apricot, grapeseed, or sesame oil. To this add about 40 drops of pure essential oil, which will give the massage oil a wonderful and therapeutic aroma. Shake well to blend the ingredients before using. Store your oil in a cool, dark place when it's not in use.

MOUTHWASHES AND GARGLES

Gargles and mouthwashes are made by preparing a standard tea, allowing it to cool, swishing it around in the mouth or gargling it, and then spitting it out. (For a gargle to be effective, it should be continued for 5 minutes.)

POULTICES

A poultice is a soft mass of herbs applied directly to the skin. Crush the fresh or dried herbs first, then mix them with hot water, apple cider vinegar, olive oil, or castor oil. If you are using dried herbs you can add a bit of cornmeal or freshly ground flaxseed to thicken the paste. Use a sufficient amount of herbs to cover the area needing attention. Apply the poultice to that area, using a cloth to hold it in place if necessary.

Poultices may be applied several times a day or in a succession during one sitting.

SALVES

Prepare an infused oil (see page 10). Warm the oil, if necessary, in a slow cooker (such as a Crock Pot) or a double boiler. Add $\frac{1}{8}$ cup of grated beeswax for every cup of oil. Stir gently until the beeswax has melted and combined with the oil. To test the consistency, take a small spoonful and set it in the refrigerator until it cools. If it becomes too hard, add a little more oil; if it is too soft, add a bit more beeswax. When the consistency is just right, pour the salve into clean, dry containers. Be sure to date and label the containers.

SITZ BATHS

A sitz bath is a method of treating many gynecological problems, pelvic pain, and hemorrhoids. A sitz bath is made the same way as an herbal bath (see page 8), although in this case you are localizing the benefits of the water temperature and herbs. You can take a sitz bath in a full-size bathtub or in a smaller basin. In general, the water level should be below the knees and not above the navel. Pour the hot or chilled herbal tea into the tub and soak your hip area in it for about 3 minutes.

A cold sitz bath tonifies the pelvis and bowel. Use cold-water sitz baths for back and lower organ problems such as menstrual pain, pelvic inflammatory disease, hemorrhoids, and congestion in the liver and spleen. A cold compress can be applied to the forehead to improve the effect.

A hot sitz bath increases circulation to the area and can break up congestion and relieve pain.

Sitz baths can be taken alternately hot and cold, with 3 minutes in hot water followed by 2 minutes in cold, repeating up to three times but always ending with cold. When you're finished, keep warm. These alternating baths help move toxins from the area and bring in fresh nutrients and deep healing power.

STEAM INHALATIONS

Steam inhalations can benefit conditions such as asthma, bronchitis, coughs, laryngitis, nasal congestion, and sinus infections by helping to warm, increase circulation in, and loosen mucus from the respiratory tract.

To prepare a steam inhalation, bring 1 quart of water to a boil and add 4 heaping teaspoons of herbs. Remove the pot from the stove and place it on a counter or table on a heatproof pad. Leaning over the pot, drape a towel over both your head and the pot. Breathe in the steam for about 7 minutes or so. If the water cools enough that the steam starts to dissipate, gently blowing into the herb pot will cause more steam to rise.

SUPPOSITORIES

A suppository is used to draw toxins from or soothe irritation in the vagina or rectum. To make herbal suppositories, mix together well-powdered herbs with enough softened cocoa butter to make a thick paste. Form the mixture into suppository-size shapes and refrigerate. (Molds for suppositories are sometimes available from pharmaceutical supply houses.) When the suppositories have set, insert one at night, before bedtime, in the appropriate orifice. Keep in until morning. Wear a cloth pad in your underwear to avoid staining your clothing. Store the remaining suppositories in a cool, dry location.

SYRUPS

Combine 1 ounce of herb and 1 quart of water in a saucepan, and simmer until this amount is reduced to 1 pint. Strain out the herbs. Add 1 cup of honey, which acts as a preservative, to the warm infusion, stirring over low heat until the honey is completely dissolved. Add 9 to 12 tablespoons of brandy and, if desired, 3 to 5 drops of essential oil. Stir well, then let cool. Bottle and store in a cool, dark place.

TEAS

When making tea, always start with fresh, cold

water. Since herb tea is an important aspect of healing, use pure water: distilled, spring, filtered, or from a well. Distilled water is the best medium for drawing out the therapeutic properties of the plants, as it is a more neutral medium. However, I do not recommend using distilled water that has been stored in plastic jugs, because the plastic contains xenoestrogens, substances that mimic the effects of the hormone estrogen, which may be a carcinogenic risk. The plastic also imparts a plastic flavor to the water. I also do not recommend using municipal tap waters that contain chlorine, fluoride, and other components that should be avoided.

Avoid making tea in cookware made from aluminum and copper, which are soft metals that tend to erode and may also have neurotoxic effects on the body. The best choices for kettles and other tea-making equipment are glass, cast iron, stainless steel, and enamel.

Simply bring a cup of cold water to a boil, and remove it from the heat. Add about one heaping teaspoon of herb tea per cup of water, cover and allow it to steep for ten to twenty minutes. To make a more medicinal blend, use up to one ounce of herbs per pint of water. Allow the herbs to steep for twenty minutes to several hours.

Infusions and Tisanes

Some people consider the words *infusion* and *tisane* to be synonymous, while others attribute slightly different meanings to each. The word *tisane* is derived from the Greek ptisan, "crushed barley," and originally meant barley water. Later, *tisane* came to denote a noncaffeinated herbal tea, rather than a caffeine-containing tea. Some consider a tisane to be a tea made from fresh rather than dried plant material. In more recent years, *tisane* has come to mean a tea prepared from unfermented leaves, instead of the fermented leaves of black tea. However you choose to define it, a tisane is, indeed, an herbal infusion enjoyed for its therapeutic effects.

Infusions are an ideal method for brewing tea from herb leaves, flowers, seeds, and even those roots (such as ginger, osha, and valerian) that have delicate essential oils that would be evaporated if

boiled. Before being infused, seeds should be lightly bruised in a mortar and pestle to help release their flavor and properties.

To prepare an infusion, simply bring cold water to a boil, then remove it from the heat. Add about 1 heaping teaspoon of dried herb tea per cup of water, cover, and allow it to steep for 10 to 20 minutes. To make a more medicinal blend, use up to $\frac{1}{2}$ ounce of dried herbs per cup of water, and allow the herbs to steep for 20 minutes to several hours. Strain the herbs from the liquid before serving.

Avoid oversteeping herbs, as some flavors can intensify and become rather medicinal instead of pleasant. Dont expect all herbal teas to be identical in color to the traditional black tea. Most herbal teas tend to have a more pale hue.

Overnight Jar Infusions

This is an excellent process for extracting the maximum amount of medicinal potential from an herb. It takes time but is well worth the effort. This method is more appropriate when the goal is therapeutic rather than for pleasantries, as in "Company's coming, let's have some tea."

Add about 2 ounces of dried roots or bark or 1 ounce of dried flowers, dried leaves, or seeds to the bottom of a clean half-gallon glass canning jar. Cover with boiling water and put the lid on. Allow the herbs to steep for as long as half an hour for seeds, two hours for flowers, four hours for leaves, and overnight for roots and barks. Strain out the herbs and enjoy the nutrient-rich brew.

This method is not suggested for licorice root or valerian root, which will taste too medicinal, or for slippery elm bark, which will become too mucilaginous to enjoy.

Decoctions

A decoction is the preferred method of making tea from those roots, barks, and seeds that are woodier and require more energy for their precious constituents, including minerals, to be extracted.

To brew a decoction, bring cold water to a boil. Add 1 ounce of herb per quart of water, reduce heat, cover, and simmer for about 20 minutes. For large or whole roots, you can simmer for up to an hour. Be sure to keep the heat as low as possible and the cover on, as many constituents, such as essential oils, can be lost through evaporation. After being simmered, the herbs can be strained out immediately or left to steep overnight.

Decoctions are so potent that a serving size can be much less than for an infusion. An adequate portion would be $\frac{1}{4}$ to 1 cup of tea.

Infusion-Decoctions

What if you wanted to mix an herb that needed to be infused, such as peppermint leaf, with an herb that needed to be decocted, such as cinnamon bark? In this case, you'll use a hybrid infusion. Bring the water to a boil. Add the herbs that need to be decocted, such as the cinnamon bark. Cover and simmer for 20 minutes. Then remove from the heat and add the herbs that need to be infused, such as the peppermint leaf. Cover and allow to steep an additional 10 minutes. Strain before serving.

I have been embracing the raw lifestyle, so I prefer not to apply heat to my herbs. With that in mind, these next three types of infusions, known as cold-water infusions or macerations, have become my favorite tea-making methods. They are also simple and help preserve delicate essential oils and water-soluble nutrients like vitamins B and C, which are decreased by heat.

If you desire a cold-water infusion to be sweet, some of the strained tea can be run through a blender with a bit of honey and added back to the rest of the batch.

Sun Teas

Sun teas work best with leaves and flowers. Place 1 cup of dried herbs or twelve tea bags in a glass gallon jug, fill with cool water, and allow the herbs to sit in sunlight for four to six hours. It is best to cover the top of the jar to prevent leaves and other debris from blowing into the jar. Then strain. Many believe that this method infuses the water with not only the herbs' properties but also the healing rays of the sun.

Storing Tea

If you make teas in batches larger than a cup, you'll save time and be encouraged to drink more of them. Leftover teas should be strained and stored in the refrigerator, where they'll keep for about four days. If you want to rewarm the tea, do so, but don't bring it to any higher than about 110°F to protect the tea's enzymes and constituents.

Tea is full of life force, and any microorganism that enters the tea can multiply. If there is any sign of spoilage, such as a fizziness or flatness to the taste, discard the tea and make a fresh batch.

Lunar Teas

This type of infusion is best made when the moon is full or close to full. Place 1 cup of dried herbs or twelve tea bags in a glass gallon jug, fill with cool water, and allow the herbs to sit outside under the moonlight for four to twelve hours. (Of course, if the temperature is going to drop below freezing, avoid this method, or the water might freeze and break your container.) Some people believe that this method infuses the tea with the feminine, intuitive, mystical properties of the moon.

Cold-Water Infusions

If the weather prevents you from making a sun tea or lunar tea, you can also place your herbs (1 cup of dried herbs to 1 gallon of water) in a jar, cover with cold water, cover, and allow the herbs to steep in the refrigerator for about twelve hours. Strain before serving.

TINCTURES

Tinctures are herbal extracts made with alcohol, vegetable glycerin, or vinegar instead of water. Tinctures are especially useful for extracting resins and oils from plant material, which water doesn't do very well. The liquid used to extract the herbs is known as the menstruum. The herbs being tinctured are known as the mark.

Prepare the herbs by chopping or grinding them. Put them in a glass jar and cover with the menstruum of your choice, adding enough that there is an extra inch of liquid above the plant material. Store in a cool, dry location. Shake daily. After a month, strain out the herbs, first with a strainer and then through a clean, undyed cloth, squeezing tightly. You may also wish to press the herbs through a potato ricer lined with cloth. Pour the tincture into dark glass bottles, and label and date them. Compost the spent plant material. Store the bottles away from heat and light.

Alcohol is an ideal menstruum for extracting fats, resins, waxes, and most alkaloids. It is an excellent preservative and is quickly assimilated. It must be at least 50 proof to have good preservative qualities. Vodka or brandy is a good choice. Alcohol tinctures will last for many years.

Vegetable glycerin is a useful menstruum when you are making tinctures for those who are alcohol-intolerant, for children, or for pregnant or nursing mothers. Glycerin is both a solvent and a preservative that has an effectiveness somewhere between that of water and alcohol. It is naturally sweet and can extract mucilage, vitamins, minerals, and tannins from plant material, although it doesn't extract

resins very well. It is itself slightly antiseptic, demulcent, and healing when diluted. Glycerin tinctures, known as glycerites, are usually prepared using 1 part water to 2 parts glycerin. Glycerites have a shorter shelf life than alcohol tinctures, about 1 to 3 years.

Apple cider vinegar, preferably organic, can also be used as a menstruum, and it is itself a digestive tonic. Look for a vinegar that is 5.7 percent acetic acid or thereabouts for a long shelf life. Warm the vinegar before pouring it over the herbs, and do not prepare or store the tincture in a jar with a metal lid, or the lid will rust. This type of tincture will have a shelf life from six months up to four years.

DOSAGE GUIDELINES

Dosages will depend in part on the herbs you're thinking about using. If you're using a commercial product, of course you should follow the dosage guidelines on the product packaging. If you've made your own tea or tincture, in general, one cup of tea or one dropperful of tincture qualifies as a single dose. For an acute, serious, right-there-in-your-face type of illness, one dose every hour or two would be

---

Special Situations

The general dosage guidelines discussed above are generally true for adults. However, dosages may need to be adjusted for different people or different categories of people. For example:

- Large people need more than small people.
- Women may need less than men.
- For dosages for the elderly, reduce the dose by one-fourth for those over age 65 and by one-half for those over age 70.

Through breast milk, a nursing infant can reap the benefits of the teas the mother drinks. An infant will most benefit from drinking mother's milk fifteen to thirty minutes after Mom has had her tea.

To figure out a dosage for children, you can follow one of two rules:

- Cowling's rule: Take the child's age at his or her next birthday and divide by 24. The resulting fraction is the amount of the adult dosage the child can have. For example, a five-year-old will be six at his next birthday. The number 6 divided by 24 equals $1/4$; this child should have $1/4$ of the adult dosage.
- Clark's Rule: Divide the child's weight by 150. The resulting fraction is the amount of the adult dosage the child can have. For example, for a fifty-pound child, 50 divided by 150 equals $1/3$; this child can have $1/3$ of the adult dosage.

appropriate. Except while sleeping, of course—rest is good medicine in its own right.

For a chronic health concern, one dose three or four times daily would be appropriate. Some herbalists recommend pulsing remedies for chronic conditions, which means ten days on, then three days off, in a continuing cycle. Pulsing helps the body acclimate and learn to respond even without the herbs. Another pulsing regimen is six days on, one day off, with a three-day break every two or three weeks.

When you are using herbs for therapeutic purposes, continue with the appropriate dosage for at least a week, and then evaluate your progress. If your health concern has been remedied, then you can stop taking the herb formula on a regular basis. However, you might wish to include some of it in your diet from time to time as a tonic tune-up.

Be aware that some herbs should not be combined with some medications because they can cause exacerbated or unpredictable effects. This is especially the case when you are using an herb for the same purpose as a drug. You may end up with a double dose! As general rules:

- If you're taking prescription medication, don't take any herbs that are not regarded as safe for all people without first checking with your health-care practitioner.

- If you're taking medication for a particular ailment, you shouldn't also take herbs for that ailment without first checking with your health-care practitioner.

Of course, many herbs, especially those that are nutritive and flavorful, can simply be a delight in their own right. Enjoy them whenever you like! Experience the simple pleasures in life!

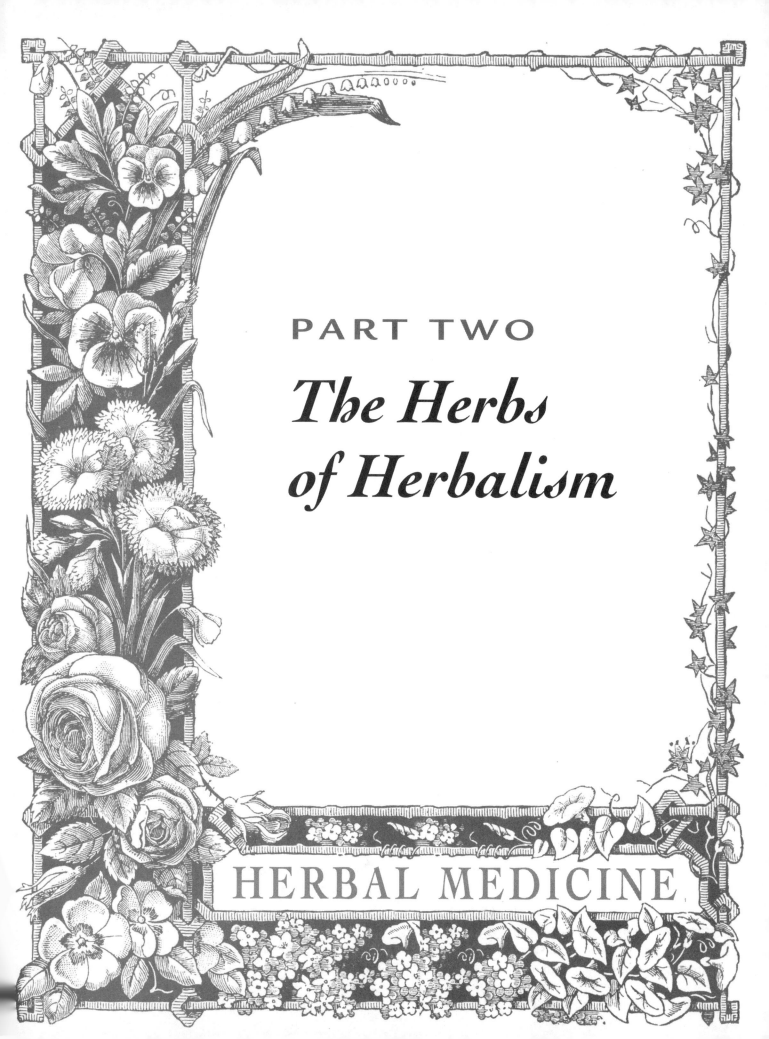

PART TWO
The Herbs of Herbalism

HERBAL MEDICINE

3. Profiles

To enable you to find the information you're looking for quickly, and to compare herb properties easily, these herb profiles follow the same outline. While comprehensive, the information in the profiles is by no means complete—and how could it be, with all the new, wonderful things we are learning about plants every day? I'll describe here the basic rationale behind each part of the outline to help you interpret the information in the profiles. Each section below corresponds to a section in each of the herb profiles.

BOTANICAL NAME

Many plants are known by more than one common name. The Linnaean nomenclature system, based on the work of Swedish botanist Carolus Linnaeus, gives to each plant a binomial, or a two-part name, consisting of the plant's genus and species name. Each species of plant is thus given a unique name that differentiates it from all other species. In this way, no matter where or in what language, we can be sure exactly which plant is under discussion.

I have included in this section the botanical names of those plants that are most commonly available commercially. This list does not always contain *every* plant that can be used medicinally. Those that are not listed, however, are so rare as to be very difficult to find or have properties aside from those that are described in the profile. Or perhaps they have yet to be discovered! I would encourage you to use only those species that are listed. If you want to use a species that is not listed, be sure to first research its properties, and consult with a qualified herbalist if

necessary to discuss how it should (and how it should *not*) be used.

FAMILY

Families are lovely, and plants have them too. Families rank just above genera in the system of biological classification. Understanding which families the different healing herbs belong to can help you begin to see the bigger web of relationships among them.

ETYMOLOGY

The meaning of a plant's name, whether its Latinized binomial or its common name, connects us to its history of use. In understanding why a plant was given a particular name, we begin to understand the nature of the plant itself.

ALSO KNOWN AS

This section lists other common names by which each plant is known, in English and in other languages. These may be useful in identifying plants discussed in older or foreign-language literature. I find it interesting to note which cultures have similar names for a plant, indicating a common history of use.

PARTS USED

This section identifies the part or parts of the plant used medicinally.

PHYSIOLOGICAL EFFECTS

Plants stimulate various actions in the body, which are listed in this section. I've given them in alphabetical order, rather than in order of strength, because different plants can have different effects on different people, and so gauging the strength of one action against another is an imperfect science.

MEDICINAL USES

This section describes the ways in which the plant interacts with the body. It includes both internal and topical uses, and it offers a list of ailments for which the plant can be a useful part of treatment. I've listed these ailments in alphabetical order because the mode and scope of treatment will depend on the practitioner and the patient; whether a plant is useful in the treatment of an ailment in a particular person will depend on that person's unique physiology and state of being. Nevertheless, thinking about the ways in which a plant could be of benefit in the treatment of various ailments can stimulate a broader questioning, exploration, and understanding of that plant's interaction with the body.

Note that when an herb is said to be used in the treatment of an ailment, "treatment" does not equate to "cure." For example, if nettles are said to be useful in the treatment of arthritis, they may alleviate its symptoms and possibly slow its progression, but they may not rid the body of it. Similarly, if ashwagandha is said to be useful in the treatment of AIDS, it will not rid the body of the disease but will, among other things, support and strengthen the immune system and nutrify the body, all of which could be tremendously beneficial for a person suffering from AIDS.

EDIBLE USES

Many of the healing herbs profiled in this book are also delicious and nourishing foods. What better way to "get your medicine" than to eat it? Of course, other foods, while edible, are not tasty and would be eaten only in emergency situations, and still others are not edible at all. You'll find all this information here in this section.

OTHER USES

Plants have long served humanity not only as medicine and food but as sources of dyes, fibers, scents, fuels, building materials, magic, and so much more. This section describes those "other" uses, ranging from historical to modern trends.

CONSTITUENTS

Here you'll find what are thought to be the important constituents, in approximate order of composition, in each plant. The list is by no means complete, as scientists are still discovering new constituents every day.

Pharmaceutical companies and much scientific research are devoted to finding the "active" constituents that cause a plant's therapeutic effects. However, many herbalists prefer to work with the whole plant, rather than isolated compounds. The many constituents a plant contains can be said to have a synergistic effect, working together in unknowable ways to produce effects that can't be re-created by using the constituents individually.

ENERGETIC CORRESPONDENCES

This section brings together Asian theories about the energy of the body with the four-element theories of ancient Greece and the planetary correspondences of Oriental philosophy and astrology.

Flavor

All the flavors we are able to sense can be broken down into five categories: sour, bitter, sweet, pungent (spicy), and salty. In Oriental medicine, each of these five flavors is associated with particular organ systems of the body. When we experience a flavor, our taste sensors send signals to our brain, which in turn induces physiological effects in the organ system linked to that flavor. In this way, through flavor, we can affect the energy and function of our bodies.

As a culture, Westerners tend to overemphasize the sweet and salty flavors. Yet leaving out flavors is like removing colors from the rainbow. All the flavors together help keep the body in balance.

The salty, sour, and bitter flavors are considered yin or cooling, with a downward-moving energy. These yin flavors tend to arise and subside quickly. The sweet and pungent flavors are usually considered yang or warming, with an upward-moving energy. These yang flavors are slower to be sensed and remain longer.

The sour, bitter, and pungent flavors are considered to have a drying energy, meaning that they help correct imbalances such as abnormal fluid buildup, swelling, and other fluid obstructions in the body. Conditions that result from dampness, such as oily skin, edema, joint swelling, yeast overgrowth, and a "heavy" or fatigued feeling, can all benefit from drying.

The sweet and salty flavors are considered moistening and can help soothe conditions resulting from a deficiency of fluids. Herbs that have a moistening effect usually contain natural mucilage and are classified as demulcent and emollient. Dry skin, dry mucous membranes, dry cough, constipation, and irritated eyes can all benefit from moistening herbs. Moistening herbs also benefit the metabolism of fluids. Dryness can be a sign of yin deficiency, and many moistening herbs help build the yin fluids of the body.

Sour

The sour flavor is cooling, drying, and astringent. Sourness usually is due to the presence of acids such as ascorbic, citric, and malic acids. It stimulates liver and gallbladder function as well as the appetite, increases saliva production, and can aid in fat metabolism. It restricts secretions such as seminal fluid, sweat, urine, blood, and diarrhea. The sour flavor is carminative, diaphoretic, and refreshing. It helps cleanse the skin and tonify tissue and may benefit conditions such as varicosities and hemorrhoids. Examples of sour herbs include lemongrass, orange peel, rose hips, and hawthorn berries. Those with diarrhea, hyperacidity, broken capillaries, or dark circles under their eyes should be careful of overdoing the sour flavor.

Bitter

The bitter taste is cooling, drying, strengthening, and draining. It also has anti-inflammatory and antibacterial effects. Most bitter herbs contain some sort of alkaloid. Bitter stimulates the small intestine, the pancreas, and digestive secretions. It strengthens the

---

What Is Chi?

Chi, also spelled qi, is a continuous flow of energy that circulates in the body and permeates the universe. It is invisible, formless, odorless, and tasteless, yet it has consciousness. It can be construed of as the Hindu concept of prana, or life force. We receive chi from the sun, the earth, and the nutrients we ingest. In the body, chi flows from one meridian point to the next, bringing energy to every body part and system. Chi is warming, protects the body from harmful influences, and is the source (not the cause) of movement. Herbs that are chi tonics promote energy circulation.

---

heart, lowers cholesterol and fevers, helps deter parasites in the body, reduces cravings for sweets, supports fat metabolism, helps strengthen those with food allergies, and helps eliminate heat and mucous, especially from the lungs. It can aid weight loss, decrease fat, detoxify the blood, and clear the mind and skin. Bitter herbs include angelica, chamomile, dandelion leaf, globe green tea, and yarrow. Bitter is beneficial for people who are lethargic, as well as those who are hot and aggressive. People who are deficient in energy, cold and dry, or suffering from ulcers should use bitter sparingly.

Sweet

The sweet flavor is regarded as a tonic, nourishing to the stomach and spleen. It usually results from the presence of carbohydrates. It helps to slow down acute symptoms and increase tolerance to stress and pain. It also is rejuvenating, builds tissue, and heals and tones muscles. It is considered energizing yet calming. The sweet flavor nourishes yin, or the fluids of the body, which helps to build up a person who is dry, has a weak immune system, and is frail. People who are dry, cold, and spacey can benefit from good-quality sweet foods, such as fruits, whole grains, and sweet herbs such as anise, fennel, licorice, and stevia.

Pungent

Pungent, or spicy, is warming and dispersing and stimulates the lungs and large intestine. It induces perspiration, stimulates the nerves, relieves nerve pain, clears chi stagnation, promotes circulation, and imparts a glow to the skin. It also stimulates hydrochloric acid production and thus aids digestion. Most pungent herbs contain some sort of essential oils that move internal energy to the surface. Many of these essential oils have antimicrobial activity. Pungent is cooling to the interior and warming to the exterior of the body. Basil, cinnamon, ginger, and mint all represent the pungent flavor and are good to use for a cold condition.

Salty

The salty flavor is cooling, softening, draining, and diuretic. It indicates the presence of mineral salts in a food. The salty flavor can help soften hardened masses in the body, such as tumors. If used in moderation it can have a moistening effect. It especially affects the nerves, kidneys, and bladder. It aids fluid metabolism, helps strengthen the nerves, opens blocked chi channels, improves circulation, awakens the mind and senses, and strengthens the heart. Craving salt excessively may indicate adrenal exhaustion. Sea vegetables such as kelp and dulse are good examples of the salty taste, as are the herb nettle and plantain.

Temperature

The temperature here refers not to degrees on a thermometer but rather to the activity of a plant: Does it heat the body, like ginger? Or does it cool the body, like peppermint? In hot conditions, such as inflammation or fever, cooling plants may be called for. In cold conditions, such as poor circulation, warming plants may be called for.

I must admit that at this time not everyone can agree on whether an herb is cold, cool, neutral, warm, or hot. As American herbalism evolves, the concept of temperature will become a more integral part of our healing tradition, with more agreement among herbal practitioners.

Moisture

Asian medicine speaks of dampness and dryness as conditions of imbalance in the body. Dampness is evidenced by swelling, edema, diarrhea, and other conditions. Dryness is evidenced by dry cough, dry skin, constipation, and other conditions. Depending on their content and predisposition to moisturize or dry, plants can help normalize the moisture state of the body. Many moistening plants contain mucilage, while many drying plants contain tannins.

Polarity

Yin and yang are vital forces that permeate the universe from the tiniest to the grandest of things. They are sometimes described as opposites but are in truth merely opposite sides of a circular contiuum, merging into one another and continuously moving in a spiral dance. They are only yin and yang in relation to each other; one does not exist without the other, and each contains aspects of the other.

In traditional Asian medicine good health is the result of a balance of yin and yang. When these forces become out of balance, health problems result. Plants with a yang nature can be used to correct yang deficiencies, while plants with a yin nature can be used to correct yin deficiencies. Yin plants are said to be cooling, while yang plants tend to be warming. But of course yin and yang are constantly in motion and never absolute, so that while an herb can be said to be yin, it may have a warming effect, and vice versa.

Planet

The association between herbs and astrology is rooted in the ancient Doctrine of Signatures. This theory, thought to have been developed by Paracelsus, an early-sixteenth-century physician, holds that as all things were created, each was marked with an energetic signature, which is revealed partially through each object's appearance, and that those signatures that resemble each other link the objects to which they belong. In terms of healing, this means that observing the color of a flower, the shape of a leaf, the growth habit of a plant, and where the plant grows could give clues about the plant's therapeutic uses. The Doctrine of Signatures also acknowledges that macrocosms such as planets can be represented in microcosms such as plants.

In this way, celestial correspondences can be established by closely examining an herb and its correspondences to the ancient, intricate field of astrology and the rich language of the zodiac.

Sun

The Sun corresponds to hot, dry energy. It is the heart of the solar system and also governs the physical heart of the human body, as well as the spinal column and eyes. The Sun governs herbs that have large golden or yellow blossoms with radiating petals that may turn toward the sun. These herbs often affect the heart and are hot and drying.

Moon

The Moon corresponds to cool, moist, and feminine energy. In plants, this energy is reflected in juice, soft leaves with a mild flavor; a preference for growing in or near water; and whitish or pale yellow flowers and fruits. The Moon governs the body's fluids, digestive secretions, breasts, and glandular and mucous membrane secretions. Moon-governed plants may affect the subconscious, soothe the stomach, and aid digestion.

Mercury

Mercury, the planet in closest proximity to the Sun, is classified as cool and dry. It governs the nervous system and the physiological mechanisms of communication, including the senses of hearing and speaking, thyroid, respiratory system, lungs, bronchi, and vocal cords. Mercury facilitates the ability to make associations and link concepts.

This planet rules mosses as well as plants that grow on trees or in the air. Mercury-governed plants often exhibit finely divided leaves or stems, resembling the bronchi of the lungs, and stems with an airy, grasslike nature. They may help relax the nervous system and improve respiration and often have a changeable flavor.

Venus

Venus is considered to be cool and moist. It is associated with love, sensual pleasures, beauty, and the arts. Venus governs the internal sexual and repro-

ductive organs, skin, nose, sense of smell, umbilical cord, neck, spine, and palate. It affects the relationships between various body systems such as the thyroid, parathyroid, and thymus glands, the kidneys, and the breasts.

Venus rules plants growing near or under the ground, such as fungi and truffles. Venus-governed plants are likely to have beautiful flowers and delicious fruits. They tend to help purify the blood, keep the sweat glands open, and calm a desire for overindulgence.

Mars

Mars is considered to be hot, pungent, and dry. It governs the adrenal glands, muscles, gallbladder, sense of taste, red blood cells, metabolism, motor nerves, rectum, eye muscles, head, left brain, and left ear. Mars is also said to govern the transmission of sexual energy from the genitals (Scorpio) to the head (Aries).

Mars-governed plants may have a phallic signature. They tend to have a strong, acrid flavor, a pungent aroma, prickles and thorns, a conical tap root, and red coloring; they also tend to grow under adverse conditions and are often biennials. Mars also governs plants that look like seaweeds yet are pioneers on land, such as lichens.

Jupiter

Jupiter is said to be warm and moist. It is associated with adventure, social order, morals, and optimism. It governs the anterior pituitary gland, liver, pancreas, sciatic nerve (the largest nerve in the body), arteries of the abdomen and legs, subcutaneous fat tissue, adrenal glands, kidneys, spleen, immune system, fibrin and oxygen levels in the blood, blood sugar levels, buttocks, genitals, feet, lungs, right ear, and semen.

Jupiter takes twelve years to travel through the Zodiac, so it is represented by long-living perennial plants. Jupiter governs large forest trees that bear catkins and represent the ability to grow in stature and understanding. Many Jupiter plants benefit the liver, increase bile flow, help balance the pancreas, and are expansive to the growth of the mind and body. Many are large and showy. They often have a sweet fragrance that promotes a positive frame of mind. Plants governed by Jupiter help promote the growth and preservation of the body, and they tend to be nutritive. On a mental level they help promote affection, intuitive understanding, and cosmic comprehension.

Saturn

Saturn is said to be cold and dry and is associated with the bitter and sour flavors. Saturn, also known as Cronus, the oldest god and lawgiver, teacher, tester, and timekeeper, represents highest achievement and perfect justice. The aging process and the health of the bones, teeth, joints, bladder, skin, knees, vagus nerve, spleen, endocardium, left auricle, anterior pituitary lobe, and blood constituents are under the dominion of Saturn.

Saturn was considered the god of time by the Romans, so slow-growing plants are under its dominion, as are long-lived woody perennials, as the planet takes thirty years to complete its journey. They include woody trees, shrubs that have annual rings, and many poisonous and narcotic plants. Saturn herbs help balance bodily fluids, dry dampness, and solidify basic structures of the body. Saturn-ruled plants often have annual rings and dark or grayish leaves or bark. Their flowers often have separated, small petals that are sometimes poisonous. Their taste may be unpleasant. They are grounding, encouraging the completion of projects and facilitating work on the material plane.

Uranus

Uranus, considered cold and dry, corresponds to dramatic, sudden, and forceful energy; originality; genius; independence; self-expression; and a desire to break away from tradition. When its energy is imbalanced, it corresponds to impatience and irresponsibility. Uranus awakens humanity to new beginnings. It represents that which is unconventional, individualistic, intuitive, and rebellious. It governs the nervous system and the electrical force that flows through its channels.

Uranus-governed herbs often grow in unusual places and may not always look the same from plant to plant. They often are hybrids and easy to transplant. They tend to have united petals to excite, stimulate, promote inspiration, energize, improve circulation, and relax the nervous system.

Neptune

Neptune, considered cold and moist, corresponds to cerebrospinal fluid, the pineal gland, and the lymph system. It governs obscure, hard-to-diagnose diseases as well as addiction, alcoholism, and schizophrenia and other psychoses.

Neptune-governed plants are mystical, sometimes psychoactive, and helpful in dreamwork, enhancing the imagination and helping to bring physical concepts to the next plane. They often grow in or near the ocean, such as algaes and seaweeds.

Pluto

Pluto, also known as Hades, is the ruler of the subconscious and underworld. It is said to be cold and moist and governs excretion and reproduction, including the colon and anus, as well as the metabolic, genetic, and chemical processes that promote health. Hidden cellular changes and tissue destruction are also under the dominion of Pluto.

Pluto-governed herbs are often found in remote places or underground. They tend to bring about dramatic change and insight and can help with sexuality and balancing the physical and spiritual aspects of a personality.

Element

The theory of the four elements arose in ancient Greece, though other cultures have similar theories about the nature of the world. It holds that all matter is made up of four basic elements: water, fire, earth, and air. Though in most plants all four elements can be found, one element tends to predominate, and that is the element identified in the herb profiles.

Water

The water element corresponds to the kidneys and bladder, sexual energy, willpower, the sense of hearing, and the emotion fear.

Fire

The fire element corresponds to the heart and small intestines, the sense of speech, and the emotions of joy and lack of joy.

Earth

Earth as an element is corresponds to the stomach and spleen, the sense of taste, and the emotions of sympathy and obsession.

Air

Air as an element corresponds to the lungs, large intestines, and the skin, communication, the sense of smell, and the emotion of grief.

CONTRAINDICATIONS

Many of the possible side effects that you'll find described over the following pages would result only if extremely large doses were used. They are unlikely to result from normal use—moderate amounts taken on occasion or for no more than a few weeks consecutively. However, there are some plants that are best used under the guidance of a qualified health-care practitioner, and others can possibly have bad results when used in cases of pregnancy, high blood pressure, and so on. I chose to be on the conservative side, rather than ignoring any possible safety issues. I hope you'll feel the same way. Remember, just because a remedy is "natural" does not mean that it is appropriate for everyone at all stages of life.

RANGE AND APPEARANCE

This is where we learn some of the herb's physical characteristics, what makes it unique from other plants, its area of origin, and, if it is a garden plant, what its requirements for cultivation are.

AGRIMONY

Botanical Name

Agrimonia eupatoria

Family

Rosaceae (Rose Family)

Etymology

The species name, *eupatoria,* was given in honor of an ancient Persian king, Mithrades Eupator, who was a renowned herbalist. The common name *agrimony* has its origins in the Greek term *argemon,* meaning "speck in the eye," a reference to the plant's traditional use as an eyewash. The common names *cocklebur* and *sticklewort* make reference to the way the plant's seeds cling to anyone who comes in contact with them.

Also Known As

Cantonese: sin hok chou
English: burr marigold, church steeples, cocklebur, garclive, philantropos, sticklewort
French: aigremoine
German: echter odermennig
Italian: agrimonia
Japanese: senkakuso
Korean: sonhakch'o
Mandarin: xian he cao

Parts Used

Entire plant, including both the aboveground portion and the root

Physiological Effects

Analgesic, anti-inflammatory, antiparasitic, antispasmodic, antiviral (mild), astringent, deobstruent, digestive, diuretic, emmenagogue, febrifuge, hemostatic, hepatic, vulnerary

Medicinal Uses

Historically agrimony was a popular European medicine for treating wounds, sprains, and bruises. In fact, it was part of a formula called Eau de Arquebusade, which took its name from that of the arquebus, a fifteenth-century heavy musket, and was used to treat bruises and sprains (you can still sometimes find this formula in the marketplace today).

Agrimony is known to cleanse and strengthen the liver, help regulate the heartbeat, and lower blood sugar levels. It is used in treatments for asthma, bladder irritation, bronchitis, cancer, coughs, cystitis, diarrhea, dysentery, incontinence, kidney stones, laryngitis, sore throat, and trichomonas. In Chinese medicine agrimony is used to mitigate excessive menstrual flow.

Recent research has shown that agrimony can increase blood coagulation when used as a wash for wounds. It is also useful as a topical wash in treatments for bruises, sore muscles, sprains, hives, and eye ailments. An agrimony poultice can help heal wounds and varicose veins. Gargling with agrimony tea can soothe a sore throat. And as a suppository, agrimony can relieve diarrhea.

As a flower essence, agrimony is helpful for those who appear cheerful but conceal mental anguish behind their smile. It helps one find true inner peace and real humor.

Edible Uses

Agrimony makes an apricot-scented tea. It is sometimes used in the making of beer and mead. The seeds can be ground and used as meal.

Other Uses

In Europe the leaves and stems of agrimony were once used to create a yellow dye.

Constituents

Polysaccharides, tannins, essential oil, flavonoids, coumarins, vitamins B and K, iron, silicon

Energetic Correspondences

- Flavor: pungent, slightly bitter
- Temperature: cool
- Moisture: dry
- Polarity: yang
- Planet: Jupiter/Venus
- Element: air

Contraindications

Agrimony should be used only in moderation, and not at all in cases of pregnancy, hypertension, constipation, or extreme dryness (as evidenced by persistent thirst, dry skin, and constipation).

Range and Appearance

Native to Eurasia, agrimony grows in all types of soils but prefers sunny slopes, sandy terrain, and poor pastureland. This perennial plant can reach a height of 12 to 28 inches. Its basal leaves form a rosette and, along with the stem leaves, are irregularly pinnate and widely spaced. The flowers, which appear from June through September, are golden yellow and grow in a long inflorescence.

ALFALFA

Botanical Name

Medicago sativa

Family

Fabaceae (Pea Family)

Etymology

The name *alfalfa* is derived from the Arabic *al-facfacah,* "father of all foods." The genus name, *Medicago,* refers to ancient Media of western Persia, where this plant is thought to have originated; the genus name could be interpreted to mean "sowed by the Medians." The species name, *sativa,* means "cultivated"; it is generally given to plants that have been in cultivation since ancient times. The folk name *lucerne,* "lamp," makes reference to the plant's bright, shiny seeds.

Also Known As

Afrikaans: lusern
Arabic: barseem higazi
Cantonese: gum fa choi
Croatian: lucerna
Danish: foder-lucerne
English: buffalo grass, Chilean clover, lucerne, purple medic, Spanish hay
Finnish: kylvomailanen
French: lucerne
German: luzerne
Greek: midiki
Hebrew: aspeset
Hindi: jungli lucerne, vilaiti gawuth
Italian: luzerna, medica
Japanese: arufarufa, murasaki, umagoyashi
Korean: ja ju gae ja ri
Mandarin: jin hua cai
Norwegian: blalucern
Polish: lucerna
Portuguese: feno-de-borgonha
Russian: al'fal'fa
Sanskrit: lasunghas
Slovenian: alfal
Spanish: alfal
Swedish: blausern
Turkish: adi yonca, kaba yonca

Parts Used

Aboveground plant

Physiological Effects

Alterative, anti-inflammatory, diuretic, galactagogue, nutritive, stomachic, phytoestrogenic, tonic

Medicinal Uses

Alfalfa is an excellent nutritive food and also improves the body's assimilation of nutrients. It is especially beneficial for people who are convalescing, and it can be used as a nutritive tonic during the second and third trimesters of pregnancy. It is so rich in chlorophyll that it is grown commercially as a source of this nutritive compound.

Alfalfa is used to treat anemia, arteriosclerosis, arthritis, blood pressure problems (high or low), bruising, celiac disease, high cholesterol, colitis, diabetes, fatigue, fever, indigestion, jaundice, menopause symptoms, menstrual problems, obesity, osteoporosis, peptic ulcers, and varicose veins. It also helps remove excess uric acid from the body.

Topically, alfalfa is used as a moistening bath herb, facial steam, hair rinse, and poultice for wounds.

Edible Uses

Alfalfa's young leaves and flowers may be eaten as salad greens or potherbs. Seed sprouts can be added to salads. Alfalfa is often added to other teas to improve their flavor and nutrient profile. Its flavor is reminiscent of the scent of summer-cut hay.

Other Uses

Where alfalfa grows wild, it is an indicator of rich soil. In their search for nutrients deep in the soil, its roots can reach 120 feet in depth. Alfalfa often is planted in fallow fields and then turned under to enrich and fix nitrogen in the soil.

When alfalfa is part of their diet, cows produce more milk and chickens lay more eggs. Green cuttings of alfalfa are said to deter bedbugs. Alfalfa has long been thought to attract prosperity.

Constituents

Chlorophyll, betaine (a digestive enzyme), electrolytes, fiber, protein, beta-carotene, vitamin C, vitamin K, folic acid, octacosanol, calcium, chromium, copper, phosphorous, manganese, iron, zinc, silicon, fluorine, electrolytes, isoflavones, coumarins, alkaloids (stachydrine), steroidal saponins (beta sitosterol, alpha spinasterol, and stigmasterol)

Energetic Correspondences

- Flavor: salty, bitter
- Temperature: cool
- Moisture: moist
- Polarity: yin
- Planet: Venus/Jupiter
- Element: earth

Contraindications

Alfalfa is considered very safe. However, there has been some concern about the safety of eating large amounts of the sprouts, which contain the alkaloid canavanine. Therefore, people with lupus or rheumatoid arthritis are encouraged to avoid eating alfalfa sprouts; the leaves and flowers, however, are safe for consumption.

Those taking blood-thinning medication should avoid using alfalfa.

Range and Appearance

Native to Asia, alfalfa was an important crop for the Arabs, who fed it to their fabled racehorses. Spanish conquistadors brought it to Chile and Mexico, where it was grown as animal fodder in the mid-1800s, earning it the nickname Chilean clover. It now can be found in cultivation or in the wild worldwide.

Alfalfa can grow in a wide variety of locales, both moist and dry, and is often found by roadsides and in fields. This perennial plant can reach a height of 2 to 3 feet. Its three-part cloverlike leaf is alternate and compound. The alternate flowers are blue, lavender, or purple; they grow in short terminal clusters and bloom from June until August. The seedpods are coiled.

ALISMA

Botanical Name

Alisma plantago-aquatica

Family

Alismataceae (Water Plantain Family)

Etymology

The genus name, *Alisma,* is thought to be of Celtic origin, meaning "water." Early botanists gave this plant the species name *plantago-aquatica,* "water plantain," because its leaves resemble those of plantain, though they are not related.

Also Known As

Cantonese: jaak sei
English: alismatis, mad dog weed, marsh drain, water plantain
Japanese: takusha
Korean: t'aeksa
Mandarin: ze xie

Part Used

Rhizome

Physiological Effects

Antibacterial, antitumor, astringent, diuretic, febrifuge, hypotensive, kidney tonic, liver cleanser, parturient, refrigerant, urinary stimulant

Medicinal Uses

In *Chinese Tonic Herbs* (Japan Publications, 1985), author Ron Teagarden notes the profound respect given to alisma in ancient Chinese classics, which state that if alisma is taken for a long time, "the eye and ear become acute, hunger is not felt, life is prolonged, the body becomes light, the complexion radiant, and one can walk upon water" (the last a reference to spiritual enhancement).

Alisma is considered a very safe diuretic, even for the elderly. It is also useful for painful, difficult, or scanty urination. It neutralizes moist heat in the body and aids in the elimination of urea and sodium. It can be used to promote fertility, to facilitate labor, and in treatments for allergies, bloating, cancer, cystitis, diabetes, diarrhea, dizziness, dysentery, edema, epilepsy, fertility, hypertension, kidney stones, labor, low libido, lumbago, premature ejaculation, nephritis, and tinnitus.

Edible Uses

The bulb can be eaten as a vegetable.

Other Uses

None known

Constituents

Triterpenoids (alisol, epiasol), asparagine, essential oil (furfuraldehyde), alkaloids, biotin, potassium, lecithin, stigmasterol, vitamin B_{12}

Energetic Correspondences

- Flavor: sweet
- Temperature: cold
- Moisture: moist
- Polarity: yin
- Planet: Moon/Venus
- Element: water

Contraindications

Though alisma is considered very safe, it is not recommended for people with cold, damp conditions such as leukorrhea or spermatorrhea. Prolonged use can irritate the intestinal tract.

Range and Appearance

Native to temperate regions of Asia, alisma grows in lowland swampy bogs and achieves 2 to 3 feet in height. Its leaves are round or heart-shaped and have defined veins. Its small white to pinkish flowers grow on panicles and bloom in summer.

ALLSPICE

Botanical Name

Pimenta dioica, P. officinalis

Family

Myrtaceae (Eucalyptus Family)

Etymology

The species name, *dioica,* indicates that the plant is dioecious, meaning that it has male and female flowers borne on separate trees. The common name *pimento* is derived from the Spanish term for pepper, *pimienta,* which the berries resemble. The fruit of the tree is known as allspice because its flavor resembles that of a combination of cinnamon, cloves, and nutmeg.

Also Known As

Arabic: bahar, bhar hub wa na'im
Danish: allehande
Dutch: piment
English: clove pepper, Jamaican pepper, myrtle pepper, newspice, pimento
Finnish: maustepippuri
French: piment, tout-epice
German: nelkenpfeffer, neugewurz, piment, pimentbaum
Hebrew: pilpel angli
Hungarian: jamaikai szegfubors, pimento

Italian: pepe di giamaica, pimento
Japanese: orusupaisu
Norwegian: allehande
Polish: ziele angielskie
Portuguese: pimenta da Jamaica
Russian: yamayski pyerts
Spanish: pimienta, pimienta gorda
Swedish: kryddpeppar
Turkish: yeni bahar

Part Used

Dried, unripe fruit

Physiological Effects

Antioxidant, antiseptic, aromatic, astringent, carminative, digestive, stimulant, stomachic, styptic

Medicinal Uses

Allspice can be used to remedy poor appetite, chills, diarrhea, dyspepsia, flatulence, indigestion, high blood sugar, and rheumatism. It aids digestion, improves protein assimilation, and prevents the buildup of gases in the upper intestinal tract. It has a very warming effect and can be beneficial when taken as a tea in cases of frostbite and hypothermia.

Applied topically, allspice has an anesthetic on sore teeth and gums. It can be added to liniments to help relieve the pain of arthritis and neuralgia.

Edible Uses

Before the arrival of Europeans, allspice was one of the most common culinary herbs of the Caribbean. The Aztecs used it to flavor chocolate. Nowadays, allspice is used to flavor cakes, carrots, chutneys, cookies, curries, custards, fish, fruit, jam, pickles, pies, soups, sweet potatoes, and stews. It is sometimes added to medicines to improve their flavor. The very best allspice comes from Jamaica.

Other Uses

In the 1800s allspice was used by the Maya for embalming their dead. Because of its light salmon color, the wood of the tree was once in such demand for the making of walking sticks and umbrellas that the tree became in danger of extinction. It has also been used to make magic wands, burned as an incense to attract prosperity, and worn in medicine bags as a protective amulet. A dish of allspice berries placed in a sick room can lift the patient's spirit and help prevent the spread of infection. Allspice essential oil is used in perfumery, mens' cologne, and mouthwash.

Constituents

Essential oils (eugenol, cineole, phellandrene), vitamin C, vitamins B_1 and B_2, beta-carotene, calcium, iron, magnesium, potassium, zinc

Energetic Correspondences

- Flavor: pungent
- Temperature: warm
- Moisture: dry
- Polarity: yang
- Planet: Mars/Venus/Uranus
- Element: fire

Contraindications

During pregnancy, avoid excessive use; moderate culinary use is permitted.

Range and Appearance

This tree is native to tropical regions of the West Indies and Central and South America. It grows up to 40 feet in height, and its branches bears corymbs of white flowers. The inferior ovary of the flower produces a green berry, which is harvested in July or August and dried in the sun, whereupon it becomes reddish brown.

ALOE

Botanical Name

Aloe ferox, *A. vera* (syn. *A. barbadensis*)

Family

Liliaceae (Lily Family)

Etymology

The name *aloe* derives from the Arabic *alloeh*,

"shiny" or "bitter," in reference to the aloe gel. The species name *vera* means "true" in Latin.

Also Known As

Afrikaans: aalwee, aalwyn
Danish: aloés, laegealoe, port
English: Barbados aloe, medicine plant
Finnish: laakeaaloe
French: aloès
Hawaiian: aloi, panini'awa'awa
Hindi: ghikanvar, guar patha
Japanese: rokai
Korean: nohwa
Mandarin: lú hui
Nepali: ghiu kumari
Polish: aloes zwycajny
Portuguese: aloes
Sanskrit: kumari
Spanish: acíbar
Thai: hang ta khe
Zulu: umhlaba

Part Used

Gel extracted from stalk

Physiological Effects

Antibacterial, antifungal, anti-inflammatory, biogenic stimulator, cholagogue, demulcent, emmenagogue, emollient, laxative, purgative, rejuvenative, vulnerary

Medicinal Uses

Aloe has long been used in medicine; references to its use as a healing agent can be found in early Egyptian, Chinese, Greek, Indian, and Christian literature. Legend has it that desire for aloe plants led Alexander the Great to conquer the island Socotra, where aloe was cultivated, in the fourth century B.C. Aloe is also thought to have been among the secret components of Cleopatra's beauty regimen.

Aloe vera gel cools heat and reduces inflammation in the body. It also helps the body slough off dead tissue, stimulates the formation of new tissue cells, and can help prevent scarring. It is used in the treatment of arthritis, bursitis, burns, constipation, dysentery, jaundice, sore throat, tuberculosis, and ulcers. Taken twenty minutes before a meal, the juice can help heal irritated digestive tissues.

Topically, aloe is used, on its own or as part of lotions, poutices, salves, shampoos, and sprays, to treat acne, boils, burns, dandruff, dermatitis, fever, hemorrhoids, herpes, insect bites, poison ivy and oak, psoriasis, rash, ringworm, scar, sunburn, and wounds.

As a flower essence, aloe vera restores inner balance in cases of exhaustion.

Edible Uses

Aloe gel/juice is edible. It is usually mixed in with juices or smoothies to improve its flavor.

Other Uses

African hunters sometimes rub aloe gel on their bodies to reduce sweating and mask their scent. The gel is sometimes applied to the nails as a remedy for nail biting; its bitter taste helps break the habit.

Constituents

Aloins, anthraquinones, polysaccharides, salicylic acids, calcium oxalate, glucose

Energetic Correspondences

- Flavor: bitter
- Temperature: cool
- Moisture: moist
- Polarity: yin
- Planet: Moon/Mars/Pluto
- Element: water

Contraindications

Avoid internal use during pregnancy. Also avoid internal use while nursing except under the guidance of a qualified health-care practitioner, as it may have an overly laxative effect on the infant. Excessive use may aggravate hemorrhoids. High doses may cause vomiting. When using aloe as a laxative, combine it with carminative herbs to prevent gripe. When using aloe topically, combine it with moisturizing ingredients to prevent dry skin.

Range and Appearance

Aloe, a perennial succulent native to Africa, is characterized by long, lanceolate, thick, and fleshy leaves that are green to gray-green in color, have a serrated margin, and ooze a water gel when broken. The leaves rise almost directly from the base of the plant; there are either no or very short stems. The pendulous flowers are borne on a spike and have a tubular yellow corolla.

Aloe prefers full sun, moderate water, and well-drained soil. It is among the easiest of houseplants to keep; in fact, it's been said that if you can't grow aloe, you should get plastic plants.

AMLA

Botanical Name

Emblica officinalis

Family

Euphorbiaceae (Spurge Family)

Etymology

The common name *amla* is thought to derive from one of the Sanskrit names for this plant, *amalaki*. The other Sanskrit common name, *dhatri,* means "nurse," in reference to the herb's many healing properties. The genus name, *Emblica,* is thought to be a Latinization of the common name.

Also Known As

English: amalaki, dharty, emblic myrobalan, Indian gooseberry

Sanskrit: amalaki, dhatri

Part Used

Fruit

Physiological Effects

Antibacterial, antifungal, anti-inflammatory, antioxidant, antiviral, aphrodisiac, astringent (when used over a short period), blood tonic, carminative, demulcent (when used over a long period), digestive, diuretic, hemostatic, hypotensive, immune tonic, laxative, nutritive, refrigerant, rejuvenative, stomachic, yin tonic

Medicinal Uses

Amla has been found to accelerate the regeneration of connective tissue and to enhance interferon production. Amla is used in treatments for allergies, anemia, asthma, bleeding gums, bronchitis, cancer, colds, colitis, constipation, debility, diabetes, dysuria, flatulence, gastritis, gingivitis, gout, hair loss, heart palpitations, hemorrhoids, hepatitis, hypertension, indigestion, jaundice, liver weakness, lung disease, osteoporosis, prematurely graying hair, scurvy, spleen weakness, tuberculosis, vertigo, vision weakness, and yeast infection. It is also used to encourage convalescence and to prevent wrinkles. And it is reputed to make people feel lighter and to promote love, longevity, and good fortune.

Amla is an ingredient in Chayvanprash, a popular five-thousand-year-old Ayurvedic tonic containing herbs, fruits, ghee, raw sugar, and honey. The herb is also an ingredient in the Ayurvedic formula Triphala, which aids in the regulation of all bodily functions, especially digestion. Amla is a traditional Ayurvedic remedy for mothers who act angrily toward their children, helping to calm their emotions. It is also used to comfort children who have lost their mothers.

For topical application, amla is an ingredient in shampoos and other hair preparations as well as massage oils. It has a calming effect when applied as a poultice to the head in cases of mental disorders.

Edible Uses

Amla can be enjoyed as a fresh or dried fruit, stewed, or in sherbets, jelly, or jam. Green amla fruits can be pickled.

Other Uses

None known

Constituents

Bioflavonoids, niacin, calcium, vitamin C, vitamin E, gallic acid, ellagic acid, tannins, polyphenols; amla is about twenty times higher in vitamin C than oranges.

Energetic Correspondences

- Flavor: sour, sweet, bitter, pungent
- Temperature: cool
- Moisture: moist
- Polarity: yin
- Planet: Venus/Moon
- Element: water

Contraindications

Avoid amla in cases of acute diarrhea or dysentery.

Range and Appearance

Native to India, amla is a small to midsize deciduous tree with feathery leaves. The flowers have a pale green hue; male and female flowers blossom on the same tree. The fruits are greenish, with six defined ridges and six seeds. Cultivated fruits weigh about 1 ounce each, while wild fruits are about half as heavy.

ANDROGRAPHIS

Botanical Name

Andrographis paniculata

Family

Acanthaceae (Acanthus Family)

Etymology

The prefix *andro* is Greek for "male"; *graphis* is also Greek and means "writing implement." The species name, *paniculata,* refers to the panicles in which the flowers grow.

Also Known As

Arabic: quasabhuva
Bengali: kalmegh
Cantonese: chyun sam ling
English: alui, creat, green chiretta, halviva, Indian echinacea, kariyat, king of bitters, thread-the-heart lotus
Hindi: kirayat
Japanese: senshinren
Korean: ch'onsimyon
Mandarin: chuan xin lian

Persian: naine-havandi
Sanskrit: kalmegha

Part Used

Entire plant, but predominantly the leaf

Physiological Effects

Abortifacient, analgesic, anthelmintic, antibacterial, antibiotic, antifungal, anti-inflammatory, antioxidant, antithrombotic, antiviral, astringent, bitter, cardioprotective, cholagogue, choleretic, depurative, diaphoretic, expectorant, febrifuge, hepatoprotective, hypoglycemic, immune stimulant, laxative, sedative, stomachic, uterine stimulant, vulnerary

Medicinal Uses

Andrographis clears heat (fever, inflammation) and detoxifies the body. It also stimulates antibodies and macrophages to counteract invading pathogens. In fact, it was used with success to treat the flu epidemic of 1919. It is used in the treatment of AIDS, bronchitis, cancer, cholera, colds, diabetes, dysentery, ear infection, *E. coli,* flu, hepatitis, herpes, HIV, kidney infection, leprosy, malaria, pneumonia, sore throat, staph infection, sinusitis, tonsillitis, tuberculosis, tumors, typhoid, and whooping cough.

Edible Uses

None known

Other Uses

None known

Constituents

Flavonoids, lactones (andrographolide, deoxyandrographolide), aldehydes, alkanes, ketones, paniculide, polysaccharides (galacturonic acid, galactose, rhamnose, arabinose)

Energetic Correspondences

- Flavor: bitter
- Temperature: cold
- Moisture: dry
- Polarity: yin
- Planet: Saturn
- Element: earth

Contraindications

A few cases of hives as a side effect have been reported. Andrographis is not recommended for use during pregnancy, as it has uterine-stimulating and abortifacient properties. Large doses have been reported to cause digestive disturbance.

Range and Appearance

Andrographis can be either an annual or a perennial shrub. It grows wild in thickets and in forests throughout southern Asia. In the fall small cymes of white terminal and auxiliary flowers appear.

ANGELICA

Botanical Name

Angelica archangelica (European angelica; syn. *A. officinalis*), *A. atropurpurea* (American angelica), *A. sylvestris*

Family

Apiaceae (Parsley Family)

Etymology

This herb is believed to have obtained the name *angelica,* or "angelic herb," because it was thought to help protect people against disease, poisoning, and witches. Legend recounts that the archangel Raphael appeared to a monk in a dream and told him that angelica would cure bubonic plague. European peasants once made garlands of angelica to place around their children's necks to protect them from illness and witches. And if a woman grew angelica in her garden, it was believed to indicate that she was not a witch, because witches were thought to avoid the plant.

The plant may also have been given this name because it blooms around May 8th, the feast day of the archangel Saint Michael.

Also Known As

Dutch: engelwortel
English: archangel, masterwort, root of the Holy Ghost, wild celery
Finnish: Väjnönputki
French: angeline, angélique
German: brustwurz, engelwurz
Italian: arcangelica
Sanskrit: choraka
Spanish: angélica, hierba del epiritu santo
Swedish: kvanne

Parts Used

Root (dried), leaf, stem, seed

Physiological Effects

Alterative, anti-inflammatory, antirheumatic, antispasmodic, aromatic, bitter, carminative, diaphoretic, digestive, diuretic, emmenagogue, expectorant, nervine, stimulant, stomachic, tonic, uterine stimulant

Medicinal Uses

As a tea angelica is used in treatments for amenorrhea, anemia, anorexia, arthritis, asthma, bronchitis, colds, colic, coughs, depression, dysmenorrhea, dyspepsia, fever, flatulence, flu, gout, irregular menses, migraine, placenta retention, poor appetite, poor circulation, and typhus. Regular use of angelica is said to promote a distaste for alcohol, and it may be beneficial in the treatment of alcoholism. Small amounts stimulate digestive secretions, and it is known to improve digestive metabolism and liver and spleen function. It also strengthens the lungs and heart. It is traditionally used to improve mental harmony and well-being.

Used in the bath, angelica can relieve muscle soreness and promote relaxation. An angelica sponge bath, using upward strokes, can aid in the treatment of victims of electric shock. Prepared as a liniment, angelica can be beneficial in cases of arthritis.

Angelica is potent even aromatically: the scent of the crushed leaves can prevent motion sickness.

As a flower essence, angelica helps build trust and bring in light and spiritual protection in life-threatening situations. It is helpful when one is facing the unknown, such as birth, death, and other passages of life. It is also helpful in treating alcoholism and nervous skin disorders.

Edible Uses

In Iceland and Lapland angelica stems are cooked as a vegetable. The stems and roots can be candied and made into syrups and jellies or added to fruitcake. They also can be used to season fish. The fresh leaves can be added to salads and soups. The dried leaves are wonderful in baked goods and fruit desserts; their sweetness makes it possible to decrease the amount of refined sugar in the recipe. The oil from the seeds and roots is used in the manufacture of Benedictine, Chartreuse, vermouth, and gin.

The herb's flavor is reminiscent of that of juniper berries, celery, and licorice.

Other Uses

In the language of flowers, angelica denotes inspiration. Angelica is traditionally burned as an incense to attract angelic presence. Its essential oil is sometimes used in perfume, and its leaf in potpourri. Native Americans in the Arkansas region used to combine angelica root with tobacco as a smoking mixture to inspire visions. Some carry angelica as a talisman for luck in gambling. And angelica leaves were once used to wrap and preserve food for traveling.

Constituents

Flavonoids (archangelone), essential oils (beta-phellandrene, pinene, limonene, caryophyllene, linalool), coumarins, acids (valerianic, angelic), caffeic acid, citric acid, fatty acids, resins, sterols, tannins, vitamin C

Energetic Correspondences

- Flavor: sweet, pungent
- Temperature: warm
- Moisture: dry
- Polarity: yang
- Planet: Sun/Jupiter
- Element: fire

Contraindications

Use only the dried root, and not the fresh root. Diabetics should use angelica with caution, as the plant can increase blood sugar levels. Large doses can affect blood pressure and respiration and can stimulate the nervous system. Avoid during pregnancy, in cases of heavy menstrual bleeding, and in conditions of excess heat, such as fever.

There is a slight possibility that angelica can increase photosensitivity in some people.

Range and Appearance

Angelica, a biennial, is native to North America and thrives in meadows, swampy areas, and marshy woods from Canada to the Carolinas. It can achieve a height of 5 to 8½ feet. Its thick, hollow stalk is purplish near its base. The large, pale green leaves are compound and triply divided. The small flowers range in color from white to yellow to green and grow in spherical umbels.

When planting angelica, keep in mind that black flies and fruit flies are attracted to it and will congregate around it, so avoid planting it under your window or by the front door.

Wild angelica looks similar to water hemlock and poison hemlock, which are toxic. When collecting angelica from the wild, take extra care not to confuse it with these two plants.

ANISE

Botanical Name

Pimpinella anisum

Family

Apiaceae (Parsley Family)

Etymology

The genus name, *Pimpinella,* is thought to be derived from the Latin *bipinnula,* "bipinnate," and indeed the leaves are arranged similarly on both sides. The species name, and many of the common names, are derived from the ancient Greek name for the plant, *anison.*

Also Known As

Arabic: yànîùsun
Dutch: anijs

Esperanto: aniz
French: anis, boucage
German: anis, anissamen
Hindi: saunf
Italian: anice
Japanese: anisu
Portuguse: erva-doce
Russian: anis
Sanskrit: shatapushpa
Spanish: anís, simiente de anis
Swedish: anis

Part Used

Seed

Physiological Effects

Antispasmodic, aphrodisiac, carminative, diuretic, expectorant, galactagogue, parturient, stimulant, stomachic, tonic

Medicinal Uses

Anise seeds are used to remedy asthma, bloating, catarrh, colic, coughs, diarrhea, flatulence, halitosis, hiccups, indigestion, insomnia, menstrual cramps, nausea, poor appetite, and whooping cough. They are sometimes added to cough syrups and lozenges because of their soothing effect on coughs and their pleasant taste.

The essential oil from the seeds is used to prevent and treat lice and scabies.

Edible Uses

The seeds, with their licorice-like flavor, improve the taste of other medicines and are used to flavor breads, cakes, cookies, fruits, soups, sauces, and pickles. They are a primary ingredient in mustaceum, an after-dinner digestive cake. They also can be eaten by themselves; they function as both a digestive aid and a breath freshener.

Many alcoholic beverages are made with anise, including Pernod, Raki, Aguardiente, Uzo, Anisette, Kummel, and Ojen.

Fresh anise leaves and stalks (before the plant has produced seed) are also edible can be added to salads.

Other Uses

The essential oil is used to flavor unpleasant medicines, toothpastes, and mouthwashes and to scent soaps. In India, anise water is used as cologne.

Stuffed in a sachet and taken to bed, anise seeds are said to prevent nightmares. Some believe that hanging a sprig of anise on one's bedpost promotes youthfulness. Anise seeds are irresistable to mice and can be used as bait to catch the rodents.

Constituents

Volatile oils (anethole, methyl chavicol), furanocoumarins, flavonoid glycosides, fatty acids, phytoestrogens, starch, protein, choline, mucilage

Energetic Correspondences

- Flavor: sweet, pungent
- Temperature: warm
- Moisture: dry
- Polarity: yang
- Planet: Sun/Mercury/Jupiter/Moon/Uranus
- Element: air

Contraindications

Avoid therapeutic doses during pregnancy except under the direction of a health-care professional.

Range and Appearance

This annual Eurasion native now grows wherever the climate is amenable; it prefers dry, light soil in full sun. The herb grows to about 2 feet in height and has feathery leaves divided into many leaflets. The umbrella-like clusters of tiny white or yellow flowers bloom in midsummer and produce small, downy, ribbed seeds in late summer.

ANISE HYSSOP

Botanical Name

Agastache foeniculum (syn. *A. anethiodora*, *Lophanthus anisatus*); sometimes also *A. rugosa* (Korean mint)

Family

Lamiaceae (Mint Family)

Etymology

The genus name, *Agastache,* means "many spiked" in Greek, referring to the numerous spikes on the plant. The species name, *foeniculum,* means "little hay" in Greek and derives from the Greek *foenum,* "fragrant hay," perhaps in reference to the delightful fragrance of this plant.

Also Known As

Cantonese: fuk heung
English: wonderhoney plant, licorice mint, lavender hyssop, giant blue hyssop
Finnish: yrtti-iiso
French: anis hysope
German: anisysop
Japanese: kakko
Korean: huo xiang
Mandarin: xiang ren hua
Swedish: anis-isop

Part Used

Aboveground plant

Physiological Effects

Antibacterial, antiemetic, antifungal, diaphoretic

Medicinal Uses

Anise hyssop is used in treatments for bloating, catarrh, colds, colic, diarrhea, fever, flu, morning sickness, nausea, poor appetite, and vomiting. It can be used as a preventive for heat stroke and summer colds. It is known to stimulate the gastrointestinal system and to clear excessive dampness in the stomach and spleen and heaviness in the chest. The Chippewa Indians included this herb in lung formulas.

The leaves are used topically as a poultice in treatments for angina, burns, fever, headache, heatstroke, and herpes.

Edible Uses

Anise hyssop has a wonderful aniselike flavor, with a hint of sassafras, and it is often used as a flavoring agent. Plains Indians used anise hyssop tea as a liq-uid sweetener. The plant's leaves are wonderful in small amounts in salads. It also can be made into a liqueur.

Other Uses

The essential oil is used in perfumery. The herb's leaf and flower can be used as breath fresheners.

Constituents

Essential oils (cinnamic aldehyde, caryophyllene, pogostol, benzaldehyde, eugenol), marrubiin

Energetic Correspondences

- Flavor: pungent, sweet
- Temperature: slightly warm
- Moisture: dry
- Polarity: yang
- Planet: Mercury
- Element: air

Contraindications

Generally considered safe.

Range and Appearance

Anise hyssop, a perennial native to North America, grows to about 3 feet in height. The roughly textured leaves are opposite, oval at the base, and pointed at the tip, with soft gray hair on the underside. The bluish purple flowers produce nectar throughout the day and attract hummingbirds, butterflies, and honeybees. The plant prefers moist conditions in open woods and prairies and along lakes, streams, and ditches.

ASHWAGANDHA

Botanical Name

Withania somnifera

Family

Solanaceae (Nightshade Family)

Etymology

The common name translates from the Sanskrit *ashva,* "horse," and *gandha,* "smells like," which alludes to the virility of a horse. The species name, *somnifera,* indicates that the herb is a soporific agent.

Also Known As

Afrikaans: geneesblaarbossie
English: Indian ginseng (though it is not related to ginseng), turragi, winter cherry, withania
German: ashvaganda
Hindi: varahakarni ("boar-eared"), vrisha ("amorous")
Zulu: ubuvimbha

Parts Used

Root (primarily), leaf, berry, seed

Physiological Effects

Root: adaptogen, anabolic, analgesic, anti-inflammatory, antioxidant, antispasmodic, antitumor, aphrodisiac, astringent, diuretic, hormone tonic, hypotensive, immune tonic, nervine, nutritive, rejuvenative, sedative, tonic, uterine relaxant
Leaf: adaptogen, antibiotic, aphrodisiac, deobstruent, diuretic, narcotic, sedative, tonic
Fruit: diuretic

Medicinal Uses

Ashwagandha's use has been recorded for at least three thousand years. It is excellent for those in convalescence. An Ayurvedic maxim says that taking ashwagandha for fifteen days imparts strength to the emaciated body, just as rain does to a crop.

The herb has many other medicinal uses, including being of benefit to those with AIDS, alcoholism, anemia, anorexia, anxiety, arthritis, asthma, bronchitis, bipolar depression, cancer, candida, cough, chronic illness, depression, dropsy, dyspepsia, edema, Epstein-Barr virus, erectile dysfunction, exhaustion, failure to thrive (in children), fever, forgetfulness, glandular swelling, graying hair, headache, hypertension, infertility, insomnia, leukoderma (localized loss of pigment in the skin), low libido, lumbago, memory loss, mental fatigue, miscarriage, multiple sclerosis, nausea, neurosis, overwork, panic attacks, premature aging, rheumatoid arthritis, seizures, low sperm count, stress, tremors, tuberculosis, tumors, and wasting diseases.

Ashwagandha is believed to maintain the immune system and is often prescribed in India to be taken along with antibiotics to prevent weakening of the immune system. It elevates iron levels in the blood, slightly decreases respiration, lowers blood pressure, relaxes smooth muscles, and, due to its flavonoid compounds, counters liver toxicity.

It works as a monoamine oxidase inhibitor, thereby increasing the availability of dopamine, a neurotransmitter. It also appears to mimic the action of the neurotransmitter GABA (gamma amino butyric acid) in relaxing the body. It is known as a *medharasayan* remedy, "a promoter of memory and learning."

A poultice of the leaves can be applied topically to reduce tumors, treat wounds, expel worms and lice, lower fever, and soothe boils and sore hands and feet. An oil infusion prepared from the plant can be used to ease a sore back.

Edible Uses

The plant has a flavor somewhat similar to that of unsweetened chocolate. Tea prepared from the plant is often flavored with spices such as cinnamon, cardamom, ginger, nutmeg, and milk. Ashwagandha powder is sometimes mixed with honey and almond butter or ghee and served on crackers.

The seeds have been used in place of rennet to curdle milk for the making of cheese.

Other Uses

The leaf is used as an insect repellent. The fruit, which is rich in saponins, is sometimes used as a soap.

Constituents

Thirty-five alkaloids (including ashwagandhine), steroidal lactones (withanolides), amino acids (tryptophan, alanine, ornothine), iron

Energetic Correspondences

- Flavor: sweet
- Temperature: warm
- Moisture: moist
- Polarity: yang
- Planet: Jupiter
- Element: fire

Contraindications

During pregnancy use ashwagandha only under the guidance of a health-care professional, as there have been some reports of the herb having abortifacient properties. Using this herb in combination with barbiturates can exacerbate their effects. The berries have caused gastrointestinal distress when consumed by children. Do not use the leaf in cases of congestion.

Range and Appearance

Ashwaghanda is native to India and the subtropical areas in the drier regions of the foothills of the Himalayas, at altitudes of up to 5,500 feet. It now grows wild from Europe to North Africa and the Middle East, often along roadsides and in fields.

This perennial plant somewhat resembles a stout potato plant but grows as large as a shrub. During its fruiting stage, the auxiliary clusters of yellow-green flowers look like miniature Chinese lanterns. As the plant reaches maturity, the calyxes become transparent, revealing orange-red berries that contain yellow seeds.

ASPARAGUS

Botanical Name

Asparagus cochinchinensis (Chinese asparagus), *A. lucidus*, *A. racemosus* (Indian asparagus)

Family

Liliaceae (Lily Family)

Etymology

The word *asparagus* comes from the Greek *asparagos,* which refers to tender shoots that can be consumed. Due to its phallic shape, the plant has long been regarded as an aphrodisiac, which can be seen in its etymology; the Ayurvedic name *shatavari,* for example, means "she who has one hundred husbands."

Also Known As

Cantonese: tin dung

English: sparrowgrass, hundred-rooted vine, many-heired vine, longevity vine, sataver
French: asperge
Hindi: sahansarmuli, satavar, shatavri
Japanese: tenmendo
Korean: ch'ônmundong
Mandarin: tien men tong
Nepali: sataavarii
Sanskrit: challagadda, shatavari
Spanish: esparrago
Thai: chuang khruea, sam sip
Vietnamese: mang tay

Part Used

Tuber

Physiological Effects

Alterative, aphrodisiac, brain tonic, cardiotonic, demulcent, diaphoretic, diuretic, expectorant, female tonic, galactagogue, kidney yin tonic, laxative (mild), lung tonic, nutritive, refrigerant, rejuvenative, reproductive tonic, sedative

Medicinal Uses

Asparagus has been known as a supreme tonic since ancient times. The Taoist classic *Embracing the Uncarved Block,* written in A.D. 300 by Ko Hung, tells the story of a man named Tu Tze-wei, who drank asparagus root tea for many years and was able to have sexual relations with eighty wives and concubines, walk a distance of fifty miles a day, and attain the advanced age of 145.

Asparagus root is used to treat acid indigestion, AIDS, cancer and the side effects of chemotherapy, chronic fever, cystitis, diarrhea, dry cough, dry skin, dysentery, Epstein-Barr virus, erectile dysfunction, female organ weakness, frigidity, gout, herpes, infertility, jaundice, kidney stones, low libido, low sperm count, menopause symptoms, poor memory, post-hysterectomy dryness, rheumatism, sciatica, tuberculosis, ulcers, and vaginal dryness. It can be used to encourage healing during convalescence. Because asparagus helps dissolve uric and oxalic acid, it benefits arthritic conditions and kidney stones. In general, it moistens and restores the entire system.

Psychologically, asparagus root is said to foster feelings of love and compassion, peace of mind, a loving nature, a good memory, and a calm spirit.

Topically, the leaves, shoots, and roots can be used as a poultice or compress to relieve muscle spasms and stiff joints. The leaves can be applied as a poultice for boils.

Edible Uses

Although only the tubers are used as internal medicine, the shoots, of course, are also edible. The young shoots can be eaten raw or cooked. The roots and shoots can be added to soups or salads. Asparagus seeds can be roasted and used as a coffee substitute.

Other Uses

Asparagus can increase the milk production of cows and is sometimes cultivated for cattle to graze on.

Constituents

Essential oil, steroidal glycoside (asparagoside), asparagine, arginine, tyrosine, flavonoids (kaempferol, quercitin, rutin), copper, iron, zinc, resin, tannin, mucilage

Energetic Correspondences

- Flavor: sweet, bitter
- Temperature: cool
- Moisture: moist
- Polarity: yin
- Planet: Venus
- Element: water

Contraindications

Do not eat raw asparagus seeds, as they can be toxic. The root is not recommended in cases of chronic diarrhea or cough with excessive clear phlegm.

Range and Appearance

Asparagus grows as a delicate perennial shrublike climbing plant in east Asian lowland jungle, woods, and shaded hillsides. It bears small ivory flowers in summer.

ASTRAGALUS

Botanical Name

Astragalus hoangtchy, A. membranaceus, A. mongolicus, (syn. A. propinquus)

Family

Fabaceae (Pea Family)

Etymology

The genus name, *Astragalus,* derives from the Greek *astragalos,* "vertebra." The Mandarin name *huang qi,* by which the plant is sometimes known in herb shops, refers to the color of the root (*huang* = "yellow") and the high esteem with which the plant is regarded (*qi* = "venerable").

Also Known As

Cantonese: beg kei
English: goat's thorn, milk vetch, yellow vetch
Finnish: kurjenherne
Japanese: ogi
Korean: hwanggi
Mandarin: huang qi

Part Used

Root

Physiological Effects

Adaptogen, adrenal tonic, antiviral, blood tonic, chi tonic, digestive, diuretic, hypotensive, immune stimulant, tonic, vasodilator

Medicinal Uses

Astragalus is one of the most widely prescribed herbs in Chinese medicine. Generally it is used not to treat any disease in particular but to enhance and balance bodily functions.

Astragalus helps increase vitality, builds the blood, normalizes the hormones, and improves circulation. It is used to bolster the *wei chi,* or the defensive immune system, helping the body to be more resistant to invasive pathogens. It increases phagocytic activity, inhibits viral replication, and increases the formation of lymphocytes. Astragalus reduces levels of T suppresser cells and enhances the function of the adrenal cortex. It is included in the database of the National Cancer Institute as an herb that can inhibit tumor growth. In a 1989 study at the Chinese Academy of Medical Sciences, patients with lung or liver cancer were given astragalus combinations during their courses of chemotherapy or radiation therapy; the one-year survival rates increased from 28% to 71% for those undergoing radiation and from 8% to 47% for those undergoing chemotherapy.

In addition to cancer recovery, astragalus is beneficial in cases of AIDS, blood loss (recovery from), bone marrow depression, frequent colds, diabetes, edema, exhaustion, hepatitis, hypertension, weakened immunity, lung weakness, night sweats, prolapsed organ, poor sperm motility, slow-healing wounds, and wasting diseases.

Edible Uses

Though the root is too tough to chew, you can tenderize it through soaking or cooking. It can be added to soups of all sorts, and it is wonderful in immune-building soups with garlic, onions, carrots, shiitake mushrooms, and miso.

Good-quality roots should have a consistent deep yellow color and a sweetish taste.

Other Uses

None known

Constituents

Polysaccharides, asparagine, calcyosin, formononetin, astragalosides, phytosterols, isomnine, kumatakenin, choline, betaine, linoleic acid, linolenic acid

Energetic Correspondences

- Flavor: sweet
- Temperature: warm
- Moisture: moist
- Polarity: yang
- Planet: Jupiter/Mars
- Element: air

Contraindications

Astragalus is not recommended in cases of severe

congestion, extreme tension, or an overactive immune system. It is generally not recommended in cases of fever and inflammation or extreme dryness (as evidenced by persistent thirst, dry skin, and constipation). It is best to avoid its use in cases of hot, toxic skin lesions and at the onset of cold and flu symptoms. It tends to hold infection in the body, so if you use astragalus during cases of infection, combine it with diaphoretic herbs.

Wild North American astragalus, often called locoweed, should not be used until further research has been done, since it may contain in its leaves toxic alkaloids that contribute to heart and lung suppression. Livestock that have consumed locoweed have been known to jump over imaginary objects, wander aimlessly, and drool excessively.

Range and Appearance

Astragalus is native to Mongolia and China, growing along forest margins and in open woodland and grassy areas. It is an upright perennial plant growing to about 2 feet in height with odd-pinnate, compound, featherlike leaves with a leaflet at the tip. The roots are usually harvested when they are four or five years old, in the spring or fall.

ATRACTYLODES

Botanical Name

Atractylodes alba, A. japonica, A. lancea, A. macrocephala

Family

Asteraceae (Daisy Family)

Etymology

The species name *macrocephala* means "big headed" in Latin, in reference to the plant's flowers. The species name *alba* means "white," in reference to the color of the root; the species name *japonica* means "of Japan," in reference to the plant's origin.

Also Known As

Cantonese: paak sat
Japanese: byakujutsu, sojutsu

Mandarin: dong zhu
Spanish: atractylodes

Part Used

Rhizome

Physiological Effects

Anticoagulant, anti-emetic, anti-inflammatory, anti-tumor, aromatic, chi tonic, digestive, diuretic, expectorant, hepatoprotective, spleen chi tonic, immune tonic, stomachic, tonic

Medicinal Uses

Atractylodes is one of the best-known Chinese tonic herbs. It is used to remedy bloating, diarrhea, edema, excessive perspiration, exhaustion, fever, indigestion, night blindness, poor appetite, side effects of chemotherapy and radiation, and vomiting. Atracylodes helps regulate spleen function, thus improving the digestive system's ability to transport nutrients. It also helps strengthen the muscles of the legs. It is considered a supreme energy tonic.

A related species (*Atractylodes lancea,* known as black or lance-leaved atractylodes) helps dry digestive dampness.

Edible Uses

The rhizome is edible; it is most often added to immune-building soups.

Other Uses

Topically, atractylodes is used in cosmetics for treating wrinkles and dark spots on the hands and face. The essential oil is used in perfumery.

Constituents

Essential oils (atractylol, atractylone, eudesmol, hinesol), sesquiterpenes, polysaccharides, beta-carotene

Energetic Correspondences

- Flavor: bitter, sweet
- Temperature: warm
- Moisture: dry
- Polarity: yang
- Planet: Sun

- Element: fire

Contraindications

Atractylodes is not recommended in cases of bleeding ulcers, dehydration, or yin deficiency with heat symptoms.

Range and Appearance

Atractylodes is a perennial herb found in the mountain valleys of northern Asia. It bears large, scaled, egg-shaped buds that bloom in autumn; the blossoms resemble sea anemones. The plant prefers well-drained soil in full sun to partial shade.

BACOPA

Botanical Name

Bacopa monnieri

Family

Scrophulariaceae (Figwort Family)

Etymology

The genus name is believed to be Aboriginal in origin. The common name *brahmi* is derived from that of Brahma, the Hindu god of creation.

Also Known As

English: brain plant, herb of grace, herpestris
   monniera, thyme-leaved gratiola, water hyssop,
   white hyssop
Finnish: pikkubakopa
German: kleine fettblatt, wasserysop
Hindi: brahmi, mandukaparni
Sanskrit: brahmi, nirabradhmi
Spanish: culebra
Swedish: litet tjockblad
Thai: phak mi

Part Used

Aboveground plant

Physiological Effects

Adaptogen, antidepressant, antifungal, anti-inflammatory, antioxidant, antirheumatic, antiseptic, antispasmodic, anxiolytic, bronchial dilator, cardiotonic, carminative, diuretic, immune tonic, laxative, nervine, nervous system tonic, rejuvenative, sedative

Medicinal Uses

In Ayurvedic medicine, bacopa is considered *medhya rasayan,* an herb that benefits the mind and spirit, and it has long been used to calm restlessness in children. It is a nourishing brain, nerve, and kidney tonic. It enhances neurotransmitter function and increases production of calming serotonin. It helps protect the synaptic functions of the nerves in the hippocampus, which is considered the seat of memory. It also increases protein synthesis and brain-cell activity. It has also been found to help chelate heavy metals out of the body.

Bacopa is used in the treatment of ADD, ADHD, Alzheimer's disease, anxiety, asthma, bronchitis, depression, diarrhea, epilepsy, hoarseness, hyperactivity, hypertension, insomnia, irritable bowel, learning disability, memory loss, mental illness, pain, restlessness, stress, and ulcers.

Topically, a poultice made from the leaves and applied to the appropriate area can relieve symptoms of rheumatism or asthma.

Edible Uses

Not generally considered edible, except as tea.

Other Uses

Bacopa has been used in the Hindu culture to consecrate newborns in the hope of "opening the door of Brahma," thus increasing intelligence. Because bacopa thrives in water, it is a popular aquarium plant.

CONSTITUENTS

Flavonoids, amino acids (alpha-alanine, glutamic acid, serine, aspartic acid), d-mannitol, beta-sitosterol, saponins (bacopaside I, bacopaside II), betulinic acid, wogonin, oroxindin, alkaloids (brahmine, herpestin, nicotine)

Energetic Correspondences

- Flavor: bitter, sweet
- Temperature: cool
- Moisture: moist
- Polarity: yin
- Planet: Moon/Mars/Saturn
- Element: water

Contraindications

Bacopa is generally regarded as safe, even for children. Not enough is currently known about its use during pregnancy, however, so for now it is best to avoid its use then. Take care not to confuse bacopa with gotu kola, which is also known as *brahmi.*

RANGE AND APPEARANCE

Bacopa is a semi-aquatic perennial creeping herb that can form mats. It has rounded, succulent leaves and small blue, white, or purplish flowers. Bacopa prefers muddy shores and wetland areas. It is believed to be native to India but grows throughout tropical regions of the world.

BALM OF GILEAD

Botanical Name

Populus balsamifera, P. candicans, P. gileadensis, P. nigra

Family

Salicaceae (Willow Family)

Etymology

The genus name, *Populus,* is the classical Latin name for this family of trees. The species name, *balsamifera,* derives from the Latin for "balsam-bearing."

Also Known As

English: balm poplar, balsam poplar, black cottonwood, hackmatack, Mecca balsam, tacamahac
Finnish: kartanoppeli
French: peuplier baumier, tremble
German: balsam-pappel, östliche, zitterpappel
Italian: piopo
Swedish: balsampoppel
Turkish: ak kavak

Part Used

Leaf bud

Physiological Effects

Alterative, analgesic, anodyne, antifungal, anti-inflammatory, antiscorbutic, antiseptic, bitter, diuretic, expectorant, fcbrifuge, stimulant, vulnerary

Medicinal Uses

The resinous leaf buds clear inflammation, cool and moisten the skin, encourage tissue repair, thin mucus secretions, and increase circulation to the respiratory system. Due to their salicin content, the buds can be used for many of the same things that aspirin is used to treat. They have long been used internally to treat bronchitis, coughs, laryngitis, sore throat, tonsillitis, and urinary tract infections.

Topically, the leaf buds are helpful in the treatment of skin ailments. They were used by Native Americans to treat sores, and in the 1970s Russian physicians had success using the leaf buds in a clinical trial to treat bedsores and postoperative abscesses. The leaf buds also can be used in poultices or compresses in the treatment of arthritis, rheumatism, burns, eczema, and psoriasis.

Edible Uses

The dried inner bark, which is best if collected in the spring, can be ground into a powder and used as a flour; it is often used in combination with other flours. The catkins, though bitter, can be consumed raw or cooked. The sap can also be ingested, as an emergency food source.

Other Uses

The fragrant resin is used in the manufacture of perfume, soap, and potpourri. The sap can be used as an adhesive glue. The roots are used to make baskets and string. The wood ashes are mixed with oil to make a soap; the white inner bark is also used to make soap. The fluffy seed coverings can be used to stuff pillows. The shoots of the plant can be soaked in water to make a hormonal rooting solution that will encourage other plant cuttings to root. The wood warps easily if exposed to water but is used to make crates and boxes. A yellow dye is made from the leaf buds.

Constituents

Phenolic glycosides (salicin), populin, essential oils (arcurumene, bisabolene, cineole, farnesene), gallic acid, tannins

Energetic Correspondences

- Flavor: bitter, pungent
- Temperature: cold
- Moisture: moist
- Polarity: yin
- Planet: Saturn/Uranus/Jupiter/Venus
- Element: water

Contraindications

Extended use of this plant can reduce the production of breast milk, so pregnant or nursing women should avoid it. Those sensitive to aspirin should use this plant with caution, as it contains compounds similar to those found in aspirin.

Range and Appearance

Balsam poplar is a deciduous tree that attains a height of 50 to 70 feet and has heart-shaped leaves and smooth gray bark. In spring, the tree's catkins release tiny seeds covered in hairlike cottony threads. The buds should be collected in early spring, after they have formed but before the leaves inside them have developed. The tree is dioecious, meaning that male and female flowers grow on different plants.

Balsams poplars can be found in forests around the world, including North America, South America, India, Africa, and Siberia.

BAPTISIA

Botanical Name

Baptisia alba, B. tinctoria

Family

Fabaceae (Pea Family)

Etymology

The genus name, *Baptisia,* comes from the Greek *baptein,* "to dye." The species name, *tinctoria,* also refers to dyeing, deriving from the Latin word for the process, *tinctura.* The common name *indigo* is derived from the Latin *indicum,* "from India."

Also Known As

English: American indigo, clover broom, false indigo, horsefly weed, indigo broom, indigo weed, prairie indigo, rattle brush, shoofly, wild indigo, yellow broom
Finnish: keltaetelänherne
French: indigo sauvage
German: baptise
Swedish: gul färgväppling

Parts Used

Root, leaf

Physiological Effects

Alterative, antibiotic, anti-inflammatory, antiseptic, antiviral, astringent, emmenagogue, laxative, purgative, stimulant

Medicinal Uses

Baptisia was an important remedy for the Native American peoples, and it became a popular remedy among Eclectic physicians in the early 1900s. The Eclectics considered it an ideal "epidemic remedy," appropriate for rapid progression of infectious states with dark-colored mucous membranes, a constant feeling of drowsiness, foul-smelling secretions (breath, urine, stool, and sweat), and possibly difficulty in swallowing.

Baptisia has been used with success to treat boils, cancer, chronic cystitis, chronic fatigue, diptheria, dysentery, fever with chills, flu, gangrene, herpes, immunization reactions, lymphatic obstruction, malaria, mononucleosis, pharyngitis, scarlet fever, spinal meningitis, swelling, sore throat, tissue necrosis, tonsillitis, toxemia, typhoid, typhus, venereal disease, and infections of the ear, nose, throat, and respiratory system. Its high polysaccharide content helps stimulate phagocytosis, thus stimulating the immune system, and so it is beneficial in cases of chronic infection. It especially affects the glandular and lymphatic systems, helping to clear toxins from the body. It also helps clear heat and reduces inflammation.

Topically, baptisia can be applied as a poultice to treat boils, eczema, gangrene, staph infection, tumors, and wounds. It can be used as a mouthwash or gargle to eliminate gingivitis, pyorrhea, sores, or soreness in the throat. It also can be used as a douche to treat cervical ulceration, leukorrhea, or vaginitis.

Edible Uses

The young shoots (less than 10 inches in height) can be prepared like asparagus. (If consumed when more mature, however, they will have strong cathartic properties.)

Other Uses

Baptisia is well known for its use in dyeing. The leaves of the plant contain indican, a colorless glucoside that oxidizes in water to form a blue hue, and they were used to dye the uniforms of both British and American soldiers during the time of the American Revolution.

Constituents

Polysaccharides, isoflavones, alkaloids (baptitoxin), glycosides (baptin), oleoresin, coumarins

Energetic Correspondences

- Flavor: bitter, pungent
- Temperature: cool
- Moisture: dry
- Polarity: yin
- Planet: Saturn
- Element: earth

Contraindications

Large doses are emetic and can be purgative. The plant is not recommended for use during pregnancy, and it is not recommended for long-term use by anyone except under the supervision of a qualified health-care practitioner.

Range and Appearance

Baptisia is a perennial North American plant that thrives in poor, dry soil and grows to a height of about 3 feet. It has cloverlike alternate leaves. Its half-inch-long flowers appear in clusters in July and August; *B. tinctoria* bears bright yellow flowers, while *B. alba* bears white flowers. The plant bears a bluish black fruit in an oblong pod.

BASIL

Botanical Name

Ocimum spp., including *O. americanum* (American basil), *O. basilicum*, *O. citriodorum* (lemon basil), *O. gratissimum* (tree basil), *O. minimum* (bush basil), *O. tenuiflorum* (holy basil)

Family

Lamiaceae (Mint Family)

Etymology

The genus name, *Ocimum,* is derived from the ancient Greek word *okimon,* "smell." The species name *basilicum* and the common name *basil* originate from the Greek *basilikon phuton,* "kingly," "valiant," or "royal herb." The Sanskrit name *tulasi* comes from that of Tulasi, wife of Vishnu, who took on the form of this herb when she came to earth.

Also Known As

Afrikaans: basilikum
Arabic: habaq, raihan
Armenian: shahasbram
Bulgarian: bosilek
Czech: bazalka
Danish: basilikum
Dutch: basilicum, koningskruid, vol mynte
English: Saint Josephwort
Esperanto: bazilio
Estonian: basilik
Farsi: reihan
Finnish: basilika
French: basilic, basilique
German: basilienkraut, basilikum, königskraut
Greek: vasilikos
Hebrew: bazilikum, rehan
Hindi: tulsi
Hungarian: bazsalikom
Icelandic: basilika
Indonesian: indring, kermangi
Italian: basilico
Japanese: bajiru
Korean: pasil
Malay: kemangi
Mandarin: jiu ceng ta, lui le
Nepali: tulsi patta
Nigerian: efirin wewe
Norwegian: basilikum
Polish: bazylia wonna
Portuguese: alfavaca, manjeriacão
Romanian: busuioc
Russian: bazilik
Sanskrit: krishnamula (*O. tenuifolia*), tulasi
Spanish: albahaca
Swahili: mrihani
Swedish: basil, basilkört
Thai: horapa, krapau
Turkish: feslegen, peslen
Vietnamese: e' do'
Yiddish: basilik

Parts Used

Leaf

Physiological Effects

Antidepressant, anti-inflammatory, antioxidant, antiseptic, antispasmodic, carminative, circulatory stimulant, diaphoretic, digestive, emmenagogue, expectorant, febrifuge, galactagogue, nervine, sedative

Medicinal Uses

Basil stimulates the lungs, warms the body, calms the stomach, and dries dampness. It is used in the treatment of acne, asthma, anxiety, bronchitis, colds, constipation, coughs, depression, diarrhea, drug overdose or withdrawal, dysentery, exhaustion, flatulence, headache, nausea, rheumatism, stomachache, and vomiting. It can be used to encourage the expulsion of the placenta after birthing.

Topically, basil is used as a poultice to treat insect bites, acne, and ringworm. It can be made into a gargle or mouthwash to treat thrush or into an eyewash to treat tired eyes. The essential oil can be added to massage oils to soothe sore muscles. Basil also has an energizing aromatherapeutic effect, released by crushing the leaves, using basil as a bath herb, or using the essential oil.

As a flower essence, basil helps one put aside things that no longer serve one's purpose and promotes humanitarian motives, self-nurturing, and integrity. It improves the outlook of high achievers who feel inadequate.

Edible Uses

Basil leaf is a supreme culinary herb used in cuisines around the world. (Although *O. tenuiflorum* is not widely used because of its strong medicinal flavor.) In Thailand, the seeds of some basil species are used as a culinary thickening agent. Basil is also one of the ingredients in the liqueur Chartreuse.

Other Uses

In ancient India basil was considered sacred to Vishnu and his incarnation as Krishna. It was held in such high esteem that it was used in court to swear upon, and basil water was used to bathe the dead. It was believed that no leaf of this herb should be taken without a reason or a prayer for forgiveness. And the ancient Indians weren't the only ones to use basil in sacred death rituals: the ancient Egyptians used it as an embalming herb.

In many cultures, basil is considered an herb of protection and one to attract prosperity and luck. In some parts of Mexico, for example, basil carried in one's pocket is thought to attract money and to keep a lover faithful. And in Italy, a woman places a pot of basil on her balcony to signify that she wants to see her lover.

Basil essential oil is often included as an aromatic and healing agent in soaps, shampoos, and perfumes. The dried herb can be burned as an incense, while the plant can be used as a strewing herb. In the garden, basil acts as a natural insect repellent; in the home, keeping a pot of basil on the table repels flies, mosquitoes, and cockroaches.

Constituents

Essential oils (cineol, estragol, eugenol, lineol, linalool, methyl cinnamate), caffeic acid, monoterpenes, sesquiterpenes, tannins, beta-carotene, vitamin C

Energetic Correspondences

- Flavor: pungent, bitter
- Temperature: warm
- Moisture: dry
- Polarity: yang
- Planet: Mars/Jupiter
- Element: fire

Contraindications

Generally regarded as safe.

Range and Appearance

Native to Africa and Asia but now grown as a garden herb worldwide, basil is a bushy annual growing to about 2 feet in height. The deep green leaves are oval and opposite, borned on a square stem. The small white flowers bloom in spikes at the ends of the stem. In the garden, basil prefers full sun, well-draining soil, and moderate water.

BAY

Botanical Name

Laurus nobilis

Family

Lauraceae (Laurel Family)

Etymology

The genus name, *Laurus,* is Latin, meaning "to praise." The species name, *nobilis,* is also Latin and means "noble" or "notable." The common name *bay* derives from the Latin *baca,* "berry," in reference to the tree's purplish black fruits.

Also Known As

Arabic: ghàr
Armenian: tapni derev
Bulgarian: dafinov list, lavrovo durvo
Cantonese: yuht gwai

Croatian: lovor
Czech: bobkyovy', vavrín
Danish: laurbaer
Dutch: laurier
English: bay laurel, laurel, sweet laurel
Estonian: harilik loorberipuu
Farsi: barg-e-bu
Finnish: laakeripuu
French: laurier, laurier d'Apollon
German: edler lorbeerbaum, lorbeer,
    suppenblätter
Greek: dhafni
Hebrew: aley dafna
Hungarian: albertlevél, babér
Icelandic: lárvioarlauf
Italian: alloro, lauro franco, lauro poetico,
    lauro regio
Japanese: gekkeiju
Korean: pei, rorel-bei
Lithuanian: lauras
Mandarin: yue gui, yueh kuei
Polish: lisc laurowy
Portuguese: loureiro
Romanian: dafin
Russian: lavr
Serbian: lovorov list
Spanish: bahia, laural
Swedish: lager
Thai: bai krawan
Turkish: defne agaci
Ukranian: lavr
Vietnamese: lá nguyêt quê
Yiddish: lorber

Part Used

Leaf

Physiological Effects

Antifungal, antiseptic, aromatic, astringent, carminative, circulatory stimulant, diaphoretic, stimulant, stomachic, tonic

Medicinal Uses

Bay leaf strengthens and tonifies the digestive system and aids digestion and the assimilation of food. It has been used to treat arthritis, atherosclerosis, bronchitis, colic, cramps, delayed menses, flatulence, flu, indigestion, memory loss, and poor circulation.

An infusion of bay leaf can be added to the bath as a treatment for sore muscles, to a hair rinse for dandruff, and to a hand soak for nail fungus. Bay leaf also can be prepared as a poultice to treat bronchitis, coughs, and chest complaints.

The essential oil is often added to massage oils and liniments for use in cases of headache, sprains, and arthritis.

As a flower essence, bay helps release suppressed emotions, increases vitality, and brings spirituality to the physical level.

Edible Uses

Bay leaf is a classic culinary herb and is used to flavor myriad dishes. The whole, dried leaves are usually too tough to eat and have sharp edges that can lodge in the throat, so remove them from dishes or teas before serving.

Other Uses

Ancient Greeks and Romans regarded bay as a symbol of victory and nobility. Olympic athletes, poets, scholars, and military heroes received wreaths of bay to place on their heads. Roman senators wore bay chaplets on their heads (though perhaps this was to cover their bald spots). To this day we still use the term *baccalaureate,* "laurel berries," to signify the completion of a bachelor's degree. We also bestow the term *laureate* upon a poet as a term of honor and respect for his or her work.

Bay leaf repels cockroaches, fleas, moths, and other bugs. The essential oil can be used in topical insect repellents, and placing bay leaves in food canisters can repel bugs from them. When placed in clothing, books, or other fiber items, bay can help prevent damage from a variety of vermin. Placing bay leaves in lard helps prevent it from becoming rancid. The wood is used to build cabinets and make bowls.

Bay leaf is also held in high regard in magical traditions. For a wish to be granted, for example, it can be inscripted on a bay leaf, which is then burned as incense. A sprig of bay placed under a bed pillow is said to enhance clairvoyance. And to ensure their continued union, lovers may pick a twig, divide it in half, and each keep one half.

Bay in Myth

Mythology recounts that Apollo relentlessly pursued the nymph Daphne until the gods had mercy upon her and turned her into a bay laurel tree. Apollo was inconsolable and decreed that the bay tree would remain green all year round. Apollo then wore a laurel of bay leaves on his head in memory of Daphne.

Constituents

Essential oils (geraniol, cineol, eugenol, linalool, carvacrol, terpenes), calcium, magnesium, phosphorous, B-complex vitamins, tannins

Energetic Correspondences

- Flavor: sweet, slightly bitter
- Temperature: warm
- Moisture: dry
- Polarity: yang
- Planet: Sun/Mars/Neptune
- Element: fire

Contraindications

Bay is generally considered safe. American bay (*Umbellularia californica*), however, is poisonous, so make sure you are using the correct species. Just because a plant is called bay does not mean it is safe to consume.

Range and Appearance

Native to the Mediterranean region, bay trees grow with great variation, some with a single shoot, and others with multiple ones. The young leaves are smooth and pale green. A single tree may produce leaves of differing shapes; usually they are 1 to 3 inches long and $\frac{1}{2}$ to 1 inch wide. The tree can grow from 6 to 25 feet in height. The fruits are dark purple to black, each about $\frac{1}{2}$ inch in diameter.

BAYBERRY

Botanical Name

Myrica cerifera

Family

Myricaceae (Wax Myrtle Family)

Etymology

The genus name, *Myrica*, derives from the classical Greek name for the tamarisk plant, which is a close relative. The species name, *cerifa*, derives from the Greek *keros*, "wax bearing."

Also Known As

English: bog myrtle, candleberry, sweet gale, tallow shrub, vegetable tallow, waxberry, wax myrtle
Finnish: suomyrtti
French: arbre a cire, cirier
German: gagelstrauch, washgagel, washmyrte
Italian: albero della cera, pianta della cera
Persian: darshishaan, kandula
Sanskrit: katiphala
Spanish: arrayan, brabantico
Swedish: pors
Turkish: mom agaci

Parts Used

Bark, root bark

Physiological Effects

Alterative, antibacterial, anti-inflammatory, antioxidant, antiseptic, astringent, cholagogue, circulatory stimulant, diaphoretic, diuretic, expectorant, febrifuge, hepatoprotective, sialogogue, stimulant, styptic

Medicinal Uses

Bayberry cleanses the mucous membranes and restores mucous secretions to normal, cleanses the circulatory system, promotes lymphatic drainage, and tonifies the tissues. It was an important ingredient in composition powder, a cure-all remedy popularized in the early nineteenth century by North American herbalist Samuel Thompson. Today, bayberry is used in treatments for colds, colic, colitis, diarrhea, dysentery, epilepsy, fever, flu, irritable bowel syndrome, leukorrhea, menorrhagia, sore throat, tonsillitis, and varicose veins.

Topically, bayberry can be used as a tooth powder in treatments for spongy, bleeding gums and toothache; as a gargle for canker sores, sore throat, and tonsillitis; as a poultice for sores; as a rinse to stop hair loss; as a compress for varicose veins and hemorrhoids; or as a douche for leukorrhea. Bayberry powder can be used as a snuff to relieve nasal congestion.

Edible Uses

The bark and root bark are not generally considered edible, except as tea. The fruits are edible, however, whether raw or cooked, though they are small and have little flesh. The leaves are sometimes used as a flavoring agent, much like bay leaves; they should be removed before serving.

Other Uses

The leaves can be used in sachets and potpourris to repel insects; they also produce a green dye. The berries are a common ingredient in aftershaves and hair tonics, and they also are used to season meat. Wax from the berries has long been used to make soap, cosmetics, and candles; when the berries are boiled in water, the wax floats to the surface and is skimmed off. Four pounds of berries yields about 1 pound of wax.

Constituents

Phosphorous, sulfur, vitamin C, essential oil, triterpenes (taraxerol, taraxerone, myricadol), flavonoids (myricitrin), phenols, starch, myrica waxes (palmitic acid, stearic acid, myristic acid), lignin, albumen, gum, tannins, gallic acid

Energetic Correspondences

- Flavor: pungent
- Temperature: warm
- Moisture: dry
- Polarity: yang
- Planet: Venus/Sun/Mercury
- Element: fire/earth

Contraindications

Avoid bayberry during pregnancy. It is contraindicated for excessively hot conditions such as inflammation. Large doses may be emetic and may aggravate flatulence or cause stomach distress. People who suffer from hay fever may find the condition aggravated by bayberry pollen.

Range and Appearance

Bayberry is a perennial evergreen shrub that reaches a height of 2 to 4 feet, though it has been known to grow up to 40 feet tall. It is native to the eastern part of the United States. It grows in dry woods, fields, and thickets near sandy swamps. The leaves are shiny, green, and lanceolate. The catkins are yellow, forming drupes of berries that are first green and then greenish white.

BIRCH

Botanical Name

Betula spp., including *B. alba* (white birch), *B. lenta* (cherry birch), *B. nana* (dwarf birch), *B. nigra* (black birch), *B. pendula* (silver birch), *B. populifolia* (gray birch)

Family

Betulaceae (Birch Family)

Etymology

The word *birch* is believed to come from the Sanskrit *bhurga*, meaning "tree whose bark can be written on." It may also derive from the Old English *beorht*, "bright," in reference to the glowing white bark. The genus name, *Betula*, is the Latin name for this type of tree.

Also Known As

Danish: birk
English: lady of the woods
Finnish: koivu
French: arbe de la sagesse, bouleau
German: birke, weissbirke
Italian: betula

Russian: belaya bereza
Spanish: abedul
Swedish: biork, björk

Parts Used

Leaf bud, leaf, inner bark

Physiological Effects

Analgesic, anodyne, antibacterial (leaves), anti-inflammatory, anthelmintic, antirheumatic, antiseptic, aromatic, astringent, bitter, diaphoretic, diuretic, febrifuge, stimulant

Medicinal Uses

Birch clears toxins, softens deposits, relieves pain, and stimulates kidney function. It is used medicinally to treat arthritis, boils, cholera, diarrhea, dysentery, fever, gout, headaches, intestinal worms, kidney stones, and rheumatism. Birch bark is being investigated for its anticancer potential, with a focus on its betulinic acid content.

Topically, birch is used as a poultice in treatments for acne, bruises, burns, eczema, and wounds. It can be used as a bath herb to heal skin eruptions, as a liniment to mitigate the effects of rheumatism, and as a shampoo or hair rinse to stimulate hair growth.

Birch essential oil is used in salves and medicated soaps for the treatment of eczema and psoriasis. The essential oil also can be diluted and used as a soothing gum rub for teething infants. Curiously, what is called the essential oil of wintergreen is usually made from birch. Birch and wintergreen have similar chemistry, fragrance, and topical analgesic properties, but true wintergreen is rarely available as an essential oil.

As a flower essence, birch helps open perceptions and expands cosmic consciousness, improving peace of mind.

Edible Uses

The inner bark can be used to make birch beer. It also can be dried and ground into flour or cut into thin strips and boiled as noodles. The young leaves and catkins can be eaten fresh in salads. The sap of the tree can be made into wine, syrup, or vinegar.

Other Uses

Birch bark has been used as paper; in ancient times it was used to make clothing, shoes, and containers. The fresh leaf wards off bugs and was once used as a strewing herb, and smaller birch branches were used for broom handles. A tar made from birch is used to waterproof leather. The sap is distilled and used to treat mange in animals. As birch wood is full of air pockets and thus very buoyant, it was used to make canoes by some Native American peoples. It is used today to make plywood and furniture. In Russian and Finnish saunas, people strike their bodies with birch branches to stimulate circulation, while Laplanders carve statues from birch wood.

Constituents

Vitamins B and C, magnesium, potassium, saponins, essential oil (methyl salicylate), betulinic acid, tannin, flavonoids (hyperoside, luteolin, quercitin), bitter principle, glycosides

Energetic Correspondences

- Flavor: pungent, bitter
- Temperature: warm
- Moisture: moist
- Polarity: yin
- Planet: Venus/Jupiter/Saturn/Sun
- Element: water

Contraindications

Generally regarded as safe.

Range and Appearance

Birch flourishes in cold, moist environments, areas where other plant life may be sparse, and thus is considered a symbol of reawakening. There are at least sixty species in the genus, native to Europe, Asia, and North America. Birch trees are deciduous and can attain a height of up to 50 feet. They have a silvery white bark. The small leaves are alternate, toothed, and simple; they are bright green during the warmer months and turn yellow in autumn. The trees are monoecious and bear catkins of flowers: male flowers are thin and hang down, while female flowers are smaller and more erect. The fruits have a central axis with many small scales and are scattered by the wind.

BLACKBERRY

Botanical Name

Rubus spp., including *R. arcticus* (arctic bramble), *R. canadensis* (smooth blackberry), *R. fruticosus* (European blackberry), *R. laciniatus* (cut-leaf blackberry)

Family

Rosaceae (Rose Family)

Etymology

The genus name, *Rubus,* is the Latin name for this type of berry plant. The folk name *bramble* is derived from the Old English word bræmel, "prickly."

Also Known As

Danish: brombaer
Dutch: braam
English: blackberry, bramble, dewberry, gout berry
French: murier, ronce commune
German: brombeere
Italian: mora, rova
Portuguese: amora-preta
Spanish: zaezamoras
Swedish: björnbär

Parts Used

Leaf, root bark, fruit

Physiological Effects

Leaf, root, root bark: alterative, astringent, blood tonic, diuretic, hemostatic, nutritive, refrigerant, tonic, uterine tonic, yin tonic
Fruit: antioxidant, antiscorbutic, astringent, tonic

Medicinal Uses

Blackberries are closely related to raspberries, being in the same genus. They can be differentiated by the fact that blackberries bear larger, black or purplish berries and have longer, thornier canes that appear greenish white in their first year. Most herbalists agree that blackberry plants share common uses, as detailed here, and red raspberry plants share their own common uses, as detailed in the profile of raspberry (see page 246).

Blackberry leaf was recommended for therapeutic use as early as the first century, by Dioscorides. The leaf helps clear heat, reduces inflammation, cools fever, and dries dampness. It is of benefit in cases of anemia, bleeding, cholera, diarrhea, dysentery, fever, gout, hemorrhoids, and infertility.

The berries are considered to be a blood-building tonic and are beneficial in cases of anemia. With their antioxidant content, they are also a powerful anticancer and antitumor remedy. They also can be made into a delicious syrup to alleviate diarrhea in children.

The root bark is considered to have the strongest medicinal action. It can be used in treatments for diarrhea, dysentery, internal bleeding, and leukorrhea.

Topically, blackberry leaf is used as an astringent for oily skin, to treat wounds, as a mouthwash for sores and weak gums, and as a gargle for sore throat. The leaves can be applied as a poultice to relieve the pain and itchiness of insect bites and to shrink hemorrhoids.

As a flower essence, blackberry is helpful for those who find it difficult to initiate projects and those who are hampered by lethargy and inertia. It helps remove creativity blockages, allows hidden talents to blossom, and calms fear of death. It is particularly beneficial for those who do dream work, meditate, or practice visualization.

Edible Uses

The berries are a beloved fruit wherever they are grown. They can be consumed raw or cooked in pies, tarts, and jams. They also can be made into liqueurs, wine, and brandy.

The leaf and root bark are not generally considered edible, except as tea.

The fruit yields a bluish dye. A fiber obtained from the stem can be used to make twine.

Other Uses

None known

Constituents

Leaf, root, root bark: tannins, gallic acid, saponins (villosin), iron
Fruits: vitamin C, niacin, pectin, sugars, anthocyanins, flavonoids (kaempferol, quercitin)

Energetic Correspondences

- Flavor: leaf, root, root bark—bitter; fruit—sweet, sour
- Temperature: leaf, root, root bark—cold; fruit—neutral
- Moisture: leaf, root, root bark—dry; fruit—neutral
- Polarity: yin
- Planet: Venus/Mars
- Element: water

Contraindications

Overindulgence in the berries can cause constipation or diarrhea and can inhibit menstrual bleeding. Those with sensitive stomachs may find the high tannin content of the leaves and root to cause nausea or vomiting.

Range and Appearance

Blackberry is believed to be native to both Europe and North America. This perennial plant is found most often growing in hedges and open woods. It has woody stems up to 16½ feet long, with large hooks (thorns). The leaves are palmate with three to five rounded, toothed leaflets. The five-petaled flowers can be white or pink.

BLACK COHOSH

Botanical Name

Actaea racemosa (formerly *Cimicifuga racemosa*)

Family

Ranunculaceae (Buttercup Family)

Etymology

The former genus name, *Cimifuga,* is from the Latin *cimicus,* "insect," and *fugare,* "to drive away," in reference to the plant's ability to drive off insects. The species name, *racemosa,* refers to the racemes of flowers. The common name *black cohosh* makes reference to the dark color of the rhizome; *cohosh* is Algonquin for "rough with hairs," in reference to the bumpy texture of the rhizome.

Also Known As

English: bugbane, black snakeroot, rattle root, squaw root
French: racine d'actee a grappes
German: schwarze schlangenwurzel, traubiges wazenkraut
Spanish: cimifuga negra, cohosh negro
Swedish: spjutsil verax

Parts Used

Rhizome, root

Physiological Effects

Alterative, anti-inflammatory, antirheumatic, antispasmodic, antitussive, astringent, cardiotonic, central nervous system depressant, circulatory stimulant, diaphoretic, diuretic, emmenagogue, expectorant, hypoglycemic, hypotensive, muscle relaxant, parturient, sedative, vasodilator

Medicinal Uses

Black cohosh, a member of the United States Pharmacopoeia from 1820 until 1926, was used in that time to treat scarlet fever, smallpox, and whooping cough. It was an ingredient in the famous Lydia Pinkham Vegetable Compound for "female complaints."

Black cohosh is a popular women's herb. Many Native American tribes, including the Cherokee, Delaware, Iroquois, Penobscot, and Winnebago, have used it to ease childbirth. It is known to help restore healthy menses and to soothe irritation and congestion of the cervix, uterus, and vagina. It also improves circulation in general and lowers blood pressure by temporarily dilating blood vessels.

Black cohosh is used in the treatment of anxiety (related to menopause), arthritis, asthma, bronchitis, colitis, convulsions, debility, depression, dysmenorrhea, dyspareunia (painful sexual intercourse), headache, heart palpitations, hyperhidrosis, hysteria, insomnia, irritability, menopause symptoms (including hot flashes), mood swings, night sweats, premenstrual syndrome, rheumatism, sciatica, tinnitus, tuberculosis, vaginal atrophy, vaginal dryness, vertigo, and whooping cough. It can also be used to induce labor or the menstrual cycle (under the supervision of a qualified health-care practitioner).

Topically, black cohosh can be used as a poultice to treat snakebite.

As a flower essence, black cohosh helps those who are in abusive and addictive relationships. It aids one in building up the courage to confront rather than retreat and to transform the negative; it also helps bring balance to negative situations.

Edible Uses

Black cohosh rhizomes and roots are not generally considered edible, aside from as tea. The leaves can be eaten when cooked, but they are more of a survival food, rather than a suggested wild edible.

Other Uses

The plant, whether in the garden, fresh, or dried, can be used as a bug repellent.

Constituents

Calcium, magnesium, potassium, zinc, vitamin E, triterpene glycosides (acetin, cimicifugoside), phytoestrogens, isoflavones, isoferulic acid, essential oil, tannins, resin (cimicifugin), salicylates

Energetic Correspondences

- Flavor: bitter, pungent
- Temperature: cool
- Moisture: dry
- Polarity: yang
- Planet: Pluto
- Element: earth

Contraindications

Avoid during pregnancy and while nursing, except under the guidance of a qualified health-care practitioner. Avoid also in cases of heart conditions. Excess use can irritate the nervous system and cause nausea, vomiting, headache, and low blood pressure. Unlike pharmaceutical hormone replacement therapy, black cohosh is considered to be a menopause tonic that is safe for women with estrogen-dependent cancers, uterine bleeding, fibrocystic breast disease, endometriosis, liver disease, gallbladder disease, or pancreatitis. Recently concern has arisen regarding the effect of this herb on the liver over the long term; further research is under way to investigate this issue.

Range and Appearance

Native to North America, black cohosh is a hardy perennial that prefers moist or dry woodland environments. It grows from 3 to 8 feet in height. The large, toothed leaflets are pinnately compound. The tiny white flowers grow in long spires and bloom from late summer through early fall.

Black cohosh is at risk of becoming endangered in the wild, so instead of wildcrafting, consider cultivating your own supplies. When purchasing black cohosh products, be sure they are made only from cultivated stock.

BLADDER WRACK

Botanical Name

Fucus vesiculosus

Family

Fucaceae (Seaweed Family)

Etymology

The genus name, *Fucus,* derives from the Greek *phukos,* "seaweed." The common name *bladder wrack* refers to the bladderlike air pods (vesicles) that help keep this plant afloat on the ocean.

ALSO KNOWN AS

English: black tany, cutweed, dyer's fucus,

kelpware, lady wrack, paddy tang, popping wrack, red fucus, rockwrack, sea oak, sea spirit, seaweed, seawrack, vraic

Finnish: rakkolevä

French: fucus, laminaires

German: blasentang

Italian: quercia marina

Japanese: kombu

Spanish: encina de mar, fuco verigoso

Swedish: blåstång

Part Used

Entire plant

Physiological Effects

Alterative, antibacterial, antibiotic, anticarcinogenic, antioxidant, antitumor, demulcent, diuretic, emollient, endocrine tonic, expectorant, laxative, nutritive

Medicinal Uses

Bladder wrack has a generally softening, draining, nourishing effect on the body. It also increases the body's rate of metabolism and promotes the cleansing and clearing of toxins, including radioactive strontium 90. Bladder wrack is used in the treatment of anemia, asthma, candida, catarrh, constipation, cough, cysts, edema, fatigue, goiter, heartburn, high cholesterol, hormonal imbalance, hypertension, hypotension, hypothyroidism, lymph node enlargement, nail weakness, obesity, rheumatism, and tumors. Because bladder wrack helps stimulate a sluggish metabolism, it can be helpful as part of a weight-loss program. It also can be used as a breast cancer preventive and to encourage convalescence.

Topically, bladder wrack can be used as a compress or oil to ease arthritic joints and bruises or as a bath herb to encourage the breakdown of cellulite or to soothe sore muscles.

Edible Uses

Bladder wrack can be eaten raw or cooked. It is rich in minerals and can improve the digestibility of fiber-rich foods, such as beans. It has a salty flavor and can be used as a seasoning.

Other Uses

Bladder wrack is often included in lotions for its skin-softening qualities and in shampoos and hair conditioners for its rich mineral content. The plant also makes a wonderful garden fertilizer.

In magical traditions, bladder wrack is associated with psychic ability, protection, and wealth.

Constituents

Alginic acid, fucoidan, carrageenan, calcium, chromium, germanium, iodine, iron, phosphorous, potassium, bromine, magnesium, manganese, selenium, silica, zinc, mucopolysaccharides, mannitol, alginic acid, kainic acid, laminine, histamine, zeaxanthin, protein, beta-carotene, vitamins B_2 and B_{12}, vitamin C, vitamin D, vitamin E

Energetic Correspondences

- Flavor: salty
- Temperature: cool
- Moisture: moist
- Polarity: yin
- Planet: Venus/Neptune/Moon
- Element: water

Contraindications

Avoid bladder wrack in cases of hyperthyroidism or general weakness and coldness. Overuse can produce goiterlike symptoms. Those on a low-sodium diet or using thyroid medication should consult with a qualified health-care professional before using kelp therapeutically.

Range and Appearance

Bladder wrack, though classified as a brown algae, is light yellow to olive green in color. It consists of thin, leathery, branching fronds with a distinct midrib that reach 2 to 3 feet in length. The plant usually has oval bladders that exist in pairs, though the bladders may be missing in places where the plants are heavily pounded by surf. Bladder wrack is found on the northern coasts of the Atlantic and Pacific oceans, including the Baltic and North seas. It is commonly attached to submerged rocks between the high- and low-tide marks.

If you are wildcrafting kelp, for maximum nutritional value collect plants that are still growing in the ocean rather than ones that have washed up on the shore. Avoid collecting kelp from polluted waters.

BLESSED THISTLE

Botanical Name

Cnicus benedictus (formerly *Carduus benedictus, Carbenia benedicta*)

Family

Asteraceae (Daisy Family)

Etymology

The genus name, *Cnicus,* comes from the Greek *knicos,* meaning thistle or safflower. The species name, *benedictus,* was bestowed in honor of Saint Benedict, who founded the religious order that bears his name.

Also Known As

Afrikaans: karmedik

English: blessed cardus, blessed thistle, cardin, holy thistle, lady's thistle, Saint Benedict's thistle, spotted thistle

Finnish: karvasohdake

French: chardon bénit

German: benediktendistel, bitterdistel, kardobenedikte

Italian: cardo santo

Spanish: cardo bendito

Swedish: kardbenedikt

Part Used

Aboveground plant

Physiological Effects

Alterative, anti-inflammatory, antiseptic, aromatic, astringent, bitter, cholagogue, digestive, diaphoretic, diuretic, emmenagogue, expectorant, febrifuge, galactagogue, hemostatic, vulnerary

Medicinal Uses

Blessed thistle has a long history of use in folk medicine. In Greek folk medicine, blessed thistle was used to treat malaria. During the Middle Ages, it was believed to cure smallpox and the plague. In *Much Ado About Nothing,* one of Shakespeare's characters advises, "Get you some of this distilled *Carduus benedictus* and lay it to your heart: it is the only thing for a qualm." The Zuni Indians used it to treat venereal disease. The herb has also seen use, by the Quinalt Indians and others, as a contraceptive agent.

Blessed thistle stimulates digestive secretions, dries damp phlegm, improves memory, and lifts the spirits. Its essential oil has shown activity against *Staphylococcus faecalis, S. aureus, Nycobacterium phlei,* and *Candida albicans.* It is recommended (in the form of a tea) for adolescent females and menopausal women with low hydrochloric acid secretions. It is also used to help detoxify the body, particularly of drug and alcohol residues. It can be used to treat ague, alcoholism, anorexia, appetite loss, cancer, catarrh, colic, constipation, depression, flatulence, headache, hepatitis, indigestion, jaundice, memory problems, menorrhagia, menstrual cramps, and tumors.

Topically, blessed thistle can be used in a salve to treat boils, shingles, and wounds and to help stop bleeding.

Edible Uses

The young leaves can be added to salads, and the young flowerheads can be eaten like the hearts of artichoke, to which the plant is related. The tops can be added to aperitif wines.

The root is used as a potherb.

Other Uses

Blessed thistle has been used as cattle fodder in Scotland. European folklore holds that growing the plant outside the home promotes love, peace, and harmony. It is sometimes carried in medicine bags as a purifying talisman.

Constituents

Calcium, iron, magnesium, manganese, sesquiterpene lactones (cnicin), bitter glycosides, tannin, mucilage, antibacterial agents

Energetic Correspondences

- Flavor: bitter, pungent, sweet
- Temperature: cool
- Moisture: neutral
- Polarity: yang
- Planet: Mars
- Element: fire

Contraindications

Avoid during pregnancy and in cases of ulcers. Large doses can cause stomach irritation and vomiting.

Range and Appearance

Blessed thistle is believed to be native to the Mediterranean and Eurasia. An annual, it often grows in wasteland areas and achieves a height of about 2 feet. It has brown, densely hairy stems and compound basal leaves with triangular leaflets, which are white veined and prickly. The upper leaves form a cuplike shape around the flowers, which are yellow with violet streaks.

BLOODROOT

Botanical Name

Sanguinaria canadensis

Family

Papaveraceae (Poppy Family)

Etymology

The genus name, *Sanguinaria,* derives from the Latin *sanguis,* "blood," and *anguina,* "snakelike." The species name, *canadensis,* refers to the plant's origin in northeastern North America.

Also Known As

English: Indian paint, red pucoon, red root, sanguinaria, sweet slumber, tetterwort
Finnish: lumikki
French: sang dragon
Swedish: blodört

Part Used

Rhizome

Physiological Effects

Alterative, anesthetic, antibacterial, cathartic, diuretic, emetic, escharotic, emmenagogue, expectorant, febrifuge, odontalgic, sedative, stimulant, tonic

Medicinal Uses

Bloodroot was widely used by Native Americans to treat, among other things, cancer, skin ailments, and snakebite. It was listed in the United States Pharmacopoeia from 1925 to 1965. The herb offers many benefits to gum tissues: it interferes with bacteria's ability to convert carbohydrates into a gum-eating acid, and it also blocks an enzyme that acts to destroy collagen in the gum tissue, thereby reducing plaque buildup. It is used in the treatment of arthritis, asthma, bronchitis, cancer, croup, fever, intestinal dryness, laryngitis, phlegm buildup, rheumatism, tuberculosis, tumors, vaginal dryness, and whooping cough.

Topically, bloodroot can be made into a salve to treat cancer, eczema, fungal infection, nasal polyps, plaque buildup, ringworm, and warts. It is often included in toothpastes and mouthwashes for its ability to lessen tooth sensitivity and reduce plaque buildup and tooth decay. It also can be made into a gargle to relieve sore throat, a snuff to treat nasal polyps, or a wash (made with vinegar) to treat athlete's foot.

Edible Uses

Not generally regarded as edible, aside from as tea.

Other Uses

When harvested, bloodroot exudes an orange-red sap that was traditionally used as a ceremonial body paint by Native Americans. A red dye is made from the rhizome. In magical traditions, the root is carried to attract love.

Constituents

Isoquinoline, alkaloids (sanguinarine, berberine, whelidonine, chelerythrine)

Energetic Correspondences

- Flavor: bitter
- Temperature: hot
- Moisture: dry
- Polarity: yang
- Planet: Mars
- Element: fire

Contraindications

Bloodroot is best used under the guidance of a qualified health-care practitioner. Use only very small doses internally, as large doses can cause vomiting, faintness, a burning sensation in the stomach, and temporary paralysis; excessive doses may be deadly. Avoid both topical and internal use during pregnancy, while nursing, and in cases of glaucoma.

The fresh root is somewhat caustic and can cause skin irritation.

Range and Appearance

Native to North America, bloodroot is an early spring wildflower found most often in moist, shady woodlands. The single, short-lived white flower appears before the plant's leaves and has seven to sixteen petals and a waxy consistency. The leaves at first are wrapped around the flower bud and then open into a palmate shape with deep grooves.

BLUE COHOSH

Botanical Name

Caulophyllum thalictroides

Family

Berberidaceae (Barberry Family)

Etymology

The genus name, *Caulophyllum,* derives from the Greek *kaulos,* "stem," and *phullon,* "leaf," in reference to the manner in which the plant's stems appear to be continuations of its leaves. The common name *cohosh* is an Algonquin term meaning "rough with hairs," in reference to the texture of the rhizome.

Also Known As

English: beechdrops, blueberry root, blue ginseng, papoose root, squaw root, yellow ginseng
French: cohost bleu
German: blauer hahnenfuss, frauenwurzel, stengelblett
Russian: steblelist moshny
Spanish: caulofilo, cohosh azul

Part Used

Rhizome

Physiological Effects

Anthelmintic, anti-inflammatory, antirheumatic, antispasmodic, diaphoretic, diuretic, emmenagogue, nervine, parturient, tonic, uterine tonic

Medicinal Uses

Blue cohosh was used by several Native American tribes for gynecological concerns. The Fox, Menominee, and Ojibwa peoples used it to relieve menstrual cramps. The Cherokee and Potawatomi used it to facilitate birthing, to bring on overdue labor, and to encourage expelsion of the placenta. The herb was also used as a contraceptive agent. It was widely used by the Eclectic physicians of the late 1800s and 1900s and was included in the United States Pharmacopeia from 1882 till 1905 as a labor stimulant.

The herb is known to tonify uterine tissues. When used during delivery it helps stretch the neck of the uterus and increases the strength of labor contractions, making labor easier. In addition, blue cohosh has long been used in treatments for arthritis, bladder irritation, epilepsy, hypertension, hysteria, irregular menses, menstrual cramps, premenstrual tension, rheumatism, and spasms.

Edible Uses

The rhizome is not considered edible, aside from as tea. The roasted seeds have seen use as a coffee substitute, though they should not be eaten raw, as they are mildly toxic.

Other Uses

Some Native American peoples used blue cohosh as a protective charm for children.

Constituents

Calcium iron, potassium, alkaloids (methylcystine, caulophylline, anagyrine, baptifoline, laburine magnoflorine, quninolizidine), saponins (caulosaponin, caulophyllosaponins), phytosterol (daucosterol), resin, gum, starch

Energetic Correspondences

- Flavor: bitter, sweet
- Temperature: warm
- Moisture: dry
- Polarity: yang
- Planet: Mars/Venus
- Element: fire

Contraindications

Use only the dried root, as the fresh plant may cause dermatitis and the berries are toxic. Avoid its use during pregnancy until the onset of labor or until labor is overdue, and then use only under the guidance of a qualified health-care professional. Long-term use or large doses can cause spastic contractions, tachycardia, hypertension, respiratory depression, nausea, vomiting, uncoordination, pupil dilation, and joint pain. As blue cohosh can increase blood supply to the pelvis, it should not be used in cases of heavy menstrual bleeding.

Range and Appearance

Blue cohosh, a perennial, grows throughout the United States in open woods, in moist lowlands, near running streams, and in other locations that offer rich soil and shade. The plant has one or more stems with several compound leaves and reaches a height of 1 to 3 feet. It is blue-purple when young and blue-green when mature, while the inconspicuous six-petaled flowers, blooming from mid-spring until early summer, are yellowish green. The globular seeds are blue in color and resemble small grapes.

BOLDO

Botanical Name

Peumus boldus

Family

Monimiaceae (Lemonwood Family)

Etymology

The common name *boldo* and species name *boldus* is thought to derive from *boldu*, the name given this plant by the Araucan tribe of Chile. The genus name, *Peumus,* is thought to derive from *peumo,* the name given to a similar tree by the Mapuche tribe of Chile.

Also Known As

English: boldina, boldu
French: boldu
German: chilensicher boldobaum
Turkish: boldu ag

Parts Used

Leaf, root, bark

Physiological Effects

Alterative, anthelmintic, anti-inflammatory, antioxidant, antiseptic, antispasmodic, aromatic, cholagogue, choleretic, demulcent, digestive, diuretic, febrifuge, hepatoprotective, laxative, liver stimulant, stomachic, sedative, urinary antiseptic, vermifuge

Medicinal Uses

Boldo increases gastric secretions, aids in the elimination of uric acid, and improves circulation. It also functions as a liver tonic: folklore tells of a flock of sheep recovering from liver problems after grazing on a hedge of boldo. The herb was formerly used in place of quinine. Today it is used in the treatment of cystitis, gallbladder pain, gallstones, gonorrhea, hepatitis, jaundice, obesity, and urinary tract infection.

Topically, boldo can be prepared as a compress or used as a bath herb to relieve arthritis pain.

Edible Uses

Boldo's aromatic fruit pulp is edible. The herb is also used to flavor alcoholic beverages.

Other Uses

The bark is used for charcoal making and leather tanning. The essential oil is used in soaps and perfumes.

Constituents

Flavonoids, glycosides (phyllirine), saponin, alkaloids (boldine, isocorydine, N-methyllaurotetanine, norisocorydine), essential oils (p-cymene, 1-8-cineole, ascaridole, linalool, eucalyptol)

Energetic Correspondences

- Flavor: bitter
- Temperature: cool
- Moisture: dry
- Polarity: yin
- Planet: Saturn
- Element: earth

Contraindications

The powdered leaf can cause sneezing. Large doses can cause vomiting. Avoid during pregnancy, while nursing, and in cases of bile duct obstruction or acute cases of gastrointestinal irritation. Use only as needed, and not as a daily supplement.

Range and Appearance

Native to Chile, boldo is now naturalized in the Mediterranean region. It is an evergreen shrub, from 15 to 20 feet high, with opposite, sessile, leathery leaves that have a lemony fragrance. Each leaf is about 2 inches long and become reddish brown when dried. The flowers are light yellow and about $\frac{1}{2}$ inch long. The fruit is orangish green and contains a single seed.

BONESET

Botanical Name

Eupatorium perfoliatum

Family

Asteraceae (Daisy Family)

Etymology

The name *boneset* comes from the time when this plant was used to treat the flu, known as break-bone fever for the bone pain it caused, in the early part of the twentieth century. *Eupatorium,* the genus name, is derived from that of Mithrades Eupator, a first-century Persian king who was also a famed herbalist. The species name, *perfoliatum,* refers to the leaves, which appear to be perforated by the stem.

Also Known As

English: agueweed, boneset, crosswort, feverwort, Indian sage, sweating plant, tedral, thorough-stem, thoroughwort, vegetable antimony, wild Isaac, wood boneset

French: eupatoire perforée, herbe à la fievre, herbe parfaite

German: durchwachsdost, virginischer walddosten

Spanish: rompe zaraguey, alba haquilla, hierba de chiva, Santa Maria

Part Used

Aboveground plant

Physiological Effects

Aperient, antispasmodic, astringent, bitter, carminative, diaphoretic, emetic, expectorant, febrifuge, immune stimulant, laxative, stimulant, tonic

Medicinal Uses

Boneset was a beloved herb of Native Americans, including the Menominee, Iroquois, Creek, and Alabama tribes, who used it for treating fever. The Native Americans shared its use as a flu remedy with the Pilgrims, and the plant was later widely used by Africans and Europeans in the New World. During the Civil War, Confederate soldiers used boneset to treat fevers and also to treat malaria when quinine was in short supply. Boneset was widely used in medical practice through the late nineteenth century, including as a treatment for typhoid and yellow fever.

Boneset promotes sweating, thus helping to clear heat and toxins from the body. The sesquiterpene alkaloids in the leaves increase appetite and, in larger amounts, are anthelmintic. Boneset boosts the body's resistance to both bacterial and viral infections, perhaps due to its polysaccharide content, which increases white blood cell production. In vivo studies indicate that the plant exhibits some anti-tumor activity. It is often used in the treatment of allergic rhinitis, arthritic and rheumatism pain, bronchitis, catarrh, chest colds, coughs, dyspepsia, fever, flu, herpes I and II, tapeworm, and typhoid. Inhaling the vapors is of benefit in cases of catarrh.

The cold infusion is tonic and mildly laxative. The warm infusion is more diaphoretic.

Topically, boneset tea can be used as a wash to lower fever.

Edible Uses

Not generally considered edible, except as tea.

Other Uses

Chippewa hunters called deer by rubbing boneset roots with milkweed to create a whistling sound.

Constituents

Sesquiterpene lactones (eupafolin, euperfolitin), polysaccharides, flavonoids (kaempferol, quercitin, hyperoside, rutin), glucoside (eupatorin) diterpenes, gallic acid, sterols, essential oil

Energetic Correspondences

- Flavor: bitter, pungent
- Temperature: cold
- Moisture: dry
- Polarity: yin
- Planet: Saturn
- Element: water

Contraindications

Large doses can cause vomiting, trembling, weakness, drooling, stiffness, and diarrhea. It is best to use boneset for no more than five days in a row.

Range and Appearance

Boneset, a native American perennial, grows in low, moist areas. It has erect hairy stems that reach a height of 2 to 5 feet. Its wrinkled, narrow leaves are marked with yellow resin dots and are united at the base. The flowers have purplish white coloring.

BORAGE

Botanical Name

Borago officinalis

Family

Boraginaceae (Borage Family)

Etymology

The word *borage* is thought to derive from the Celtic *borrach*, "courage," or perhaps from the Arabic *abu 'buraq*, "father of sweat," in reference to the plant's diaphoretic properties. However, some claim that the name might be derived instead from the Latin *borra*, "rough hair," in reference to the hairy leaves and stems.

Also Known As

Arabic: lisaan ath-thaur, himhim
Bulgarian: porech
Cantonese: lauh leih geuih
Czech: borec, brotnák
Danish: hjulkrone
Dutch: bernagie, komkommerkruid
English: bee bread, bugloss, burrage, star flower
Estonian: harilik kurgirohi
Farsi: gavzaban
Finnish: kurkkuyrtti, purasruoho
French: bourrache officinale
German: boretsch, gurkenkraut
Greek: borantsa, vorago
Hebrew: borag

Hungarian: borágó, borragofu
Icelandic: hjólkróna
Italian: borragine, borrana
Japanese: boriji, ruridisa
Korean: poriji
Lithuanian: agurkle
Mandarin: bo li ju, liu li ju
Norwegian: agurkurt
Polish: ogórecznik lekarski
Portuguese: borragem
Romanian: limba mielului
Russian: ogurechnaya trava
Serbian: borac, volujsko uvo
Spanish: borraja, borrega
Swedish: gurkört
Turkish: hodan
Ukrainian: ohirkova trava
Yiddish: buritsh

Parts Used

Leaf, flower, seed oil

Physiological Effects

Leaf and flower: adrenal tonic, anti-inflammatory, antirheumatic, aperient, decongestant, demulcent, diaphoretic, diuretic, emollient (flower), febrifuge, galactagogue, laxative (mild), refrigerant, sudorific (leaf)
Seed oil: anti-inflammatory

Medicinal Uses

Borage leaves, flowers, and seed oil moisten yin, clear heat, and reduce inflammation. The leaves and flowers have long been used in treatments for bladder infection, bronchitis, catarrh, colds, convalescence, coughs, depression, fevers, grief, hypertension, pleurisy, pneumonia, and worry. The oil from the seeds is used in the treatment of arthritis, dermatitis, eczema, menstrual and menopausal problems, obesity, psoriasis, and rheumatism.

Topically, borage leaves and flowers are used as a compress on sore eyes, a poultice for inflammations, bruises, and eczema, and a salve for rashes. They can be prepared as a facial mask or bath herbs to soothe dry skin or as a gargle to relieve sore throat. The oil

from the seeds can be massaged into the fingers as a treatment for Raynaud's phenomenon.

As a flower essence, borage is used to lighten depression and discouragement. It helps bring joy, optimism, enthusiasm, and good cheer, improves confidence and courage, and dispels sadness in the face of danger and troubles.

Edible Uses

Borage flowers (with the prickly sepals on their backs removed) can be eaten fresh in salads, candied, or used as edible garnishes for pastries and cakes, punches, ice cubes, and the like. The flowers are also sometimes used as a food-coloring agent. The young leaves taste like cucumbers; the fresh leaves are more flavorful than the dried ones. They can be chopped small and added to salads; mixed with yogurt for a refreshing chilled soup; or added to cooling summer drinks like lemonade.

The roots are also edible and in the past were used as a flavoring for wine.

Other Uses

In 1597 herbalist John Gerard quoted in his writings an old saying, "Ego borago gaudia semper ago," meaning "I, Borage, always bring courage." In fact, the flowers have long been used to bolster courage (perhaps the fact that they nourish the adrenal glands explains why). In medieval times the flowers were embroidered on the mantles of knights and jousters to give them courage, and they were also floated in drinks given to Crusaders as they took their leave. They were also sneaked into the drinks of prospective husbands to give them the courage to propose.

Constituents

Leaf and flower: mucilage, tannin, saponins, essential oil, alkaloids (pyrrolizidine, lycopsamine), essential fatty acids, vitamin C, calcium, potassium
Seed oil: linoleic acid, gamma-linolenic acid

Energetic Correspondences

- Flavor: slightly sweet, salty, pungent
- Temperature: cold

- Moisture: moist
- Polarity: yang
- Planet: Jupiter
- Element: air

Contraindications

The leaf contains pyrollizidine alkaloids, which are possibly toxic; use the leaf only in moderation unless further research negates the danger of these alkaloids. Avoid the leaf during pregnancy and while nursing.

Range and Appearance

Borage, native to Eurasia and northern Africa, is a bristly plant growing to a height of 1 to 2½ feet. The stems are round and hollow with prickly white hairs. The juice of the stems is cucumber scented. Borage is an annual, though it self-sows easily, with bright blue star-shaped flowers with brown anthers. After pollination, the flowers turn pink. Borage thrives well in poor soil, in full sun to partial shade. In the garden, borage attracts bees and repels tomato worms.

BUCHU

Botanical Name

Agathosma betulina (formerly *Barosma betulina,*
  Diosma betulina)

Family

Rutaceae (Citrus Family)

Etymology

The genus name, *Agathosma,* derives from the Greek *agathos,* "pleasant," and *osme,* "smell." The word *buchu* derives from the Khoikhoi (Hottentot) name for the plant, *bookoo.*

Also Known As

Afrikaans: boegoe
English: bucco, bookoo, buchu, bucku, diosma
French: buchu, diosme

German: buchublatter, duftstrauch, starkduft
Italian: diosma
Khoikhoi (Hottentot): bookoo
Spanish: buchu
Turkish: diozma

Part Used

Leaf

Physiological Effects

Anti-inflammatory, antiseptic, aromatic, astringent, carminative, diaphoretic, digestive, diuretic, kidney stimulant, stimulant, tonic, urinary antiseptic, uterine stimulant, vulnerary

Medicinal Uses

Buchu is widely used by the Khoikhoi (Hottentot) peoples of southern Africa, where the plant grows wild. Buchu helps remove uric acid accumulations, improves circulation to the urogenital systems, and dries mucus. Its diasphenol content has an antibacterial effect. The leaf is used to treat bladder infection and inflammation, bloating, cystitis, edema, flatulence, gout, hematuria, indigestion, kidney stones, leukorrhea, nephritis, polyuria, prostate inflammation, rheumatism, and yeast infection.

Topically, buchu leaf can be used as a poultice to treat bruises and as a douche to treat leukorrhea and yeast infection.

Buchu Tea: When making a tea with buchu leaves, do not boil them, or else the essential oils will be inactivated.

Edible Uses

Buchu is not generally considered edible, aside from as tea. It is sometimes used to flavor brandy and cassis.

Other Uses

The leaves are mixed with oil as a perfume in Africa. The essential oil has an odor similar to that of black currant and is used in perfumery.

Constituents

Vitamin C, beta-carotene, calcium, chromium, magnesium, zinc, sulfur, essential oils (barosma, camphor, diosphenol, limonene pulegone, menthone), flavonoids (diosmin, hesperidin, quercitin, rutin), mucilage

Energetic Correspondences

- Flavor: bitter, pungent
- Temperature: warm
- Moisture: dry
- Polarity: yin
- Planet: Venus/Moon
- Element: water

Contraindications

Avoid buchu during acute inflammatory conditions, as well as during pregnancy and while nursing. Large amounts can cause nausea and vomiting. It is not unusual for a person who has been drinking buchu tea to have his or her urine become scented like buchu, although this is not harmful in any way.

Range and Appearance

Native to southern Africa, buchu grows in rocky, hilly valleys. It is a woody shrub, from 1 to 4 feet tall, with many twigs covered with oil glands. The leaves are flat, opposite, and about 1 inch long. The flowers are pink and single.

BUCKBEAN

Botanical Name

Menyanthes trifoliata

Family

Menyanthaceae (Bogbean Family)

Etymology

The genus name, *Menyanthes,* comes from the Greek, meaning "moon flower" and/or "month," denoting the duration of the flowers' blooming period. However, buckbean often blooms for up to three months!

The species name, *trifoliate,* refers to the three leaflets.

Also Known As

Dutch: bocks, boonan

English: bean trefoil, bitterworm, bogbean, buckbean, bog-hop, bog nut, marsh clover, moonflower, treefold, water shamrock, water trefoil

Finnish: raate

French: herbe à canards, menianthe, menyanthe trifolie, trefle d'eau

German: bitterklee, fieberklee, sumpfflee

Italian: scarfano, trefoglio d'acqua, trifoglio fibrino

Swedish: vattenklöver

Turkish: su yoncasi

Parts Used

Aboveground plant, rhizome

Physiological Effects

Alterative, antirheumatic, bitter, cathartic, cholagogue, deobstruuent, diuretic, emetic, febrifuge, laxative, stomachic, tonic

Medicinal Uses

Buckbean was once considered a panacea in Europe. The leaf was included in the United States Pharmacopoeia from 1820 to 1842 and in the National Formulary from 1916 to 1926.

Buckbean stimulates digestive secretions, clears heat, and promotes bowel action and lymph and bile flow. It has been used to treat amenorrhea, arthritis, constipation, dropsy, fever, gout, lack of appetite, muscle pain, and rheumatism.

The leaf is used as a poultice to treat swelling, sores, herpes, sore muscles, and glandular inflammation.

Edible Uses

In Scandinavia, the root is eaten as a vegetable; as the root is bitter, it is usually cooked in several changes of water to make it more palatable. Some Europeans infuse the root in wine. The Inuit tribe grinds the root into flour. In Sweden, the leaf is used as a substitute for hops in making beer.

Other Uses

Buckbean leaves are sometimes smoked in place of tobacco. And in the Victorian language of flowers, buckbean signifies calm repose.

For travelers crossing a marshy area, the presence of buckbean marks a firm bed and safe footing.

Constituents

Vitamin C, rutin, iron, iodine, manganese, alkaloids (meliatine, gentianin, gentialutin), anthraquinone derivatives (emodin, chrysophanol), gluciside (menyanthin), tannins, saponins

Energetic Correspondences

- Flavor: bitter
- Temperature: cool
- Moisture: dry
- Polarity: yin
- Planet: Moon/Neptune
- Element: water

Contraindications

Large doses of buckbean can cause vomiting and diarrhea and can overstimulate the sympathetic nervous system. The fresh leaf is more emetic than the dried leaf. Buckbean is not recommended in cases of acute intestinal inflammation.

Range and Appearance

Buckbean, native to Eurasia, is an aquatic plant that grows in marshy or boggy areas in northern temperate areas. The stem stays immersed in water, while the leaves and flowers grow above water level. The plant has three thick leaflets and five-petaled, rose-colored flowers that grow in clusters and have a silky white fringe. The fruits are beanlike capsules.

Buckbean is considered an endangered species in some regions.

BUGLEWEED

Botanical Name

Lycopus americanus, L. europaeus, L. virginicus

Family

Lamiaceae (Mint Family)

Etymology

The genus name, *Lycopus,* derives from the Greek *lykos,* "wolf," and *pous,* "foot," in reference to the shape of the rhizomes.

Also Known As

English: gypsywort, Paul's betony, sweet bugle, water bugle, water horehound
French: chanvre d'eau, lycope d'Europe, pied de loup
German: wolfstrapp, wolfsuss
Italian: marrobio acquatico
Spanish: menta de lobo

Part Used

Aboveground plant

Physiological Effects

Antitussive, aromatic, astringent, bitter, cardiotonic, diuretic, hemostatic, hypoglycemic, laxative, narcotic (mild), nervine, peripheral vasoconstrictor, sedative

Medicinal Uses

Bugleweed reduces the activity of iodine, the activity of an overactive thyroid, and blood levels of thyroid hormones. It also lessens mucus discharge and contracts tissue to a more firm, solid state. It quiets the pulse, calms the spirit, and increases the strength of the heartbeat. It is used to treat anxiety, catarrh, cough, enlarged thyroid, Grave's disease, hyperthyroidism, thyroid inflammation, and nervous heart palpitations.

Bugleweed is considered a mild remedy. It may work best in the early stages of illness or in combination with allopathic medicines.

Topically, bugleweed is sometimes used as a liniment or poultice to treat bruises and snakebite and to stop bleeding.

Edible Uses

The young shoots can be consumed fresh in spring salads. The roots are edible raw or cooked, but they are not very tasty and are considered only a survival food.

Other Uses

A black dye can be made from the plant.

Constituents

Magnesium, tannins, lithospermic acid, lycopine, phenolic derivatives (caffeic acid, chlorogenic acid, ellagic acid, rosmarinic acid), essential oil, resin

Energetic Correspondences

- Flavor: bitter, pungent
- Temperature: warm
- Moisture: dry
- Polarity: yin
- Planet: Venus/Mercury
- Element: earth

Contraindications

Avoid bugleweed during pregnancy. To avoid excessive dryness, combine the plant with demulcent herbs.

Range and Appearance

Bugleweed is native to Eurasia but is naturalized to North American and can be found growing throughout the northern hemisphere in damp areas with full sun to partial shade. This perennial can achieve a height of 12 to 36 inches. It has lanceolate, parallel leaves. The hermaphroditic flowers are white with a purple spot and are borne in the axils of the leaves.

BUPLEURUM

Botanical Name

Bupleurum chinense (syn. *B. scorzoneraefolium*), *B. falcatum, B. fruticosum, B. rotundifolium*

Family

Apiaceae (Parsley Family)

Etymology

The genus name, *Bupleurum,* derives from the Greek *bous,* "ox," and *pleuron,* "rib."

Also Known As

Cantonese: chai wu ("kindling of the barbarians")
English: hare's ear, thoroughwax, thorow wax
German: sichelblättriges, hasenohr
Italian: bupleuro
Japanese: saiko
Korean: siho
Mandarin: bei chai hu

Part Used

Root

Physiological Effects

Alterative, analgesic, antibacterial, anti-inflammatory, antiviral, carminative, chi regulator, choleretic, diaphoretic, febrifuge, hepatoprotective, sedative, smooth muscle relaxant, sudorific, tonic

Medicinal Uses

Bupleurum increases energy, promotes circulation to the liver, strengthens the lungs, stomach, and intestines, warms the torso, brings fresh chi into the upper part of the body, and clears internal heat. It boosts the immune-system response, in part by improving adrenal function, stimulating interferon activity, and stimulating the body's natural production of corticosteroids, thus relieving inflammation. It has long been used in Oriental medicine to improve conditions that begin on the surface but linger for a long time.

Bupleurum is used to treat amenorrhea, alcohol and drug abuse (by helping clear the liver of old emotions), anger, asthma, bloating, cancer, capillary weakness, cirrhosis, colds, coughs, depression, dizziness, epilepsy, fever, flatulence, grief, hemorrhoids, hepatitis, irregular menses, irritability, irritable bowel syndrome, liver stagnation, malaria, moodiness, organ prolapse, pain, premenstrual syndrome, respiratory congestion, and tumors.

Edible Uses

The roots are not generally considered edible, aside from as tea. The young white shoots and leaves can be consumed as vegetables.

Other Uses

The old, dry plant is used for kindling. Hence the Chinese prefix *chai,* meaning firewood.

Constituents

Phytosterols (furfurol, bupleurumol, stigmasterols), triterpene glycosides (saikosides), saponins (sapogenin, daikogenin), oleic, linoleic, palmitic and stearic acids, polysaccharides, essential oil (ketone), flavonoids (rutin)

Energetic Correspondences

- Flavor: pungent, bitter
- Temperature: cool
- Moisture: dry
- Polarity: yin
- Planet: Saturn
- Element: earth

Contraindications

Avoid bupleurum in cases of liver fire rising, such as fever and headache, red and irritated eyes, or high blood pressure. Bupleurum is very drying, so avoid long-term use in cases of weakness or anemia. Combining it with lycii berries or dong quai counteracts some of its drying effect. Long-term use may cause dizziness.

Range and Appearance

Bupleurum is a perennial, native to Asia, that grows on sunny slopes, in waste areas, and along roadsides. Its flexible, slender stem bears oval leaves at the base and smaller, more narrow, falcate (curving like a sickle) leaves higher up. It bears small yellow flowers growing in compound umbels. The root is light red in color.

BURDOCK

Botanical Name

Arctium lappa, A. minus

Family

Asteraceae (Daisy Family)

Etymology

The genus name, *Arctium,* derives from the Greek *arktos,* "bear," a reference to the shaggy burrs. The species name, *lappa,* is derived from a Greek word meaning "to seize," in reference to the clinginess of the seeds. The common name *burdock* is derived from the French *beurre,* "butter," and the English word *dock,* meaning leaves; French women would wrap their cakes of butter in leaves of burdock to transport it to the marketplace.

Also Known As

Cantonese: ngau gon ji
English: bardane, beggar's buttons, clotburr, cockle
   buttons, gypsy rhubarb, happy major, hardock,
   hareburr, hurr burr, love leaves
Finnish: isotakianen
French: bardane, rhubarbe du diable
German: klette
Italian: bardana, lappola
Japanese: gobo, goboshi
Korean: ubanja
Mandarin: shu nian
Russian: lophuh, repeinik
Spanish: bardana
Swedish: stor kardborre

Parts Used

Root, seed, leaf (topically)

Physiological Effects

Root: adaptogen, alterative, antibacterial, antifungal, anti-inflammatory, antitussive, aperient, aphrodisiac, cholagogue, choleretic, demulcent, diaphoretic, diuretic, expectorant, febrifuge, galactagogue, laxative (mild), nutritive, rejuvenative

Seed: alterative, antiphlogistic, depurative, diaphoretic, diuretic

Medicinal Uses

During the Industrial Revolution, burdock was used as a medicine to help people cope with pollution or, as John Kelton said in 1870, "the constant deterioration of the blood from impure air and exhaustion by day, bad ventilation at night and want of attention to ordinary requirements of life."

As an anti-inflammatory demulcent agent, burdock root soothes and clears internal heat. It improves the elimination of metabolic wastes through the liver, lymphs, large intestines, lungs, kidneys, and skin. Japanese research indicates that burdock root contains desmutagens, substances that deactivate cancer-causing agents. Burdock is used to treat abscesses, acne, anger, boils, cancer, candida, chicken pox, cough (unproductive), cystitis, dandruff, diabetes, eczema, edema, fever, gonorrhea, gout, HIV, hives, hypoglycemia, indigestion, irritability, jaundice, keratosis, lumbago, lymphatic congestion, measles, mumps, obesity, pain, premenstrual syndrome, prostate inflammation, psoriasis, rheumatism, smallpox, sore throat, staph infection, syphilis, tonsillitis, urinary inflammation, and uterine prolapse. It makes an excellent spring detoxification or fasting tea. The juice of the root can be consumed to rid the body of scabies and mites.

Topically, burdock root can be used as a bath herb to relieve sore joints and gout. A compress made from the root or leaf can be used to treat boils, bruises, glandular swellings, knee swellings, sprains, and tumors. The leaf can also be bruised and applied topically to eradicate ringworm. The root can be prepared as a hair rinse or oil to prevent dandruff and hair loss and as a facial toner in cases of oily skin.

Edible Uses

Young burdock leaves can be cooked in several changes of water and eaten as a potherb—but do not expect them to be delicious. The young stalks (harvested before flowering) may be peeled and eaten raw or cooked as a vegetable. Burdock root can be added to soup, salad, stir-fries, and sukiyaki. The root also can be roasted and used as a coffee substitute.

Other Uses

Burdock has been used as a protective agent to dispel negativity when burned as an incense.

Constituents

Root: vitamin C, calcium, iron, magnesium, potassium, zinc, polyacetylenes, chlorogenic acid, taraxosterol, arctigen, inulin, lactone, essential oil, flavonoids, tannin, mucilage, resin
Seed: essential fatty acids, arctigenin, arctiin

Energetic Correspondences

- Flavor: root—bitter; seed—pungent
- Temperature: cool
- Moisture: dry
- Polarity: yin
- Planet: Venus/Jupiter/Saturn/Pluto
- Element: water

Contraindications

Avoid burdock seeds during the first trimester of pregnancy, during the later stages of measles, and in cases of open sores. And take care to avoid the sharp spines when working with the seeds.

If you are collecting in the wild, avoid confusing burdock with rhubarb, which has similar-looking but toxic leaves.

Range and Appearance

Burdock is a biennial plant that is native to Eurasia but now also grows throughout North America. It thrives in waste areas, by roadsides, and in damp areas. It has large, wavy, heart-shaped leaves and a stem that grows from 3 to 6 feet tall. The flowers are purple globes followed in the fall by burrs with a profusion of hooked prickles. Burdock's taproot is deep, slender, and 10 to 30 inches long, with a dark outer skin; it is ideally collected in the summer or fall of the plant's first year or in the spring of the plant's second year.

Burr Inspiration: The Swiss inventor George de Mestral, who invented Velcro, was inspired to his creation by the burdock burrs that stuck to his dog after a walk. The "sticking" mechanism of Velcro is modeled after the profusion of tiny curved hooks on the burrs.

BUTTERBUR

Botanical Name

Petasites hybridus (formerly *Tussilago hybrida,* syn. *P. vulgaris*)

Family

Asteraceae (Daisy Family)

Etymology

The common name *butterbur* refers to the use of the large leaves to wrap up cakes of butter before the days of refrigeration. The genus name, *Petasites,* derives from the Greek *petasos,* the name of a type of broad-brimmed felt hat worn by shepherds, again a reference to the plant's large leaves.

Also Known As

English: blatter dock, bog rhubarb, bogshorn, butterdock, capdockin, flapper dog, langwort, pestilence wort, plague flower, sweet coltsfoot, umbrella plant
Finnish: etelänruttojuuri
French: chapeau-du-diable, herbe aux teigneux
German: pestwurz, pestilenzenwort
Italian: bardana, farfaraccio
Swedish: skråp
Turkish: kel-tou

Part Used

Root

Physiological Effects

Analgesic, antispasmodic, astringent, cardiotonic, diaphoretic, diuretic, emmenagogue (mild), expectorant, stimulant, tonic, vulnerary

Medicinal Uses

Butterbur relaxes smooth muscle spasms. The petasin content blocks leukotrine biosynthesis and inhibits inflammatory histamines. Butterbur is used in the treatment of asthma, bronchitis, colds, dysmenorrhea, fever, hay fever, incontinence, kidney stones, migraine, stammering, ulcers, urinary tract spasms, and urinary tract infection.

Topically, the fresh leaf and flower can be used as a poultice in the treatment of wounds and skin sores and as a wash for itchy skin.

Edible Uses

Butterbur can be used to make cordials. The young leaves, petioles, and inflorescences are edible; however, their flavor is strong and they need to be soaked or cooked in several changes of water. *Petasites japonica,* also known as fuki, is cultivated and consumed as a vegetable in Japan.

Other Uses

Butterbur's leaves are so large that they have been used as umbrellas or sunshades. The leaves sometimes are dried and smoked. Butterbur is sometimes planted near beehives to produce early spring food sources for bees.

Constituents

Inulin, pectin, pyrrolizidine alkaloids (senecionine, interrimine, senkirkine, petastine, neopetasitine), sesquiterpene lactones (petasalbin, furanopetasin), essential oil (petasine), mucilage, tannins

Energetic Correspondences

- Flavor: pungent, slightly sweet, bitter
- Temperature: warm
- Moisture: moist
- Polarity: yin
- Planet: Sun/Venus
- Element: water

Contraindications

Use with caution due to the pyrrolizidine alkaloid and sesquiterpene lactone content, which may contribute to liver damage. Commercial butterbur products that have had the pyrrolizidine alkaloids removed are now available. Avoid butterbur during pregnancy and while nursing.

Range and Appearance

Butterbur, a perennial native to Europe, grows in marshy areas and streamsides. Like its close relative, coltsfoot, butterbur leaves appear before its flowers. The flowers grow in cylindrical clusters and range from pale pink to red or purple in color. The plant is dioecious, meaning some plants carry male flowers, while others carry female flowers. The male flowers are shorter than the female ones. The leaves can be as long as 3 feet; they are coarse and heart shaped, with a whitish down on their underside.

BUTTERNUT

Botanical Name

Juglans cinerea

Family

Juglandaceae (Walnut Family)

Etymology

The genus name, *Juglans,* derives from the Latin *jovis glans,* "nut of Jupiter," in reference to the belief that the gods lived off walnuts.

Also Known As

English: lemon walnut, oilnut, white walnut
German: butternuss
Spanish: nogal ceniciento

Part Used

Inner bark

Physiological Effects

Alterative, anthelmintic, antimicrobial, antiparasitic, astringent, cathartic, cholagogue, febrifuge, laxative (mild), purgative, rubefacient, tonic, vermifuge

Medicinal Uses

Butternut bark was used by pioneers to treat fever and arthritis during the time of the Revolutionary War, when patent medicines were scarce. It is a gen-

tle purgative and a gentle treatment for chronic constipation. It is an effective and safe remedy for intestinal worms, even in children. It is one of the few laxative herbs that can be used safely during pregnancy. It is used in the treatment of arthritis, cancer, cholesterol, constipation, dysentery, headache, hypercholesterolemia, liver stagnation, parasites, rheumatism, and skin diseases.

Edible Uses

The nuts are edible raw or cooked, and they are often used in baked goods. The sap of the tree can be made into a sweet syrup.

Other Uses

Butternut wood is softer than that of black walnut, but like walnut, it has been used in woodworking, notably to make cabinets, instrument cases, and furniture. The husks of the nut and bark yield an orange or yellow dye.

Constituents

Naphthaquinones (juglone, juglandin, juglandic acid), essential oil, tannins

Energetic Correspondences

- Flavor: bitter
- Temperature: cold
- Moisture: dry
- Polarity: yang
- Planet: Sun
- Element: fire

Contraindications

Large doses can be mildly cathartic.

Range and Appearance

Butternut is native to eastern and central North America. It can reach a height of 40 to 60 feet. The flowers are yellowish green and bloom from spring through early summer. The tree is dioecious, meaning male and female flowers are borne on the same tree: male flowers drooping as catkins and female flowers growing in short spikes. The ovalish nut has a very hard shell and can be difficult to crack.

CACAO

Botanical Name

Theobroma cacao

Family

Steruliaceae (Cacao Family)

Etymology

The genus name *Theobroma* derives from the Greek *theos,* "god," and *broma,* "food," thus meaning "food of the gods." The species name *cacao* is the Olmec name for the plant. The common name *chocolate* derives from an Aztec name for this plant, *chócolatl.*

Also Known As

English: cacaotier, chocolate, cocao, food of the
   gods, devil's food, theobroma
Finnish: kaakao
German: kakaobaum
Portuguese: cacau
Swedish: kakao

Part Used

Seed

Physiological Effects

Aphrodisiac, antioxidant, cardiotonic, diuretic, emollient, laxative, nervous system stimulant, nutritive

Medicinal Uses

Cacao increases levels of serotonin and endorphins in the body. It gives a short-term boost in energy and, when consumed in its whole, raw from, is beneficial for the teeth, as it contains tannins that inhibit dental decay. It also contains phenylethylamine, a compound that is naturally occurring in the brain in trace amounts and is released when we are in love, peaking during orgasm. Cacao also contains theobromine, a compound that dilates the coronary artery, increasing blood flow to the heart. Cacao seed is used in the treatment of anemia, angina, appetite loss, asthma, and insufficient breast milk.

Edible Uses

The cacao seed is certainly edible, as history has proven. The Aztecs were the first to prepare cacao as the delicous cocoa beverage enjoyed around the world today. Cocoa was the "love tonic" of Montezuma II, who is reputed to have drunk some fifty cups daily before visiting his harem of six hundred women. In 1502 the returning crew of Columbus brought cacao beans back to Europe, and in 1550 nuns came up with the idea of adding sugar and vanilla, leading to what we now regard as chocolate. Most commercial chocolates today, however, have a low cacao content and contain sugar and hydrogenated oil.

The fruits of the cacao tree also are edible and contain a delicious white pulp.

Other Uses

Cacao beans were once used as a currency in the Yucatan. Montezuma is said to have paid his soldiers, laborers, and civil servants in cacao beans, and they continued to be used as a form of currency in Mexico until 1887.

Cacao is valued for its nourishing oils and antioxidant properties, and it is often used in soaps, skin-care products, hair-care products, and cosmetics and as a base for boluses and suppositories.

Constituents

Vitamin E, B complex vitamins, chromium, copper, iron, magnesium, phosphorous, potassium, amino acids (arginine, phenylalanine, tryptophan, tyramine, tyrosine), phenylethylamine, anandamide, dopamine, serotonin, xanthines (caffeine, theobromine, trigonelline), flavonoids (epicatechin, catechin, procyanidins), essential oil, sucrose, glucose, mucilage, oleopalmitostearin, tannins, sugars (sucrose, dextrose)

Energetic Correspondences

• Flavor: bitter
• Temperature: warm
• Moisture: dry
• Polarity: yang
• Planet: Mars/Uranus
• Element: fire

Contraindications

In some cases cacao may cause heartburn or an allergic reaction. Since it contains caffeine, it should be used only rarely by pregnant women and can aggravate insomnia, anxiety, irritability, and breast cysts. Cacao also contains oxalic acid, which can inhibit calcium absorption and promote kidney stones.

Range and Appearance

The cacao tree, native to Central and South America, grows to 15 to 20 feet in height in the wild, though when under cultivation it is kept shorter. The large leaves are oblong to oval in shape, simple, alternate, and leathery, with a sharp point and entire margins. The small, white to pink flowers grow in clusters of ten to twenty-five. The podlike fruit is produced all year long but takes five to six months to ripen. It is a thick-skinned oval capsule that is yellow, green, or red in color.

CALAMUS

Botanical Name

Acorus americanus, A. calamus, A. gramineus

Family

Araceae (Arum Family)

Etymology

The genus name, *Acorus*, derives from the Greek *coreon*, meaning "pupil of the eyes," as calamus was once used to treat eye problems. The species and common name *calamus* derives from the Greek *calamos*, meaning "reed canes." The common name *singer's root* references the fact that singers once used calamus to numb and clear phlegm from the throat, allowing them to sing for extended periods.

Also Known As

Afrikaans: makkalmoes
Cherokee: ooyadali ustiga amayuti ehi ("little blade that lives at the water's edge")
English: gladdon, myrtle flag, sedge, singer's root, sweet flag
French: acore vrai, jonc odorant, roseau aromatique
German: ackerwurz, kalmus, magenwurz
Italian: calamo aromatico
Japanese: shobu
Korean: ch'angp'o
Mandarin: chang pu
Sanskrit: vacha
Spanish: calamo
Zulu: ikalamuzi

Part Used

Unpeeled rhizome

Physiological Effects

Analgesic, antibacterial, antispasmodic, antitussive, aphrodisiac, aromatic, bitter, brain tonic, carminative, decongestant, diaphoretic, digestive, emetic, emmenagogue, expectorant, febrifuge, hallucinogen (in large amounts), hypotensive, laxative, nervine, central nervous system stimulant, rejuvenative, sedative, spleen tonic, stimulant, stomachic, tonic, vasodilator, vulnerary

Medicinal Uses

Calamus helps dry dampness, expel phlegm, and curb infection. It has an antihistaminelike effect on hay fever and colds. Small amounts reduce stomach acidity, while larger doses can increase gastric secretions. During the Crimean War calamus was recommended to soldiers as a treatment for malaria, as quinine was in short supply. Today, calamus is used in the treatment of anorexia, appetite loss, arthritis, asthma, bronchitis, catarrh, colic, cough, diarrhea, dysentery, dyspepsia, epilepsy, fatigue, fever, flatulence, gastritis, headache, heartburn, hypochondria, hysteria, laryngitis, memory loss, mental illness, rheumatism, sinusitis, and speech problems. It also aids in recovery from stroke and detoxification from anesthetics.

Small amounts of the root are given to children in Ayurvedic medicine to enhance their intelligence and to adults in Oriental medicine to "calm the spirit."

Topically, powdered calamus can be used as a snuff to relieve nasal congestion (this may cause sneezing, which will open respiratory passages), as a deodorant for feet, or as an antiseptic healing agent for wounds. In Ayurvedic medicine calamus root is prepared as a douche or enema to deter fungal overgrowth. The root also can be used in the bath or as a compress to relieve back pain and headache. It can be smoked to deter tobacco cravings and to mitigate the negative effects of smoking marijuana. It also can be chewed to relieve teething pain. A tincture of the root can be applied topically to eliminate skin parasites. Diluted calamus essential oil is used in massage oils to treat paralysis and rheumatism.

Edible Uses

The rhizome is edible; it and the leaf can be candied and used as breath fresheners. Calamus leaf buds and inner stems can be eaten raw. The leaves have been used to flavor milk in making puddings and custards. And in India calamus ghee (clarified butter) is used as a therapeutic condiment.

Other Uses

Calamus has been used as a strewing herb and in incense and sachets for its pleasant aroma, and the essential oil has been used to flavor pipe tobacco. Mongolians planted calamus near watering holes to purify the water for horses. Native Americans were known to hold a piece of calamus root in their mouths when running long distances to increase their endurance. In large amounts the root has psychoactive effects; the poet Walt Whitman wrote many poems while under its influence.

In magical traditions, having a small piece of calamus root in all corners of the kitchen gives protection against hunger and poverty.

Constituents

Choline, eugenol, camphor, tannins, acorin

Energetic Correspondences

- Flavor: bitter, pungent, sweet
- Temperature: warm
- Moisture: dry
- Polarity: yin

- Planet: Sun/Uranus/Moon
- Element: water

Contraindications

Calamus contains beta-asarone, which when isolated may be carcinogenic. However, calamus has been used in India for thousands of years with no reports of cancer being attributed to its use. North American varieties do not contain beta-asarone and are considered safest.

Use calamus for no longer than a month at a stretch, and preferably under the guidance of a qualified health-care professional. Avoid during pregnancy.

Range and Appearance

Native to North America (*A. americanus*) and temperate and tropical Asia (*A. calamus* and *A. gramineus*) but now naturalized in many other places, calamus is a perennial aquatic herb that grows in damp areas and along streams. The light green to yellowish leaves cluster from the rhizome in a parallel fashion. The leaves, growing to about 4 feet in height, are lanceolate, with their bases enclosing the stem. Yellowish green flowers form a fleshy inflorescence and grow out at an angle about halfway up the stalk.

CALENDULA

Botanical Name

Calendula officinalis

Family

Asteraceae (Daisy Family)

Etymology

The genus and common name is derived from the Latin *calendae,* meaning the first day of the month, perhaps in reference to the fact that calendula opens as the sun rises and can be found blooming in some part of the world every month. The species name, *officinalis,* refers to the plant being an official herb of the apothecaries in Europe.

Also Known As

English: bull's eye, garden marigold, gowan,
   holigold, Mary bud, pot marigold, ruddles
Finnish: kehäkukka
French: fleurs de tous les mois, souci, souci
   des jardins
German: goldblume, ringelblume, sonnenwende
Italian: fiore d'ogni, oculus Christi, solis sponsa
Sanskrit: zergul
Spanish: claveton, flameniquillo
Swedish: ringblomma, solsocka

Part Used

Flower

Physiological Effects

Alterative, antibacterial, antifungal, anti-inflammatory, antispasmodic, antiviral, astringent, calmative, choleretic, demulcent, diaphoretic, immune stimulant, vulnerary

Medicinal Uses

Calendula clears congestion, dries dampness, promotes the healing of tissue, curbs infection (by stimulating white blood cell production), and clears toxins and inflammation. In vitro studies confirm that calendula inhibits the growth of *E. coli,* staph, and some protozoas. It also increases peripheral circulation. It is an ideal herb for infections that have been trapped in the body for a long time. A twelfth-century herbal recommends calendula to "improve eyesight, clear the head, and encourage cheerfulness." Today, calendula flowers are used to treat candida, cervical irritation, chicken pox, conjunctivitis, glandular swellings, hemorrhoids, herpes, infection, lymph inflammation, measles, mumps, smallpox, staph infection, stomach inflammation, thrush, and ulcers.

Topically, calendula promotes the formation of granulation tissue. It is used in skin creams for its nourishing, scar-preventing, and anti-inflammatory properties. It is popular in salves for the treatment of boils, bruises, bunions, burns, chapped skin, cradle cap, diaper rash, eczema, hemorrhoids, herpes, inflammation, insect bites, sprains, sunburn, varicose veins, and wounds. It is excellent in the bath to relieve skin inflammation and in sitz baths to relieve hemorrhoids. It can be prepared as a hair rinse to get rid of dandruff, stem hair loss, and soothe scalp irritation. It can even be prepared as a douche to treat trichomonas and as a foot soak for athlete's foot. Diluted calendula tincture can be as a nasal wash for sinus infections, as an eyewash for conjunctivitis, and as a mouthwash for gingivitis. A couple of drops of warmed calendula-infused oil can be dripped into the ear to treat earache.

As a flower essence, calendula is helpful for those who listen only superficially and speak hurtfully and argumentatively. It helps increase understanding and receptivity and encourages warmth, sensitivity, and better communication.

Edible Uses

Calendula flower is both colorful and edible, and its petals have been used as a substitute for saffron to color butter, rice, desserts, and egg dishes. The flowers and leaves can be eaten fresh in salads. The flowers can also be added to liqueurs as a dyeing agent.

Other Uses

Calendula can be used as a hair rinse to bring out highlights in blonde hair.

Constituents

Iodine, manganese, potassium, saponins, caretonoids (carotene, lycopene, calendulin, lutein), flavonoids, polysaccharides, mucilage, bitter principle (calendulin), phytosterols, polysaccharides, essential oil, resin

Energetic Correspondences

- Flavor: bitter, pungent
- Temperature: slightly cool
- Moisture: dry
- Polarity: yang
- Planet: Sun/Venus
- Element: fire

Contraindications

Generally regarded as safe.

Range and Appearance

Calendula is native to Eurasia but grows worldwide. It is grown as an annual, biennial, or perennial depending on weather conditions. It has hairy leaves and orange, daisylike flowers. It prefers open sunny areas, and like sunflowers, its flowers often turn to face the path of the sun. Calendula is useful in the garden in that it attracts pollinators and discourages Mexican bean beetles.

CALIFORNIA POPPY

Botanical Name

Eschscholtzia californica, E. mexicana

Family

Papaveraceae (Poppy Family)

Etymology

The genus name, *Eschscholtzia,* was given in honor of J. F. Eschscholtz (1793–1831), an Estonian physician and naturalist who explored the Pacific Coast with Russian explorer Otto von Kotzebue.

Also Known As

English: flame flower, gold poppy
French: coquelicot de Californie
Italian: papavero Californiano
Spanish: amopola de California, copa de oro ("cup of gold"), dormidera ("drowsy one")

Part Used

Aboveground plant

Physiological Effects

Analgesic, anodyne, antispasmodic, febrifuge, hypnotic, nervine, sedative, soporific

Medicinal Uses

Although it does not contain opiates, this poppy is a skeletal relaxant that encourages restoration of the nervous system, and it is nonaddictive. The Cahuilla Indians once used the plant as a sedative for babies. Today, it is used in the treatment of anxiety, bedwetting (due to stress), insomnia, headache, overexcitability, pain, restlessness, stress, and toothache.

Topically, California poppy can be used as a compress to relieve pain.

As a flower essence, California poppy encourages awakening to one's abilities and spiritual potential by fostering inner listening and self-responsibility. It helps prevent fanatacism about spirituality and psychic phenomena.

Edible Uses

Native Americans sometimes ate the leaves after boiling them or roasting them on hot stones, yet they are extremely bitter. The seeds can be sprinkled into salads or baked goods.

Other Uses

Native Americans sometimes used the pollen as a cosmetic. Spanish Californians boiled the leaves in olive oil, then added perfume to make a hair dressing. Marijuana users sometimes smoke this when their herb of choice is unavailable.

Constituents

Flavonoids (rutin, zeaxanthin), alkaloids (protopine, allocryptine, berberine, sanguinarine)

Energetic Correspondences

- Flavor: bitter
- Temperature: cool
- Moisture: dry
- Polarity: yin
- Planet: Sun/Mercury
- Element: air

Contraindications

Avoid in cases of depression. Excess use can cause one to feel hung over in the morning.

Range and Appearance

California poppy, a perennial or hardy annual, is native to the southwestern United States; in fact, it is the state flower of California. It grows wild in sunny areas, reaching a height of 1 to 3 feet. The basal leaves are finely dissected and have a bluish hue in the spring. The flowers are usually orange, though they can sometimes be purple or yellow; they carry four petals and close at night. The seedpods are long and pointed, sometimes described as resembling carpet needles.

CARAWAY

Botanical Name

Carum carvi

Family

Apiaceae (Parsley Family)

Etymology

The common name *caraway* and the species name, *carvi,* derive from the ancient Arabic name for this plant, *karawya.*

Also Known As

Arabic: karauya
Armenian: chaman
Bulgarian: kim
Burmese: ziya
Cantonese: gohy leuih ji
Croatian: kim
Czech: kmin
Danish: kommen
Dutch: karwij
English: carvies, Roman cumin
Estonian: harilik köömen
Finnish: kumina
French: carvi, cumin des pres
German: kümmel, wiesenkummel
Greek: karo, karvi
Hebrew: kravyah
Hindi: gunyan, shia jeera
Hungarian: kömenymag
Icelandic: kumen
Italian: carvi, cumino dei prati
Japanese: karuwai
Korean: kaereowei
Mandarin: ge lü zi
Norwegian: karve
Polish: kminek

Portuguese: alcaravia
Romanian: chimion
Russian: tmin
Sanskrit: karavi
Serbian: kim
Spanish: alcaravea
Swahili: kisibiti
Swedish: kummin
Thai: hom pom
Turkish: frenk kimyonu
Ukrainian: kmyn
Vietnamese: ca rum
Yiddish: kiml

Part Used

Seed

Physiological Effects

Antiseptic, antispasmodic, aromatic, astringent, carminative, circulatory stimulant, digestive, diuretic, emmenagogue, expectorant, galactagogue, stomachic, stimulant, vermifuge

Medicinal Uses

Caraway calms spasms and prevents fermentation in the digestive tract, relieves uterine and intestinal cramping, and improves circulation; it is used as a calming herb for a wide variety of gastrointestinal problems, and it is an excellent herb to use for children's digestive problems. It aids in the digestion of starches. It is often added to laxative teas to reduce gripe. It can be made into a tea to relieve respiratory congestion. Eating a few seeds not only freshens the breath but also relieves shortness of breath caused by travel to a high elevation. Caraway is used to treat amennorrhea, belching, bronchitis, Crohn's disease, colic, cramps, digestive distress, dysmenorrhea, flatulence, hiccups, hysteria, memory loss, nausea from chemotherapy, rheumatism, and pleurisy.

Topically, caraway works as a rubefacient and anesthetic. The seeds, together with the leaves, can be used as a poultice to treat bruises. The diluted essential oil or powder can be applied to relieve toothache. The essential oil can be used in mouthwashes and gargles as an antiseptic and breath-freshening agent.

Edible Uses

Caraway seed is widely used in German, Austrian, and Dutch cuisine, including cabbage dishes, cheeses, crackers, pickles, rye breads, liqueurs, soups, and roasted apples. The leaves may be chopped and added to salads. Caraway root is also edible as a vegetable, much like parsnips. The alcoholic beverages Kümmel and Aquavit and some spiced wines are flavored with caraway.

Other Uses

Caraway was used as a form of currency in sixth-century Persia.

Constituents

Calcium, iron, magnesium, protein, fatty acids, flavonoids, essential oils (arvene, carvone, limonene), linoleic acid, oleic acid, polysaccharides, tannins, coumarins, resin

Energetic Correspondences

- Flavor: pungent
- Temperature: warm
- Moisture: moist
- Polarity: yang
- Planet: Mercury/Moon/Sun
- Element: water

Contraindications

Generally regarded as safe.

Range and Appearance

Caraway is a biennial native to Eurasia but now cultivated worldwide in temperate regions. It prefers full sun in rich soil. The leaves are glabrous and bipinnate. The flowers are white to pinkish umbels, followed by oblong grooved seeds.

CARDAMOM

Botanical Name

Elettaria cardamomum

Family

Zingiberaceae (Ginger Family)

Etymology

The genus name, *Cardamomum,* is from the Greek *kardamon,* "peppergrass," and *anomon,* "fragrant spice plant."

Also Known As

Afrikaans: gemmer
Arabic: habbahan, hal
Armenian: shooshmir
Bulgarian: kardamom
Cantonese: chan jai yan
English: grains of paradise, green cardamom, Malabar cardamom
Esperanto: kardamomo
Estonian: kardamon
Finnish: kardemumma
French: cardamome
German: kardamom
Greek: kakoules, kardamo
Hebrew: hel
Hindi: elaci, ilaichi
Icelandic: kardimomma
Italian: amomo
Japanese: byakuzuku, shukusha
Korean: paektugu
Mandarin: bai dou kou, pai-tou, sha ren (seeds and pod), yang chun sha, yi jih ren
Nepali: sukmel
Norwegian: kardemomme
Polish: cardamomo
Russian: kardamon
Sanskrit: ela
Spanish: cardamomo
Swahili: iliki
Swedish: kardemumma
Thai: luke krawan
Tibetan: sugmel
Turkish: hemame, hiyl, kakule
Vietnamese: trúc sa
Yiddish: kardemon

Part Used

Seed

Physiological Effects

Antiseptic, antispasmodic, aphrodisiac, aromatic, astringent, carminative, digestive, diaphoretic, expectorant, kidney yang tonic, mucolytic, sialagogue, stimulant, stomachic, tonic

Medicinal Uses

Cardamom is used in Asian medicine to strengthen the bones and sinews. It is also known to strengthen the heart and lungs and reduce stomach acidity, and it is said to stimulate the mind and impart joy, clarity, and mental alertness. It is also considered to be an aphrodisiac. Cardamom is used in the treatment of anorexia, appetite loss, asthma, bloating, bronchitis, catarrh, celiac disease, colds, colic, congestion, cough, cramps, depression, diarrhea, dysentery, enuresis, erectile dysfunction, emphysema, fainting, fatigue, fetal restlessness, fever, flatulence, halitosis, headache, heartburn, indigestion, kidney stones, laryngitis, lung congestion, malabsorption, morning sickness, polyuria, poor circulation, premature ejaculation, spermatorrhea, stomachache, vomiting, and weak chi.

> **Note:** Cardamom is currently the third most expensive spice in the world as each seed must be hand picked. As cardamom seeds' volatile essential oils evaporate easily, it is best to buy the whole seeds, then remove the outer covering and grind them as needed.

Edible Uses

Cardamom is widely used in cuisines around the world, notably Indian, Arabic, Asian, Ethiopian, German, and Scandinavian. When added to grains it enhances the digestibility of their phytic acid content; it also improves the digestibility of milk and dairy products. It has a pleasant, sweet flavor, reminiscent of that of eucalyptus and pine, and it can be used to improve the flavor of bitter herbs.

Other Uses

Cardamom was a favored ingredient in ancient love potions. The seed is sometimes added to smoking blends. In Arabic cultures, serving cardamom to a guest is a sign of hospitality. The seed is also a great breath freshener; people chew it after drinking alcohol or garlic to conceal their indulgence. The essential oil of cardamom is used to scent perfume and massage oils and as an insect repellent.

Constituents

Essential oils (borneol, camphor, carvone, cineole, eucalyptol, limonene, linalool, methone, terpinine, sabinene), caprylic acid

Energetic Correspondences

- Flavor: pungent, slightly bitter, sweet
- Temperature: warm
- Moisture: dry
- Polarity: yang
- Planet: Sun/Mercury/Venus
- Element: fire/water

Contraindications

Generally considered very safe. Avoid in cases of ulcers.

Range and Appearance

Cardamom is a perennial, native to Asia, growing 6 to 10 feet tall. The leaves are dark green and lanceolate, with silky, paler undersides. Small yellow flowers spread along the ground above the rhizome. The seeds' capsules are irregular in shape and grayish brown in color. Each capsule contains four to eight seeds.

CASCARA SAGRADA

Botanical Name

Rhamnus cathartica (common buckthorn),
    R. frangula (alder buckthorn), *R. purshiana*

Family

Rhamnaceae (Buckthorn Family)

Etymology

The genus name, *Rhamnus,* derives from the Greek *rhamnos,* "branch" or "spiny shrub." The species name, *purshiana,* was bestowed in honor of botanist Frederick Pursh, who first described this plant in his 1814 *Flora America Septentrionalis.* The name *cascara sagrada* is Spanish for "sacred bark"; the name was given by Spanish-Americans who observed the plant's use by the Native Americans.

Also Known As

English: bearwood, bitterbark, buckthorn, chittambark, coffeeberry, mountain cranberry, persiana, sacred bark
German: amerikanische faulbaumrinde
Russian: joster, krushina

Part Used

Bark (dried and aged)

Physiological Effects

Alterative, astringent, bitter tonic, cathartic, cholagogue, digestive, emetic, hepatic, laxative, nervine, purgative, stomachic, tonic

Medicinal Uses

Casacara sagrada promotes bowel action, moves stagnation, clears heat, cleanses the liver and gallbladder, and stimulates bile flow. It stimulates peristalsis and increases the secretions of the colon, liver, pancreas, and stomach. It is the most widely used laxative in the world, and it was included in the United States Pharmacopoeia in 1890. Small doses are restorative, medium doses are laxative, and large doses are cathartic. In addition to its use as a laxative to relieve constipation, cascara sagrada is used to treat anal fissures, arthritis, cirrhosis, colitis, dyspepsia, flatulence, gallstones, gout, hemorrhoids, indigestion, jaundice, and worms.

To prevent gripe it is best to combine this herb with a carminative herb such as fennel, anise, ginger, or peppermint. The best time to use cascara sagrada as a laxative is before bed, so that its effects can take place the next morning.

Topically, cascara sagrada can be used as a wash to heal herpes lesions.

Edible Uses

The bark is not generally considered edible, except as a tea; its flavor is nauseatingly bitter. The thin fruits can be eaten as emergency ration, though they are slightly toxic if eaten in quantity.

Other Uses

The bitter tea or tincture of the bark can be applied to the fingernails to discourage one from biting them. A green dye is made from the bark. The light, soft wood is used to make tool handles and fence posts.

Constituents

Calcium, iron, sulfur, anthraquinones (emodin, cascarosides, frangulin, isomodin, chrysophanol), tannin, glycosides, resins, lipids

Energetic Correspondences

- Flavor: bitter
- Temperature: cold
- Moisture: dry
- Polarity: yin
- Planet: Saturn
- Element: earth

Contraindications

Never use fresh cascara sagrada bark. The bark must be aged at least one year to reduce its griping effect. Some age it for as long as six years. Long-term use can deplete the body of electrolytes, including potassium, and weaken intestinal muscles. Excess use can cause nausea, vomiting, and bloody diarrhea. Avoid during pregnancy, while nursing, in children under twelve, and in cases of abdominal pain of unknown cause, ulcer, intestinal obstruction, irritable bowel, Crohn's disease, appendicitis, or acute hemorrhoids. Should the plant cause excess gripe, the antidote is charcoal capsules.

Cascara sagrada is not considered habit forming, but it still is best used on occasion rather than daily; if used over an extended period the bark's effect on the body lessens, requiring that more be used, increasing the possibility of negative effects.

Range and Appearance

Casacara sagrada is a small (seldom over 30 feet in height) deciduous tree. Native to the North American Pacific Coast, the tree grows in moist, low, coniferous forest habitats. The dark green leaves are alternate, finely toothed, slightly pubescent underneath, and roundish at the base. The ends can be sharp or blunt. Clusters of hermaphroditic whitish green flowers bloom in the spring. The cascara fruits are small black globes, each containing two or three seeds.

In recent times overharvesting has reduced the number of these trees; try to be sure any cascara sagrada you use has been harvested responsibly.

CATNIP

Botanical Name

Nepeta cataria

Family

Lamiaceae (Mint Family)

Etymology

The genus name, *Nepeta,* derives from that of Nepeti, a Roman town where this herb was cultivated. The common name *catnip* refers to the attraction cats have for nipping this plant. Its smell has an effect similar to that of the pheromones that cats secrete, and it seems to affect them as an aphrodisiac and euphoric. About two-thirds of cats respond to catnip by sniffing, drooling, licking, rolling, stretching, rubbing, and so on.

Also Known As

English: catmint, catnep, catswort, field balm, nep
Finnish: kissanminttu
French: chataire, herbe aux chats, népéta des chats
German: echte katzenminze, katzenkraut, nept
Italian: cataria, erbi dei gatti
Sanskrit: zufa
Spanish: calaminta, cataria, menta de gato, nebada, yerba del gato, yerba gatera
Swedish: kattmynta

Part Used

Leaf

Physiological Effects

Anodyne, antidiarrheal, antispasmodic, aromatic, astringent, carminative, diaphoretic, digestive, emmenagogue, febrifuge, mucolytic, nervine, refrigerant, sedative, stomachic, tonic

Medicinal Uses

Catnip contains nepelactones, which are both analgesic and sedative and affect the opioid receptor sites of the body. Catnip moves chi, relaxes the nerves, and calms inflammation. This is an excellent children's herb and will help calm them through the trials of teething, colic, and restlessness. When given for colds and fevers, it helps the patient get the rest he or she needs. Early American settlers believed it would make kind people become meaner, and the dried roots were fed to hangmen and executioners.

Catnip was entered into the United States Pharmacopoeia from 1842 to 1882 and into the National Formulary from 1916 to 1950. Today, catnip is used to treat amenorrhea, anxiety, bronchitis, chickenpox, colds, colic, convulsions, delayed menses, diarrhea, dyspepsia, fever, flatulence, headache, hives, hyperactivity, hysteria, indigestion, insomnia, measles, menstrual cramps, mental illness, motion sickness, pain, pneumonia, restlessness, scarlet fever, smallpox, stomachache due to nerves, teething pain, toothache, and worms.

Topically, catnip can be used as a bath herb to relieve stress, colic, and teething pain or as a compress or poultice to treat pain, sprains, bruises, hemorrhoids, or toothache. It can be used as a hair rinse to relieve scalp irritations and get rid of dandruff, a lotion to treat acne, a liniment to alleviate arthritis or rheumatism symptoms, an enema to cleanse the colon, a salve to soothe hemorrhoids, or an eyewash to relieve inflammation, allergy symptoms, or bloodshot eyes.

As a flower essence, catnip helps those who see spirituality and sexuality as forces that cannot be reconciled. It helps those who are fearful of sexuality yet drawn to illicit sexual behavior and helps harmonize body, mind, and spirit.

Edible Uses

Young catnip leaves can be made into pesto or added to sauces or salads. The leaves can also be used as a meat rub for flavoring. Before Chinese tea became popular in the West, catnip tea was a common beverage.

Other Uses

The leaves have been smoked as a euphoric and to stop hiccups. The essential oil is used in perfumery. The dried herb tied up in an old sock makes a great catnip toy for cats; a sachet of dried herb can be placed in bedpillows to help induce sleep. The scent repels rats and many insects.

Constituents

Calcium, magnesium, chromium, B-complex vitamins, vitamin C, essential oils (cavracol, citronellol, geraniol, nepetol, nepelactone, pulegone, thymol), iridoids, tannins

Energetic Correspondences

- Flavor: pungent, bitter
- Temperature: cool
- Moisture: dry
- Polarity: yin
- Planet: Venus/Moon
- Element: water

Contraindications

Large doses of the tea can be emetic. When smoked the herb is mildly hallucinogenic, although no toxicity has been reported. It is not recommended for use during pregnancy

Range and Appearance

This perennial, native to Eurasia, grows in moist, disturbed sites, such as along roadsides, old buildings, and streambeds. The erect stem is square and hairy. The leaves are grayish green, opposite, oval or heart shaped, strongly toothed, and whitish underneath with a dentate margin. The clusters of white to light pink or purplish dotted flowers grow in terminal clusters.

In the garden, catnip is best grown from seed, because it tends to draw more attention from neighborhood felines when transplanted. Hence the saying, "If you set it, cats will eat it. If you sow it, cats won't know it."

CAT'S CLAW

Botanical Name

Uncaria guianensis, U. tomentosa

Family

Rubiaceae (Madder Family)

Etymology

Cat's claw has clawlike spines on its stems, hence the name. The genus name, *Uncaria,* derives from the Latin *unus,* "hook."

Also Known As

English: garabato, garbato casha, hawk's claw, paraguayo, rangaya, samento, tambor huasca, toron, una de gavilan, ungangui
Spanish: uña de gato ("cat's claw")

Parts Used

Inner bark, bark, root, stem, hook, leaf

Physiological Effects

Antibacterial, anti-inflammatory, antimutagenic, antioxidant, antirheumatic, antitumor, antiviral, depurative, diuretic, hypotensive, immune stimulant, vermifuge

Medicinal Uses

Cat's claw has been used by native peoples of South America for at least two thousand years. It is most closely associated with the Asháninka, Cashibo, and Campa tribes of the Peruvian rain forest.

Research on this plant is very recent. Cat's claw is known to increase the number and activity of phagocytes, macrophages, lymphocytes, and leukocytes—all important components of the immune system. It also inhibits blood platelet aggregation and cleanses the intestinal tract. It is used in the treatment of abscess, acne, AIDS, allergies, arthritis, asthma, bed-wetting, bone pain, brain tumors, bronchitis, bursitis, cancer, candida, chemotherapy and radiation side effects, chronic fatigue, cirrhosis, colitis, Crohn's disease, cysts, depression, diabetes, diverticulitis, dysentery, environmental illness, fatigue, fever, fibromyalgia, gastritis, gonorrhea, gout, growing pains, hay fever, hemorrhage, herpes, iritis, irregular menses, irritable bowel, leaky bowel syndrome, leukemia, lupus, neurodermatitis (itching with emotional origins), parasites, premenstrual syndrome, prostatitis, rheumatism, shingles, tumors, ulcers, and urinary tract infection. It also is used to aid in recovery from childbirth and to prevent strokes. Some South American natives even used it as a contraceptive, where large amounts are taken consecutively for three months to cause sterility for three to four years.

Topically, cat's claw can be used as a salve, compress, or poultice to treat athlete's foot, fistula, fungal infection, hemorrhoids, herpes, shingles, or wounds. It also can be made into an eyewash to treat conjunctivitis.

Edible Uses

The stem yields a clear liquid that is refreshing to drink.

Other Uses

None known

Constituents

Quercetin, rutin, polyphenols, proanthocyanidins, catechin, oxindole alkaloids (alloisopteropodine, alloptropodine, isopteropodine [except in *U. guianensis*], rhynchophylline, uncarine), hirsutine, quinovic acid, triterpenes, phytosterols (beta-sitosterol, stigmasterol, campesterol), tannins

Energetic Correspondences

- Flavor: bitter
- Temperature: warm
- Moisture: dry
- Polarity: yang
- Planet: Mars
- Element: fire

Contraindications

Avoid cat's claw while attempting to conceive, during pregnancy, while nursing, and in children under three. Those taking ulcer medications or immune-suppressing drugs should not use cat's claw; those anticipating or recovering from organ or bone-marrow transplant should likewise avoid it.

A possible side effect from large amounts of this herb is diarrhea. Some people will experience a "healing crisis" or worsening of their symptoms before benefits are realized.

Range and Appearance

Cat's claw is a woody liana (vine) growing up to 100 feet in length; when fully grown a single vine can weigh more than a ton. It is native to the Amazon, where it can be found in old second-growth forests, especially in Peru. The leaves are simple and ovate, with a few secondary veins along the midvein. The flowers of *U. tomentosa* are yellow-gold in color, while those of *U. guianensis* are white or reddish orange.

CATUABA

Botanical Name

Erythroxylum catuaba

Family

Erythroxylaceae (Coca Family)

Etymology

The genus name, *Erythroxylum*, derives from the Greek *erythros*, "red," and *xylon*, "wood." *Catuaba* is an indigenous name for the tree.

Also Known As

Spanish: caramuru, chuchuhuasha, pau de reposta, piratancara, tatuaba

Part Used

Bark, root

Physiological Effects

Analgesic, antibacterial, antiseptic, antiviral, aphrodisiac, brain tonic, central nervous system stimulant, tonic, vasodilator, vasorelaxant

Medicinal Uses

Among the Minas people of South America a saying exists, "Until a father reaches sixty, the son is his; after that, the son is catuaba's," in reference to the herb's renowned aphrodisiac qualities. It benefits both women and men as an aphrodisiac, in part by enhancing sexual desire by decreasing stress. Catuaba is used to treat agitation, anxiety, erectile dysfunction, exhaustion, hypochondria, insomnia, low libido, poor memory, and skin cancer.

Though it is in the same family as coca (from which cocaine is derived), catuaba does not contain cocaine alkaloids.

Edible Uses

Not generally considered edible, aside from as tea.

Other Uses

None known

Constituents

Essential oils, alkaloids, tannins, phytosterols, cyclolignans, ioimbina

Energetic Correspondences

- Flavor: pungent
- Temperature: warm
- Moisture: dry
- Polarity: yang
- Planet: Mars
- Element: yang

Contraindications

No reports of toxicity exist. However, until further research has been done, catuaba is not recommended during pregnancy.

Range and Appearance

Catuaba is a medium-size tree of vigorous growth. It bears yellow and orange flowers and a small, ovalshaped, dark yellow fruit that is not edible. It grows in the Amazon, mainly in Brazil.

CAYENNE

Botanical Name

Capsicum spp., including *C. annuum,*
  C. frutescens

Family

Solanaceae (Nightshade Family)

Etymology

The genus name, *Capsicum,* derives from the Greek *kapto,* "to bite," in reference to the spicy flavor. The common name *cayenne* is taken from that of a French Guiana town of the same name on the northeast coast of South America.

Also Known As

Arabic: fulful alahmar
Armenian: gdzoo bghbegh
Bulgarian: chili
Cantonese: laaht jiu
Croatian: feferon
Czech: pálivá paprika
Danish: chili
English: African pepper, bird pepper,
  chile, chili, red pepper
Estonian: kibe paprika
Finnish: chilipippuri
French: piment, poivre rouge
Greek: piperi kagien, tsili
Hebrew: paprika harifa
Hindi: lal mirch
Hungarian: ördögbors
Indonesian: cabé, lomok
Japanese: kaienpeppa, togarashi
Korean: kaien gochu, kochu
Lithuanian: kajeno pipirai
Mandarin: la jiao
Nepali: rato khursani
Portuguese: pimentão
Romanian: ardei iute
Russian: kajenskij perets
Sanskrit: katuvira, marichiphala ujjvala
Serbian: feferon, kajena-biber

Spanish: pimento

Swahili: pilipili hoho

Thai: prik chifa, prik khee nu

Tibetan: sipen marpo

Turkish: toz biber

Vietnamese: ot

Yiddish: ferferl

Part Used

Fruit

Physiological Effects

Alterative, anthelmintic, antioxidant, antiseptic, antiviral, aphrodisiac, astringent, carminative, counterirritant, diaphoretic, expectorant, hemostatic, sialagogue, stimulant, thermogenic, tonic

Medicinal Uses

Cayenne stimulates the brain to secrete endorphins and improves circulation by preventing blood platelet aggregation. It helps to relieve pain, not only due to the endorphin release it stimulates but also when used topically (always in diluted form) by helping to block the transmission of substance P, a neuropeptide that transports pain messages to the brain. It also opens congested nasal passages.

Cayenne is used in the treatment of arthritis, asthma, atherosclerosis, bleeding, chills, colds, cough, dysentery, flu, high cholesterol, migraine, and obesity.

Applied topically, cayenne is very effective as a styptic for bleeding wounds. It (or an extract of one of its constituents, capsaicin) is a common ingredient in lotions and creams designed to relieve pain in arthritic joints, sprains, shingles, and bruises. Cayenne can also be prepared as a gargle to relieve sore throat.

As a flower essence, cayenne helps those who feel immobilized, unable to make a decision or to make progress. It encourages self-motivation.

Edible Uses

Cayenne peppers are edible, though how edible they are depends on a person's tolerance for their heat. Cayenne is widely used as a seasoning.

Cooling the Fire

If you find the flavor of cayenne too scorching, water won't help. Instead, drink milk or beer (whichever is closer) to quell the fire.

Other Uses

Putting a bit of cayenne between your shoes and socks on a cold winter's day helps keep the feet warm.

Constituents

Beta-carotene, vitamin C, vitamin K, manganese, capsaicin, capsanthine

Energetic Correspondences

- Flavor: pungent
- Temperature: hot
- Moisture: dry
- Polarity: yang
- Planet: Sun/Mars
- Element: fire

Contraindications

Avoid large doses during pregnancy and while nursing. Cayenne is not advised for people who sweat profusely and suddenly. When handling cayenne, keep away from eyes, and wash hands afterward. The seeds can be especially hot.

Range and Appearance

Native to the Americas, cayenne has many varieties, which can grow as annuals or perennials and as small herbs or small shrubs. The plant features simple five-lobed leaves and usually white flowers. The fruit is long, twisting, and red to orange-red. In the garden cayenne enjoys full sun and can tolerate dry conditions.

CELERY

Botanical Name

Apium graveolens

Family

Apiaceae (Parsley Family)

Etymology

The genus name, *Apium,* is thought to derive from the Latin *apis,* "bee," as bees relish this plant. The species name, *graveolens,* means "heavy, penetrating odor" in Latin. The common name *celery* derives from the Greek *selinone,* "parsley."

Also Known As

Arabic: karafs
Armenian: lakhod garos
Croation: celer
Dutch: selderij
English: marsh parsley, salary, small ache, smallage
Finnish: ruokaselleri
French: achte, achte des Marias, celeri
German: sellerie, cellerie, wassweppich
Hebrew: carpas reychani
Hindi: bari ajmud
Hungarian: zeller
Italian: accio, appio, sedano, seleno
Japanese: oranda mitsuba, serori
Mandarin: ch'in
Norwegian: hageselleri
Persian: karafs
Portuguese: aipo
Russian: syel'derey
Sanskrit: ajmoda
Spanish: apio
Swedish: selleri
Thai: khuen chai
Turkish: kereviz

Part Used

Seed

Physiological Effects

Alterative, antifungal, anti-inflammatory, antirheu-matic, antispasmodic, anthelmintic, aphrodisiac, aromatic, carminative, deobstruent, diuretic, emme-nagogue, galactagogue, hypotensive, nervine, seda-tive, stomachic, sudorific, tonic, urinary antiseptic

Medicinal Uses

Celery seed reduces inflammation, clears heat and toxins (including uric acid), cleanses the liver and kidneys, and softens deposits. One of its con-stituents, butylidenephatalide, is known to stimulate the menses. Celery seed is used to treat arthritis, asthma, bronchitis, dizziness, fever, flatulence, gout, incontinence, insomnia, kidney stones, nervousness, neurological disorders, obesity, and rheumatism.

Topically, celery seed is used as a soak to relieve the symptoms of gout and arthritis.

Edible Uses

Celery seed is a common culinary herb. The seeds are also used both to make celery salt and as a flavoring agent in salt-free diets. The seeds are known to aid in the digestion of protein. The stem, or, more accu-rately, the petiole, is the ever popular vegetable cel-ery; when consumed, it can lower blood pressure and lower uric acid levels in the body, which is of benefit in cases of gout or arthritis. The root (known as celeriac) is also edible and also can help lower blood pressure. Celery leaf is usually trimmed from the stalks, but it is edible; in fact, there is a popular celery-leaf soda known as Dr. Brown's Cel-Ray.

Other Uses

Celery seeds are sometimes used in sleep pillows. The essential oil of the seeds is used in perfumery.

Constituents

Calcium, iron, zinc, luteolin, furancoumarins, essen-tial oil (apiol, d-limonene, selinene), flavonoid gly-cosides, asparagin, butylidenephatalide

Energetic Correspondences

- Flavor: bitter, sweet
- Temperature: cool
- Moisture: moist
- Polarity: yang

- Planet: Mercury
- Element: fire

Contraindications

Large amounts of celery seed may increase photo-sensitivity; avoid using the essential oil topically before going outside. Use only in moderation during pregnancy, as large amounts could have an abortifacient effect. Avoid celery seed in cases of kidney inflammation.

Range and Appearance

Celery, believed to be a native of the Mediterranean region but widely naturalized, grows as an annual or biennial, reaching a height of about 3 feet. It has leafy stems, pinnate or bipinnate leaves, and umbels of white flowers. The seeds form in the second year and are oval to globular in shape.

CENTAURY

Botanical Name

Centaurium erythraea (formerly *Erythraea centaurium*), *C. exaltatum* (desert centaury), *C. umbellatum*

Family

Gentianaceae (Gentian Family)

Etymology

The genus name, *Centauriam,* and common name *centaury* derive from the Greek *kentauros,* "centaur," in reference to the centaur Chiron, half human, half bull, who according to legend used the plant to heal himself from an arrow wound poisoned with the blood of the Hydra.

Also Known As

English: bitter bloom, bitter herb, bitter clover, Christ's ladder, feverwort, filwort, rose pink, thousand guilder herb, wild succory
Finnish: isorantasappi
French: centaurelle, chironee, fiel de terre, petite centaurée

German: erdgall, fieberkraut, laurinkraut, tausendguldenkraut, toter aurin (*Centaurium umbellatum*)
Italian: centaurea
Russian: zo-lo-to-ti-sia-chnik
Swedish: kustarun
Turkish: kücük kantaryon

Part Used

Aboveground plant

Physiological Effects

Alterative, antiseptic, aromatic, astringent, bitter, cholagogue, choleretic, diaphoretic, digestive, emmenagogue, febrifuge, liver stimulant, sialogogue, stomachic, tonic, vermifuge

Medicinal Uses

Centaury promotes digestion by increasing the production of pepsin and hydrochloric acid and strengthening the stomach. It clears heat, cleanses the bowels, promotes bile flow, promotes circulation, and has a tonic effect on the blood vessels. Centaury has long been used to treat anorexia, appetite loss, bloating, constipation, dyspepsia, fever, flatulence, indigestion, jaundice, rheumatism, and worms.

A decoction or poultice of centaury leaves can be applied topically to treat wounds, head lice, and spots on the skin.

As a flower essence, centaury is helpful for those who are easily influenced by others and allow themselves to be treated as a "doormat."

Edible Uses

Centaury is not generally considered edible as a vegetable. However, it is used in making vermouth and other bitter digestive liqueurs. It can be taken itself as a bitter tonic about ten minutes before meals.

Other Uses

The flower yields a long-lasting, bright yellow-green dye. In ancient England centaury was considered an important magical herb that offered protection against negative energy.

Constituents

Magnesium, flavonoids, essential oil, bitter glycosides (gentiopicrine, amarogentrin), alkaloids (gentianine, gentianidine), lactone (erythrocentaurin), secoiridoids (sweroside), valeric acid, wax

Energetic Correspondences

- Flavor: extremely bitter
- Temperature: cool
- Moisture: dry
- Polarity: yang
- Planet: Sun/Venus
- Element: fire

Contraindications

Culpepper said of centaury, "The herb is so safe you cannot fail in the using of it. Take it inwardly for inward diseases, and apply it outward for outward complaints; it is very wholesome, but not pleasant to the taste." His praise aside, avoid centaury during pregnancy and in cases of heartburn or acid stomach.

Range and Appearance

In its native Europe and northern Africa, centaury grows wild as an annual or biennial in the chalky soils of rocky cliffs and dry pastures. The leaves are oval in shape and form a basal rosette. The hermaphroditic, aromatic flowers are funnel shaped and grow on a terminal cyme; they are pink, purple, and sometimes white or yellow in color.

CHAMOMILE

Botanical Name

Chamaemelum nobile (Roman chamomile; syn. *Anthemis nobilis*), *Matricaria recutita* (German chamomile; formerly *Chamomilla recutita;* syn. *M. chamomilla*)

Family

Asteraceae (Daisy Family)

Etymology

The German chamomile genus name, *Matricaria,* is derived from the Latin *matrix,* "motherly" or "womblike." The species name, *recutita,* is Latin for "bare of epidermis" or "bounce back."

The Roman chamomile genus name, *Chamaemelum,* and the common name *chamomile* derive from the Greek *khamai melon,* "ground apple," as its aroma is applelike. The common name *plant's physician* refers to the fact that chamomile improves the growth of other plants around it.

Also Known As

Danish: kamille
Duten: kamille
English: ground apple, mayweed, plant's physician
Finnish: kamomillasaunio
French: camomille, espargoutte, matricaire
German: alles zutraut ("capable of anything"), kamille, magdblume, mettran, mutterkraut
Hindi: babuna
Italian: camomilla
Norwegian: kamille
Persian: babunaj
Portuguese: camomila
Russian: romanashka
Sanskrit: babuna
Spanish: manzanilla
Swedish: kamomill
Turkish: papatye cic
Vietnamese: du'o'ng cam cuc

Part Used

Flower

Physiological Effects

Analgesic, anodyne, antibacterial, antifungal, anti-inflammatory, antihistamine, antioxidant, antiseptic, antispasmodic, aromatic, carminative, diaphoretic, digestive, emetic (in large doses), febrifuge, nervine, sedative, stomachic, tonic, vulnerary

Medicinal Uses

Since the times of ancient Greece, both types of chamomile have been used medicinally in the same ways. Chamomile moves chi, relaxes the nerves, reduces inflammation, clears toxins, and promotes tissue repair. In vitro studies indicate that it has activity against *E. coli,* strep, and staph bacteria. Part of its anti-inflammatory activity may be due to its ability to inhibit the metabolism of arachidonic acid. Chamomile also helps restore an exhausted nervous system; it is an excellent herb for people who complain about every little thing. It is also a beneficial children's herb.

Chamomile is used to treat anxiety, arthritis pain, candida, colic, convulsions, crankiness in babies, digestive distress, diverticulitis, dyspepsia, fever, flatulence, gastritis, gout, headache, heartburn, hives, hyperactivity, hysteria, indigestion, insomnia, intestinal cramping, irritability, irritable bowel, itching skin, liver stress, lumbago, menstrual cramps, migraines, morning sickness, nervousness, nightmares, pain, restlessness, rheumatism, sciatica, stress, teething pain, ulcers, and the incessant urge to urinate.

Topically, chamomile is used as a bath herb to relieve stress, soften dry skin, and calm cranky children. It can be used as a sitz bath to soothe hemorrhoids. Chamomile is excellent in salves and lotions to treat skin inflammation, including burns, dermatitis, eczema, insect bites, psoriasis, ulcers (external), and healing wounds. It can be used as a gargle to relieve sore throat, as a mouthwash to treat gingivitis, as a poultice to alleviate toothache, and as an eyewash to get rid of conjunctivitis and sties. It can even be used as a douche or enema to reduce inflammation or get rid of infection.

Edible Uses

Chamomile flowers are edible raw or cooked. They are often ingredients in various liqueurs such as vermouth and Benedictine.

Other Uses

Chamomile has a wonderful scent; it was used as a strewing herb in medieval Europe and is used even today as an incense and to flavor pipe tobaccos. Its essential oil is added to calming massage blends and cooling spritzers. The herb can be included in shampoo and conditioner formulas to highlight blond hair. Stuffed into bed pillows, it aids sleep. The flower can be rubbed onto the skin to repel insects.

In magical traditions it is said to attract love and prosperity.

Constituents

Calcium, magnesium, iodine, phosphorous, potassium, vitamin B_2, choline, essential oils (bisabolol, abol, farnasene, proazulene, terpenes, chamazulene), flavonoid (apigenin, luteolin, quercetin), levomenol, sesquiterpene lactone (nobilin), coumarins, salicylates

Energetic Correspondences

- Flavor: bitter, sweet
- Temperature: neutral
- Moisture: moist
- Polarity: yang
- Planet: Sun/Venus
- Element: water

Contraindications

Some people, especially those who are sensitive to ragweed, may be severely allergic to chamomile. It can cause contact dermatitis in some individuals. Roman chamomile is more likely to cause an allergic reaction than the German variety. On the other hand, chamomile is sometimes used to treat allergies. Use the herb with caution the first time you try it. Otherwise, chamomile is considered very safe. Avoid therapeutic dosages during pregnancy.

Range and Appearance

German chamomile, native to Eurasia, is an annual herb growing from 16 inches to $2\frac{1}{2}$ feet. The leaves are pinnate and alternate. Its flower has a sweeter taste than the Roman variety.

Roman chamomile, native to Europe and northern Africa, is an annual low-growing plant reaching only 8 to 12 inches in height. The leaves are finely divided and doubly pinnate.

The flowers of both species are golden conical disks with white florets; they look similar to daisy flowers.

Chamomile makes an excellent ground cover; it survives being walked upon. As an old saying goes, "Like a chamomile bed, the more it is trodden, the more it will spread."

CHAPARRAL

Botanical Name

Larrea divaricata, L. glutinosa, L. tridentata
   (syn. *L. mexicana*)

Family

Zygophyllaceae (Caltrop Family)

Etymology

The genus name, *Larrea,* was given in honor of Juan Antonio Hernandez de Larrea, a Spanish clergyman. The common name *chaparral* derives from the Spanish *chaparro,* "evergreen oak," which in turn derives from the Basque *txapar.*

Also Known As

English: black bush, chaparro, creosote bush,
   dwarf evergreen oak, greasewood
Spanish: gobernadora, goma de Sonora,
   hediondilla ("little stinker")

Parts Used

Leaf, stem

Physiological Effects

Alterative, antiarthritic, antibacterial, antifungal, anti-inflammatory, antioxidant, antiparasitic, antiseptic, antitumor, antiviral, bitter, depurative, diuretic, emetic (in large doses), expectorant, laxative, lymphatic cleanser, tonic

Medicinal Uses

Many Native Americans considered chaparral to be a cure-all. It was listed in the United States Pharmacopoeia from 1842 to 1942 as an expectorant and bronchial antiseptic. It cleanses the lower bowels and promotes tissue repair. It stimulates immunity by stimulating mitochondrial respiration, the process in which cells utilize food for energy. It also increases the levels of ascorbic acid (vitamin C) in the adrenal glands, one of the body's primary storage sites for this vitamin. It has long been used to treat acne, allergies, amenorrhea, arthritis, bronchitis, cancer, chicken pox, cold sores, constipation, eczema, herpes, kidney infection, leukemia, leukorrhea, melanoma, parasites, pneumonia, rheumatism, staph infection, stomach cancer, strep throat, tuberculosis, tumor, uterine prolapse, venereal disease, warts, and worms.

A wonderful massage oil to ease rheumatic limbs can be made by cooking the branches in oil and then straining them out. Chaparral can be used as a mouthwash to prevent cavities, as a hair rinse to get rid of dandruff, as a suppository to treat hemorrhoids, as a bolus to treat vaginal infections, or as a liniment, salve, or compress to treat cuts, bruises, eczema, hemorrhoids, herpes, scabies, snakebite, and warts. It also can be used as a bath herb to promote detoxification.

Edible Uses

Chaparral is not generally considered edible, aside from as tea. It was once used as a preservative for oil and food.

Other Uses

The resin from chaparral was once used to mend pottery and waterproof baskets.

Constituents

Calcium, chromium, magnesium, potassium, beta-carotene, quercetin, lignan (nordihydroguaiaretic acid), resins, essential oils, saponins

Energetic Correspondences

- Flavor: extremely bitter, salty
- Temperature: cool
- Moisture: dry
- Polarity: yin
- Planet: Saturn
- Element: earth

Contraindications

In 1992, two people using large doses of chaparral in capsule form developed nonviral hepatitis and three others developed other symptoms of liver toxicity. This led the American Herbal Products Association and the U.S. Food and Drug Administration to issue a press release warning of potential risk from use of chaparral and suggesting that sale of chaparral be suspended. After more research, there was found to be no basis for the warning, and sale of chaparral was reinstated in 1995. There are still some precautions to take, nevertheless. Avoid chaparral during pregnancy and also while nursing. Excess use may be detrimental to the liver, kidneys, and lymphs. Discontinue use in case of fever, nausea, or jaundice (such as when the whites of the eyes become yellow).

Range and Appearance

Chaparral is a perennial evergreen shrub, 2 to 9 feet tall, growing throughout northern Mexico and the American Southwest. The smooth, olive green leaves exude a strong-smelling resin that is a deterrent to predators. It produces yellow flowers, about $1/2$ inch across, that become fluffy white seed heads, much like cotton balls. The plant is very hardy. It survives drought and depleted soil well and often prevents other plants from growing close to it. Its extremely bitter taste prevents animals from grazing upon it, and it does not burn easily. And after a nuclear test bomb was exploded in Yucca Flats, Nevada, in 1962, chaparral was one of the first plants to grow back, with twenty of the original twenty-one plants in the area resprouting.

CHICKWEED

Botanical Name

Stellaria alsine, S. graminea, S. media

Family

Caryophyllaceae (Pink Family)

Etymology

The genus name, *Stellaria,* is derived from the Latin *stella,* "star, " in reference to the shape of the flower. The species name, *media,* is Latin for "medium."

Also Known As

Danish: fuglegrees
Dutch: muur
English: adder's mouth, alsine, satin flower, starweed, starwort, stitchwort, winterweed
French: langue d'oiseau, morgeline, mouron blanc, mouron des oiseaux, stellaire
German: augentrogras, gansekraut, huhnerdarm, mausedarm, sternmiere, vogelmiere
Italian: buddelina, centocchio, erba gallina, paperina, stellaria
Portuguese: alsina
Spanish: hierba pajarera, pamplina, pamplina de canaries
Swedish: våtarv
Turkish: cam out

Part Used

Aboveground plant

Physiological Effects

Alterative, anti-inflammatory, antiseptic, astringent, carminative, demulcent, discutient, diuretic, emollient, expectorant, febrifuge, laxative, liver cleanser, mucolytic, nutritive, pectoral, refrigerant, vulnerary

Medicinal Uses

Chickweed nourishes yin fluids, clears heat, reduces inflammation, dissolves plaque in the blood vessels, and clears toxins. It is traditionally given to strengthen the frail. Chickweed is used to treat appendicitis, asthma, bladder irritation, bronchitis, constipation, cough, cysts, hoarseness, obesity, pleurisy, rheumatism, thyroid irregularities, tuberculosis, and ulcers.

Topically, chickweed can be used as a bath herb to soothe dry skin and chicken pox or as compress, poultice, or salve to treat boils, burns, diaper rash, eczema, hemorrhoids, itchy skin, nettle sting, psoriasis, rheumatism, and varicose veins. The fresh juice can be applied to eyes to treat cases of infection such as conjunctivitis.

Edible Uses

Chickweed is edible raw or cooked. It can also be juiced.

Other Uses

Chickweed is considered an herb to promote weight loss. The seeds are consumed by more than thirty kinds of birds, poultry, rabbits, and pigs; in fact, at one time the herb was referred to as chickenweed.

In magical traditions, chickweed is used to attract love and maintain a relationship.

Constituents

Vitamin C, phosphorous, calcium, copper, zinc, saponins, coumarins

Energetic Correspondences

- Flavor: sweet, salty
- Temperature: cool
- Moisture: moist
- Polarity: yin
- Planet: Moon/Saturn
- Element: water/earth

Contraindications

Excess use may cause diarrhea.

Range and Appearance

Chickweed can be an annual or perennial and is native to Eurasia. It grows in moist shade in gardens, waste places, and suburban lawns. It has a weak stem with a line of white hairs on one side. The leaves change direction with each pair. The tiny white flowers are deeply cleft; they begin blooming in late winter and close in cloudy weather. The seeds are borne in shiny black capsules. Chickweed makes an excellent ground cover, as it grows outward, not upward. The plant helps the soil retain nitrogen; its existence indicates fertile soil.

CHICORY

Botanical Name

Cichorium intybus

Family

Asteraceae (Daisy Family)

Etymology

The genus name, *Chicorium*, derives from the Greek name for this group of plants, *kichoreia,* which, in turn, perhaps derives from the Egyptian *keksher.* The species name, *intybus,* is derived from the Egyptian

tybi, the name of the Egyptian month corresponding to January in the Gregorian calendar, the month when chicory leaves were most eaten in that part of the world.

Also Known As

Afrikaans: sigorei
Arabic: shikôryah
Danish: cicorei, julesalat
Dutch: suikerey
English: Belgian endive, blowball, blue daisy, blue dandelion, blue sailors, coffeeweed, endive, hendibeh, ragged sailors, succory, watcher of the road, witloof
Estonian: harilik sigur
Finnish: italiansikuri
French: barbe à capucin, chicorée sauvage, ecoubette, laidron, yeux de chat
German: chicorie, eisenkraut, sonnenbraut, weglug, wegweiss, wegwarte, wirbelkraut, zichorie
Hungarian: cikória
Italian: cicoria, radicchio
Japanese: kiku nigana
Norwegian: sikori
Polish: cykoria
Russian: tzicory
Sanskrit: kasani
Spanish: achicoria
Swedish: cikoria
Turkish: radikya
Vietnamese: rau di' êp dâng

Part Used

Root (collected before the plant flowers)

Physiological Effects

Alterative, antibacterial, antiseptic, aperient, astringent, bitter, cardiotonic, carminative, cholagogue, depurative, digestive, diuretic, febrifuge, hepatic, laxative (mild), stimulant, stomachic, tonic

Medicinal Uses

Galen, the second-century physician-herbalist, called chicory a "friend to the liver." Chicory root clears heat and toxins and also promotes bile flow. It is used to treat acne, appetite loss, boils, constipation, depression, diabetes, dyspepsia, eczema, gallstones, gastritis, gout, hepatitis, irritability, jaundice, liver enlargement, rapid heartbeat, rheumatism, and urinary tract infection.

Edible Uses

Chicory root tea was a common beverage in Europe until World War II. The root can also be eaten raw (when young), baked, or sautéed. The roots and also the flowers may be candied, and the roots are sometimes added to wine both for their flavor and their therapeutic properties. Roasting the roots caramelizes their carbohydrates; such roasted roots can be used as a coffee substitute or extender, as in "Louisiana-style coffee."

The rest of the plant is edible as well. The young leaves (gathered before flowering) can be added to salads or cooked as greens. The buds and flowers can be pickled. Chicory flowers are a beautiful edible garnish in salads and other dishes.

In France, the young white shoots are pickled and made into a salad called *barbe de capucin,* meaning "beard of the monk." The entire plant can be juiced.

Other Uses

Chicory is one of the traditional bitter herbs of Passover. The Swedish botanist Linnaeus used chicory in his floral clock, as the flowers open and close with such regularity. Cows love to graze upon chicory, but it will make their milk taste bitter if they eat it to excess. Goldfinches eat the seeds.

In magical traditions, it is carried in medicine bags to remove obstacles and promote frugality.

Constituents

Beta-carotene, vitamin B, vitamin C, vitamin K, flavonoids, choline, inulin, oligofructose, sesquiterpene lactones (lactucine, lactupicrine), coumarins, latex

Energetic Correspondences

- Flavor: bitter, sweet, salty
- Temperature: cool
- Moisture: moist
- Polarity: yang
- Planet: Sun/Mercury/Venus/Jupiter/Uranus
- Element: air

Contraindications

Excessive use can cause digestive disturbances and visual problems.

Range and Appearance

Chicory, native to Eurasia, can be an annual, biennial, or perennial. It grows in dry soil in disturbed areas and reaches a height of 1 to 3 feet. The leaves are irregularly toothed and lobed and grow alternately on the stem; the upper leaves clasp the stalk. The stem produces a milky sap when broken. The flowers are daisylike, ragged, stalkless, and a vibrant shade of blue, though occasionally a white or pink one appears. On sunny days, the petals close at noon.

CINNAMON

Botanical Name

Cinnamomum aromaticum (syn. *C. cassia*), *C. verum* (syn. *C. zeylanicum*)

Family

Lauraceae (Laurel Family)

Etymology

The genus name, *Cinnamomum,* derives from the Greek name for the spice, *kinnamomon,* which may in turn derive from the Malaysian *kay manis,* "sweet wood." The common name *cassia* is believed to derive from the ancient Hebrew *qetsilah,* which perhaps means "spice."

Also Known As

Arabic: darseen, qurfa
Cantonese: gun gwai, mauh gwai, yuk gwai
Croatian: kineski cimet
Czech: skorice cinska
Danish: kinesisk kanel
Dutch: kassie

English: cassia, sweet wood

Esperanto: cimamomo

Estonian: hiina kaneelipuu

Finnish: kassia, talouskaneli

French: cannelle, casse

German: ceylonzimt, kanel, kassie, zimtbaum

Greek: kasia

Hebrew: kasia, quassia

Hindi: dalchini

Hungarian: kasszia

Icelandic: kassía

Italian: cannella, cassia

Japanese: keishi, nikkei

Lithuanian: kininis cinamonas

Korean: yukkye

Mandarin: guan gui, yok gwai, zi gui

Polish: kasja

Norwegian: kassia

Portuguese: canela

Romanian: scortisoara

Russian: korichnoje derevo, koritsa

Sanskrit: tvak

Serbian: cimet-kasija

Spanish: canela, casia

Swahili: mdalasini

Swedish: kanel

Thai: ob choey chin, thephatharo

Turkish: yabani darcin

Vietnamese: que don, que quang

Parts Used

Bark, twig

Physiological Effects

Analgesic, anodyne, antibacterial, antibiotic, antifungal, antioxidant, antiviral, aphrodisiac, aromatic, astringent, cardiac stimulant, carminative, circulatory stimulant, decongestant, diaphoretic, digestive, diuretic, emmenagogue, expectorant, hemostatic, mucolytic, stimulant, stomachic, vasodilator, yang tonic

Medicinal Uses

Cinnamon helps dry dampness, stimulates the diges-tive tract, and has activity against staph infection and botulism. It also stimulates circulation, and its prolonged use is known to beautify the skin and promote a rosy complexion. It is especially helpful for people who are always cold and have poor circulation. It is used in the treatment of appetite loss, arthritis, bedwetting, colds, colic, cough, diarrhea, dysentery, dysmenorrhea, erectile dysfunction, fatigue, flatulence, flu, halitosis, headache, hypotension, irregular menses, lumbago, malabsorbtion, nausea, poor circulation, prostatitis, rheumatism, tuberculosis, and vision problems.

Topically, cinnamon can be used in footbaths to treat athlete's foot and as a bath herb in treatments for chills and sore muscles. As a steam inhalation it is beneficial in cases of colds, coughs, and sore throat. It can be prepared as a wash to get rid of fungal infections, such as athlete's foot. It is often included in massage oils for its warming properties, and it is often included in toothpastes for its ability to freshen breath and inhibit bacteria.

Aromatically, the pleasant scent of cinnamon stimulates the senses yet calms the nerves.

Edible Uses

During the age of exploration of the fifteenth and sixteenth centuries, cinnamon was among the most sought after of spices, and is still incredibly popular in cuisines around the world. When added to dairy dishes, it enhances their digestibility.

Other Uses

Cinnamon was used in ancient Egypt in the mummification process. It was also used in ancient times to prevent food from spoiling. In sachets it repels moths. It is sometimes included in hair rinses to highlight dark hair and in massage oils to promote sexual arousal. When burned as an incense, it is reputed to encourage love, success, and prosperity.

Constituents

Iron, magnesium, zinc, essential oils (eugenol, cinnamic aldehyde, linalool, chacicol), phellandrene, gum, tannin, catechin, mannitol, coumarins, mucilage, cinnamaldehyde

Energetic Correspondences

- Flavor: sweet, pungent, bitter
- Temperature: hot
- Moisture: dry
- Polarity: yang
- Planet: Sun/Mercury/Mars/Jupiter/Uranus
- Element: fire

Contraindications

Avoid cinnamon in cases of hot, feverish conditions; excessive dryness; hemorrhoids, dry stools, or hematuria (blood in the urine). Avoid large amounts during pregancy and, because it can decrease a mother's milk supply, while nursing. Avoid therapeutic doses for extended periods of time. Doses of more than 2 grams could cause delirium, hallucinations, and convulsions.

Range and Appearance

Cinnamomum aromaticum is native to southern China, while *C. verum* is native to Sri Lanka, but both species are naturalized and cultivated in the tropics. Both are small evergreen trees with oval oblong leaves 5 to 9 inches in length. The yellow-white flowers are borne in panicles. The flowers are followed by small purple berries that each bear a single seed.

To make cinnamon spice, the thick bark of the tree is peeled away and layers are left to dry, during which time it curls up. The dried bark is then sold in pieces or ground up.

CISTANCHES

Botanical Name

Cistanche deserticola, C. salsa, Orobanche spp.

Family

Orobanchaceae (Broomrape Family)

Etymology

The family name and the sometimes genus name *Orobanche* is from the Greek *oros,* "mountain," and *stachys,* "spike."

Also Known As

Cantonese: yak sung yan
English: broomrape, beechdrops, cancer root, epifagus, ghost plant
French: orobanche
German: erbsenwurger, sommerwurz
Italian: orobanche
Japanese: nikujuyō
Korean: yukchongyong
Mandarin: róu cóng róng

Part Used

Aboveground plant

Physiological Effects

Analgesic, aphrodisiac, astringent, demulcent, emollient, kidney tonic, laxative, hypotensive, phytoandrogenic, restorative, stimulant, yang tonic

Medicinal Uses

Ancient Chinese legend says that cistanches sprang from sperm dropped to the ground by wild stallions. Its suggestive shape, resembling an erect penis, probably led to its common use as an aphrodisiac.

Cistanches moistens the intestines, strengthens the kidneys, and helps soften hardened masses in the body. It was used by Paiute Indians to treat respiratory ailments such as colds and pneumonia, and it is also used as an aid in stroke recovery. It is beneficial in cases of angina, constipation due to dryness, erectile dysfunction, hot flashes, hypertension, incontinence, infertility (male and female), knee pain, leukorrhea, lumbago, muscle weakness, premature ejaculation, rheumatism, spermatorrhea, posturination dripping, and uterine bleeding.

Topically, cistanches is used as a poultice to relieve toothache and joint pain and to clear up skin infections caused by strep and herpes. Herbalists of North America and Europe used the powdered herb topically on skin cancers.

Edible Uses

The entire plant can be eaten raw or roasted as a vegetable.

Other Uses

None known

Constituents

Alkaloids (orobanchin), phytosterols (beta-sitos-terol), betaine, glucose, succinic acid, iridoid glyco-sides, phenylpropenoid glycosides

Energetic Correspondences

- Flavor: sweet, salty, sour, slightly bitter
- Temperature: warm
- Moisture: moist
- Polarity: yin
- Planet: Moon/Mercury/Jupiter/Pluto
- Element: water

Contraindications

Avoid cistanches in cases of diarrhea due to deficien-cy in yin, stomach chi, or spleen chi, as it can inten-sify these conditions. Do not prepare the tea with utensils made of iron, as it is believed to alter the plant's effects.

Range and Appearance

Cistanches is a parasitic perennial, nourishing itself on the roots of plants growing near it. The *Cistanche* genus is native to western China, Mongolia, Siberia, and Tibet, where it grows in dry, sandy riverbanks. The *Orobanche* genus is native to the broader Eura-sia. The plant lacks chlorophyll and has a pale appearance. Its leaves look like scales. It produces terminal spikes of white or purple five-lobed flowers.

Cistanches is endangered in the wild, mostly because of overharvesting of its preferred host plants for firewood. For this reason it should not be used indiscriminately.

CLEAVERS

Botanical Name

Galium aparine, G. trifida, G. triflorum, G. verum

Family

Rubiaceae (Madder Family)

Etymology

The species name *aparine* derives from the Greek *aparo*, "to seize," in reference to the plant's tenden-cy to catch on the clothes or fur of whoever passes close by. The common name *cleavers* also refers to the clinging properties of the plant. Ancient Greeks called it *phillantropon*, "love of man" assuming that it clung to humans out of love.

Also Known As

Dutch: walstroo
English: bedstraw, catchweed, clabbergrass, cleaverwort, clivers, clives, everlasting friendship, goosegrass, gravel grass, grip grass, loveman, maid's hair, milk sweet, poor Robin, pretty mugget, sticky willie
French: aparine, gaillet gratteron, petit muguet
German: klebenkraut, kletten-labkraut, klimme, vogelheu
Italian: aparine, attacca-veste, cappello dei tignosi, gaglio
Spanish: cuaja leche, guaco
Turkish: coban suzegi

Part Used

Aboveground plant

Physiological Effects

Alterative, anti-inflammatory, antineoplastic, aperient, astringent (mild), diaphoretic, diuretic, febrifuge, hypotensive, immune tonic, lithotriptic, lymphatic cleanser, nutritive, refrigerant, tonic, vulnerary

Medicinal Uses

Cleavers helps the body eliminate uric acid and improves the body's ability to remove catabolic wastes through its waterways. It also clears heat and inflammation and promotes tissue repair, and it is a traditional spring cleansing tonic. Cleavers is used to treat acne, appetite loss, arthritis, bedwetting, blad-der stones, cancer (juice), cystitis, dropsy, dysuria, edema, eczema, epilepsy, glandular fever, hepatitis, hypertension, kidney stones, mastitis, measles, ovar-ian cysts, prostatitis, psoriasis, scarlet fever, scrofula, scurvy (with the fresh juice), sore throat, swollen adenoids, swollen lymph glands, throat cancer, tonsillitis, tumors, ulcer, and venereal disease (with the fresh juice).

Topically, cleavers can be prepared as a compress, poultice, or salve to treat burns, cancer, eczema, poison ivy, psoriasis, sagging skin, scars, sore nipples, spider bites, stretch marks, sunburn, and wounds. It can be used as a hair rinse to treat dandruff, as a facial wash and toner to treat acne or to remove freckles, or as a mouthwash to treat canker sores and throat ulcers.

Edible Uses

Young spring cleavers greens may be eaten raw or cooked. The plant can also be juiced. The seeds are sometimes roasted and used as a coffee substitute, though they do not contain caffeine. Cleavers can be juiced. Geese, sheep, and cows all relish this plant.

Other Uses

Cleavers tea can be used as an underarm antiperspirant. Ancient Greeks wove cleavers plants together to make a sieve for straining herbs and milk, and cleavers was once used to stuff mattresses. Today, cleavers is sometimes used to curdle milk in cheese making. The root makes a red dye.

Constituents

Vitamin C, calcium, niacin, silica, glycoside (asperuloside), polyphenolic acids (caffeic acid, gallic acid), flavonoids (luteolin), coumarin, tannins

Energetic Correspondences

- Flavor: salty
- Temperature: cool
- Moisture: dry
- Polarity: yin
- Planet: Venus/Moon
- Element: air/water

Contraindications

Cleavers is not recommended in cases of diabetes, as it will increase urination. Contact dermatitis from the fresh juice is a rare occurrence.

Range and Appearance

Native to Europe, cleavers is an annual that grows in open fields and moist areas, often forming a clump with other plants. It features a single trailing square stem, 2 to 6 feet in length, that is covered with small downward-curving hooks. The leaves are whorled in circular rosettes of six to eight leaves. The tiny, white, starlike flowers grow in clusters along the leaf axils. The seeds occur in pairs.

CLOVE

Botanical Name

Syzygium aromaticum (formerly *Eugenia aromatica*)

Family

Myrtaceae (Eucalyptus Family)

Etymology

The genus name *Eugenia* was given in honor of Prince Eugene of Savoy (1663–1736). The former genus name, *Syzygium*, derives from the Greek *syzygos*, "joined together," in reference to the paired leaves of the plant. The species name *aromaticum* means "aromatic." The word *clove* is from the Latin *clavus*, "nail," in reference to the shape of the buds.

Also Known As

Arabic: kabsn qaranful
Cantonese: ding heung
Czech: hřebíček
Danish: nellike
Dutch: kruidnagel
English: carnation clove
Esperanto: kariofilo
Finnish: neilikka
French: clous de girofle, giroflier
German: gewurznelkenbaum, naegelein
Greek: garifalo
Hebrew: tsiporen
Hindi: long
Hungarian: szogfú
Italian: chiodi de garofano

Icelandic: negull
Japanese: choko
Korean: jeonghyang
Mandarin: ding xiang ding zi xiang, gong ding
  xiang
Nepali: lwang
Norwegian: nellik
Polish: gozdzik
Portuguese: cravo
Russian: gvozdika
Sanskrit: lavanga
Spanish: clavo, raja
Swahili: nejlikor
Swedish: kryddnejlika
Thai: khan plu
Turkish: karanfil
Vietnamese: dinh huong
Yiddish: negelen

Part Used

Flower bud (dried)

Physiological Effects

Analgesic, anesthetic, anodyne, antibacterial, antiemetic, antifungal, anti-inflammatory, antioxidant, antiseptic, antispasmodic, aphrodisiac, aromatic, astringent, carminative, diaphoretic, digestive, diuretic, emmenagogue, expectorant, rubefacient, stimulant, stomachic

Medicinal Uses

Clove stimulates circulation and digestion, warms the body, and disinfects the skin, liver, kidneys, and mucous membranes of the bronchials. In vitro studies show that it is effective against *E. coli,* strep, staph, and pneumococci. Cloves are used to treat altitude sickness, anorexia, appetite loss, candida, colds, colic, cough, depression, diarrhea, dysentery, dyspepsia, erectile dysfunction, flatulence, flu, halitosis, hernia, hiccups, hypotension, indigestion, laryngitis, lupus, malabsorption, parasites, poor circulation, rheumatism, sinusitis, stomach cramps, vomiting, and worms.

For topical applications the essential oil of clove is most often used. It can be applied to the area of a toothache to stop pain. It is added to toothpastes and mouthwashes as a flavoring, breath-freshening, and antiseptic agent, as it inhibits dental plaque formation. It also can be applied topically to treat warts, insect bites, and infected wounds. It is beneficial in massage oils and liniments to ease neuralgia and rheumatism.

Folklore says that sucking on two whole cloves without chewing or swallowing them helps curb the desire for alcohol.

Edible Uses

Clove is a common culinary spice. It is also used to make vanillin, or artificial vanilla. It has long been added to food as a natural preservative, and it aids in the assimilation and digestion of food.

Other Uses

Clove has a long history of use in widespread cultures. It is a wonderful breath freshener; in fact, during China's Han Dynasty (207 B.C.–A.D. 220) court visitors were required to hold cloves in their mouth when addressing the emperor, so as to not offend him with bad breath. Moluccan islanders once planted a clove tree when a child was born in the belief that it would ensure that the child would grow strong and sturdy, like the tree. Clove has long been a popular scent in men's cosmetics, and whole cloves are often added to sachets and pomanders as a natural air freshener. The essential oil is a good insect repellent. Today, much of the world's clove production goes into making kreteks, or Indonesian clove cigarettes.

In magical traditions, clove is used to promote love and prosperity. It is often burned as an incense to deter negative energy.

Constituents

Calcium, magnesium, manganese, omega-3 fatty acids, flavonoids (kaempferol, rhamnetin), vitamin C, essential oils (eugenol, caryophyllene, pinene, vanillene, furfurol), tannin, gum, lipids, wax

Energetic Correspondences

* Flavor: punget, bitter
* Temperature: hot

- Moisture: dry
- Polarity: yang
- Planet: Sun/Mercury/Venus/Mars/Jupiter/Uranus
- Element: fire

Contraindications

Avoid large amounts during pregnancy or in cases of fever or yin deficiency. Prolonged contact of the essential oil with gum tissue can be irritating.

Range and Appearance

Clove is a small perennial evergreen tree native to Asia. It has large branches covered with smooth grayish bark. The opposite leaves are about 4 inches long and 2 inches wide. The tree bears rose-colored, bell-shaped flowers that grow in bunches at the ends of the branches.

CODONOPSIS

Botanical Name

Codonopsis lanceolata, C. pilosula

Family

Campanulaceae (Bellflower Family)

Etymology

The genus name *Codonopsis* is thought to derive from the Greek *kodon,* "bell," and *opsis,* "remblance," in reference to the bell-shaped flowers. Though it is not related to ginseng, in Chinese medicine it is classified as a tonic with properties similar to those of ginseng, and so its common name *dang shen* includes the generic term for ginseng, *shen,* "spirit." *Dang* refers to the region of origin, Shang Dang, in China.

Also Known As

Cantonese: fong dong sam (*C. pilosula*), yang guk (*C. lanceolata*)
English: bellflower, dang shen, goat's tit bellflower, poor man's ginseng, relative root, woodland bonnet
Japanese: tōjin

Korean: tangsam
Mandarin: dâng shèn, shan hai luo (*C. lanceolata*), tai dang shen (*C. pilosula*), yang ju (*C. lanceolata*)

Part Used

Root

Physiological Effects

Adaptogen, aphrodisiac, blood tonic, cardiotonic, chi tonic, demulcent, depurative, digestive, emmenagogue, expectorant, galactagogue, hypotensive, immune tonic, kidney tonic, nutritive, restorative, sialagogue, stimulant, stomachic, yin tonic

Medicinal Uses

Codonopsis is often regarded to have tonifying effects similar to those of ginseng, while costing much less. It is somewhat milder than ginseng, and its effect is not as long-lasting.

The root enhances the body's resistance to disease and is traditionally given around the change of seasons or during stressful times to help people acclimate to change and be better able to resist infection. It tonifies the lungs, spleen, and chi, increases the body's production of phagocytes, and nourishes the blood, increasing the red blood cell count and blood sugar levels. It also nourishes the entire body, particularly for those who are exhausted and wasting away, suffering from chronic illness, or recovering from surgery or childbirth. It helps the body clear excess phlegm and improves the resiliency of the skin. It is also said to promote weight loss.

Codonopsis is used to treat AIDS, anemia, appetite loss, asthma, cancer, chemotherapy side effects, chronic cough, chronic fatigue syndrome, debility, diabetes, diarrhea, dyspepsia, excessive perspiration, fatigue, fever, flatulence, gastritis, heart palpitations, HIV, hyperacidity, indigestion, insomnia, memory loss, nephritis, prolapse of the uterus/rectum or stomach, radiotherapy side effects, shortness of breath, stress, ulcers, voice weakness, and vomiting. Mixed with licorice root, it is used to treat anorexia.

Topically, the root (and the leaf) can be used as a poultice to treat wounds.

Edible Uses

Codonopsis is a delicious addition to soups, stews, and grain and bean dishes. It can also be added to wine. The dried root is sometimes made into a flour.

Other Uses

The root can be given to babies to teethe on (under supervision, of course); it is sweet and hard and doesn't splinter.

Constituents

Calcium, iron, manganese, zinc, carbohydrates, protein, saponins (tangshenoside), alkaloids (codonopsine, codonopsinine), polysaccharides (inulin, sucrose, glucose), essential oil

Energetic Correspondences

- Flavor: sweet
- Temperature: warm
- Moisture: moist
- Polarity: yang
- Planet: Jupiter
- Element: water

Contraindications

Generally regarded as safe.

Range and Appearance

Native to central and eastern Asia, codonopsis is a perennial twining vine. The leaves are alternate on small branches, with four or more leaves on a cluster. The vine has bell-shaped, terminal, hermaphroditic flowers that are yellowish white on top and purple on the back portion. The stems contain a milky fluid.

COLLINSONIA

Botanical Name

Collinsonia canadensis

Family

Lamiaceae (Mint Family)

Etymology

Collinsonia is named after British botanist and merchant Peter Collinson (1693–1768). The root is very hard, hence the folk name *stoneroot*.

Also Known As

English: citronella horse balm, hardback, knobroot, knob weed, kolinsonia, ox balm, rich weed, stoneroot
French: baume de cheval, guérit-tout

Part Used

Rhizome

Physiological Effects

Alterative, astringent, diaphoretic, diuretic, emmenagogue, hepatic, sedative, stimulant, tonic, vasoconstricter, vulnerary

Medicinal Uses

Collinsonia works primarily on the venous system, helping to move congestion from the mouth, throat, lungs, bowel, anus, and mucous membranes. It also helps relieve irritation to the nerves and stimulates digestive secretions. It is used to treat benign prostatic hypertrophy, bladder stones, bronchitis, catarrh, constipation, diarrhea, dropsy, gallstones, gastritis, headache, hemorrhoids, indigestion, interstitial cystitis, laryngitis, leukorrhea, kidney stones, pharyngitis, and varicose veins.

Topically, collinsonia can be used as a wash or compress to treat bruises, burns, poison ivy/oak, sprains, and wounds. A liniment of collinsonia can be applied directly to spider veins and varicose veins to decrease swelling and strengthen the tissues. It can be used as a gargle to relieve sore throat and as a salve to relieve hemorrhoids.

Note: Avoid boiling the root, or else the plant's medicinal properties will be diminished. The root is very hard, so if you're going to grind it, proceed with caution, or you will break your grinding equipment.

Edible Uses

Not generally regarded as edible, aside from as tea.

Other Uses

None known

Constituents

Flavonoids, saponins, alkaloids, rosmarinic acid, essential oil, tannin, resin, starch

Energetic Correspondences

- Flavor: pungent, sour
- Temperature: warm
- Moisture: dry
- Polarity: yang
- Planet: Mars
- Element: fire

Contraindications

Avoid during pregnancy. Beware the aboveground portion of the plant, which can be emetic even in small amounts.

Range and Appearance

Collinsonia is a perennial, native to North America, that grows in shady, damp areas. Its square stems can grow from 2 to 4 feet in height. The large leaves are few, opposite, serrated, and ovate, with the lower ones being petiolate and the upper ones almost sessile. The flowers are greenish yellow, arranged in a terminal raceme, with a funnel-shaped corolla. The flowers have a pungent balsamic, lemonlike odor.

COLTSFOOT

Botanical Name

Tussilago farfara

Family

Asteraceae (Daisy Family)

Etymology

The genus name, *Tussilago,* is from the Latin *tussis agere,* "cough dispeller." The species name, *farfara,* is thought to be ancient Latin for "to make talkative."

Also Known As

Cantonese: fong dun fa

English: British tobacco, bull's foot, butterbur, coughwort, filius ante patrem ("son before father," as the plant flowers before the leaves appear), flower velure, foal's foot, horsehoof, owl's blanket, welcome winter flower, wolverine's foot

French: herbe de Sainte Quirain, pas d'Âne, pas de cheval, procheton, taconnet, tussilage

German: brandlattich, huflattich, hustenkraut, rosshub

Italian: farfara, farfaraccio

Japanese: kantõka

Korean: kwandonghwa

Mandarin: ko dong, kùan-dõng-hõa

Russian: mati matcheha

Sanskrit: fanjuim

Parts Used

Leaf, flower

Physiological Effects

Anti-inflammatory, antispasmodic, antitussive, astringent, bitter, bronchial dilator, cardiovascular stimulant, demulcent, diaphoretic, emollient, expectorant, immune stimulant, pectoral, respiratory stimulant, sedative, tonic

Medicinal Uses

The leaf is used primarily in Western herbalism, while the flower is used more in Asian medicine. Both have approximately the same effects and are used mainly as a cough remedy.

Coltsfoot prevents blood platelet aggregation, suppresses the triggering of bronchial spasms, dilates the bronchioles, clears heat, curbs infection, and promotes tissue repair. It is used to treat asthma, bronchitis, colds, cough, diarrhea, emphysema, flu, gastritis, hoarseness, laryngitis, shortness of breath, tuberculosis, wheezing, and whooping cough. Coltsfoot is a common ingredient in cough syrups; the flowers can be soaked in honey to make a cough-relieving honey.

Topically, the leaf can be used as a poultice to

treat insect bites, puffy eyes, sore feet, and wounds. As a facial toner or steam, the leaf has antiseptic and oil-reducing properties and is used to curb blemishes. The flower can be prepared as a soothing eyewash or as a hair rinse to treat dandruff.

Coltsfoot has been recommended as a medicinal smoke since the days of Dioscorides. It is even currently marketed in China as a remedy for smoker's cough.

Edible Uses

The fresh buds, flowers, and stems can be eaten raw or cooked. The leaves are edible but somewhat bitter; they are best when cooked in two changes of water. The mature leaves also can be dried, burned, and used as a salt substitute. The root can be cooked like a vegetable. The flowers are used in wine making.

Other Uses

Coltsfoot was introduced to North America soon after Europeans discovered the continent. Some Native American tribes came to consider the young, still-rolled-up leaves such an important salt substitute that they fought wars over it. In Scotland, coltsfoot has been used to stuff mattresses. The leaves have been used as an herbal wrap for covering and protecting food. Coltsfoot is also added to animal fodder to relieve coughs in cattle and horses. Goldfinches line their nests with the soft fuzz from the leaves.

Constituents

Vitamin C, calcium, magnesium, potassium, sodium, sulfur, zinc, flavonoids (hyperoside, isoquercetin, rutin), mucilage (polysaccharide, inulin), pyrrolizidine alkaloids, sitosterol, gallic acid, tannins, triterpenoid saponins

Energetic Correspondences

- Flavor: pungent, slightly sweet, bitter
- Temperature: warm
- Moisture: moist
- Polarity: yin
- Planet: Sun/Mercury/Venus/Jupiter
- Element: water

Contraindications

The pyrrolizidine alkaloids have been shown to have hepatotoxicity, with the potenial for causing obstructive liver damage, when fed to rats. Swedish research, however, shows that these alkaloids are inactivated when subjected to heat, such as when the herb is boiled to make a tea, nor have the alkaloids been found harmful in humans. Nevertheless, to be safe, avoid coltsfoot in cases of liver disease or a history of alcohol abuse. And until further research is done, it would be wise not to use coltsfoot during pregnancy, while nursing, or continuously for longer than six weeks.

Range and Appearance

Coltsfoot, a perennial native to Eurasia but widely naturalized, grows in zinc-rich, clayey soils in waste places and along roadsides. It grows from 4 to 12 inches tall. Its downy, grayish stems are covered with leaves resembling scales. The flowers are yellow and terminal. The leaves appear after the flowers and are large, basal, and cordate, with a serrated edge and a shape like a horse's footprint. Their underside is whitish and downy.

COMFREY

Botanical Name

Symphytum caucasicum (Causcasian comfrey), *S. officinale, S. peregrinum, S. uplandicum* (Russian comfrey)

Family

Boraginaceae (Borage Family)

Etymology

The name *comfrey* is derived from the Latin *con ferva,* "with strength." The genus name, *Symphytum,* derives from the Greek *symphytis,* "grown together," and *phyton,* "plant."

Also Known As

English: blackwort, gum plant, bruisewort, knitbone, nipbone, slippery root, walwort, woundwort

Finnish: rohtoraunioyrtti

French: consoude, grande consoude, herbe aux
coupures, oreille d'ane, sain-foin

German: beinwell, blutwurz, schmerzwurz,
schwarzwurz, wallwurz

Italian: consolida maggiore

Russian: okopnik

Spanish: suelda, consuelda, sinfito

Swedish: vallört

Parts Used

Leaf, root

Physiological Effects

Alterative, anodyne, anti-inflammatory, antirheumatic, antiseptic, astringent, biogenic stimulator, demulcent, emollient, expectorant, hemostatic, immune stimulant, lung tonic, nutritive, pectoral, refrigerant, styptic, vulnerary, yin tonic

Medicinal Uses

Comfrey has been used as a healing herb for much of human history. It was carried by the armies of Alexander the Great to treat wounds and during the Middle Ages was used to treat fractures. Comfrey moistens yin, heals irritated mucous membranes, and soothes and protects damaged tissues. It helps reduce pain, especially in the bones, tendons, and lungs. It is best known as an herb that can help regenerate cells. Today, comfrey tea is used to treat acne, arthritis, asthma, bronchitis, burns, cough, diarrhea, dysentery, eczema, fractures, gallstones, heartburn, hemorrhage, laryngitis, pneumonia, pleurisy, tonsillitis, tuberculosis, ulcers, underweight conditions, and whooping cough.

Allantoin, a biogenic stimulator that is one of comfrey's important ingredients, is used in lotions to treat dry, rough, or wrinkled skin. Comfrey is also included in lotions, poultices, and salves to treat bruises, burns, carpal tunnel syndrome, eczema, fractures, hemorrhoids, scars, sunburn, swellings, wounds, wrinkles, and varicosities. As a poultice, comfrey helps draw out splinters and infection. As a bath herb, comfrey can soothe dry skin, and it can be added to shampoos and conditioners to treat dan-

druff and dry scalp. It can be used as a gargle for tonsillitis or made into a soothing douche or enema. Comfrey powder is used to brush the teeth and as a snuff for nosebleeds.

Edible Uses

The young comfrey leaves can be eaten raw, cooked, or juiced; since the plant is hairy, it needs to be finely chopped before being eaten. The roots can be candied.

Other Uses

Comfrey baths were once given to women before marriage to restore the hymen and thus "virginity." The roots were once used as a dye plant, and the plant has long been used as animal fodder. When added to the compost bin comfrey accelerates the breakdown of organic matter.

Constituents

Vitamin B_{12}, calcium, germanium, iron, potassium, phosphorous, amino acids (tryptophan, lysine, isoleucine, methionine), mucilage (mucopolysaccharides), allantoin, inulin, alkaloids (symphytine, echimidine, asparagine), triterpenoids, phenolic acids, rosmarinic acids, sterols (sitosterol), tannin

Energetic Correspondences

- Flavor: sweet
- Temperature: cool
- Moisture: moist
- Polarity: yin
- Planet: Saturn/Neptune/Moon
- Element: water/air

Contraindications

Comfrey is recommended only for short-term use of less than six weeks, and it is not recommended for use during pregnancy or while nursing. Some of its alkaloids are pyrrolizidine alkaloids, which may cause hepatic toxicity, specifically hepatic veno-occlusive disease, in which the small and medium veins in the liver become obstructed. The root contains more of these potentially dangerous alkaloids than the leaves, and young leaves contain more than mature leaves. Prickly comfrey (*S. asperum*) has the highest levels of pyrrolizidine alkaloids of all species, while *S. officinale* has the lowest. Herbalists debate about the safety of using herbs containing pyrrolizidine alkaloids, and more research needs to be conducted to determine whether comfrey is safe for internal use. But there is no problem with using it topically.

Because comfrey causes rapid wound healing, make sure a wound is clean of any dirt before applying comfrey. Also be sure of your species; poisonings have occurred from novices collecting toxic foxglove, mistaking it for comfrey.

Range and Appearance

Comfrey, a native of Europe and northern Asia, is a perennial that grows from 1 to 4 feet tall on an angular stem. It has large lanceolate or oval leaves which are about 12 inches long with a protruding midvein. The leaves get smaller as they get higher up the stem. Both the leaves and the stems are bristly. The bell-shaped flowers grow in curled clusters and can be whitish, pink, or purplish. Comfrey is found growing in the wild in open woods, along streams, and in meadows. Once planted in a garden comfrey tends to take over and can be difficult to eradicate.

COPTIS

Botanical Name

Coptis spp., including *C. japonica*, *C. laciniata*, *C. occidentalis*, *C. sinensis*, *C. trifolia* (American goldthread)

Family

Ranunculaceae (Buttercup Family)

Etymology

The genus name *Coptis* derives from the Greek *kopto*, "to cut," alluding to the plant's deeply cut leaves. The plant's shallow root system looks like a mass of gold threads, hence one of its folk names, *goldthread*.

Also Known As

English: canker root, goldthread, mishmi bitter, mouthroot, vegetable gold, yellow root
French: savoyarde
German: niesswurz
Hindi: mamira
Italian: ruta dei prati
Mandarin: húang lían
Japanese: oren
Korean: hwangnyôn
Sanskrit: mishamitita

Part Used

Rhizome

Physiological Effects

Alterative, analgesic, antibacterial, antibiotic, anti-inflammatory, antiviral, bitter, cholagogue, febrifuge, ophthalmic, pectoral, refrigerant, stomachic

Medicinal Uses

Coptis prevents bacteria and viruses from proliferating. It also lowers fever and relaxes spasms by improving circulation. It is used in the treatment of abscess, alcoholism, dyspepsia, dysentery, fever, flu, hepatitis, HIV, jaundice, and nosebleeds.

Topically, the juice of the fresh rhizome or coptis tea can be used in the treatment of cold sores, herpes lesions, and thrush. Coptis can also be made into a douche to treat yeast or bacterial infections.

This herb often can be used interchangeably with goldenseal.

Edible Uses

Not generally considered edible.

Other Uses

The rhizomes produce a yellow dye.

Constituents

Alkaloids (berberine, coptisine), albumin, lignan

Energetic Correspondences

- Flavor: bitter, pungent
- Temperature: cold

- Moisture: dry
- Polarity: yang
- Planet: Sun/Saturn
- Element: earth

Contraindications

Avoid during pregnancy and in cases of gastric inflammation or diarrhea. Coptis is best used for short periods of time (under three weeks). Long-term use can irritate the digestive tract.

Range and Appearance

Native to the northern hemisphere, coptis is a plant of the deep woodlands, an evergreen that requires moist soil and partial shade. It has strong, wiry stems that grow to about 10 inches in height. The leaves are $\frac{3}{4}$ to $1\frac{1}{2}$ inches long, borne on long petioles, and divided into two or three parts. The plant bears hermaphroditic, pale yellow flowers.

CORIANDER

Botanical Name

Coriandrum sativum

Family

Apiaceae (Parsley Family)

Etymology

The genus name, *Coriandrum,* and the common name *coriander* are derived from the Greek for the plant, *koriannon,* whose root is *koris,* "bug," in reference to a peculiar scent coriander exudes when the leaves are crushed, which some liken to that of bed bugs.

Also Known As

Arabic: kuzbara
Armenian: kinj
Bulgarian: koriander
Cantonese: fàn yùhn sài
Czech: koriandr
Dutch: koriander
English: cilantro (in reference to the leaf), Chinese parsley, Mexican parsley
Esperanto: koriandro

Finnish: korianteri
French: coriandre cultivée
German: koriander
Greek: koliandro
Hebrew: gad, kusbar
Hindi: dhaniya
Hungarian: koriander
Italian: coriandro, coriandolo
Icelandic: koriandor
Japanese: koendoro
Korean: kosu
Mandarin: yan shi
Norwegian: koriandor
Polish: kolendra siewna
Portuguese: coentro
Russian: koriandr
Sanskrit: dhanyaka
Swahili: giligilani
Thai: pak chi
Tibetan: sona pentsom
Turkish: kisnic
Vietnamese: cây rau mùi
Yiddish: feld-gliander

Part Used

Seed (primarily), leaf (rarely)

Physiological Effects

Alterative, anodyne, antibacterial, antioxidant, antispasmodic, aphrodisiac, aromatic, carminative, cordial, diaphoretic, diuretic, nervine, stimulant, stomachic, tonic

Medicinal Uses

Humans have been using coriander for its medicinal and culinary properties for at least seven thousand years. It was one of the world's earliest cultivated spices. Coriander seeds were found in the tomb of King Tut, and the spice was mentioned in the Ebers Papyrus. Coriander was an ingredient in love potions during the Middle Ages, and it is mentioned as an aphrodisiac in *The Arabian Nights.*

Coriander seed stimulates digestion, breaks up mucus, and disperses stagnation. Coriander seed tea is used to treat allergies, amenorrhea, anxiety, appetite loss, asthma, bloating, burning pain during urination, colic, cramps, cystitis, diabetes, diarrhea, fever, flatulence, halitosis, hay fever, hernia pain, high cholesterol, indigestion, insomnia, measles, menstrual cramps, migraines, nausea, neuralgia, poor digestive assimilation, rash, rheumatism, sore throat, stomachache, and vomiting. Coriander seed is often combined with laxative herbs such as senna to curb intestinal gripe.

Topically, coriander seed can be used as a compress or poultice to treat cramps, neuralgia, and rheumatism or as an eyewash to treat conjunctivitis. Coriander seed powder helps stop hemorrhoidal bleeding.

There is some speculation that coriander leaf (cilantro) can help rid the body of heavy metals, such as lead; further research is needed to examine this theory, however. The juice of the leaves can be applied topically to soothe rashes, itchiness, and inflammation.

Edible Uses

Coriander seeds are a common spice used in preparing a wide range of dishes, including many from Latin American, Indian, Ethiopian, Arabic, and Thai and other Asian cuisines. They are often roasted to enhance their flavor. The expression *à la Greque* refers to dishes spiced with coriander seed, fennel, sage, and thyme. Gin, chartreuse, and Benedictine all contain coriander, as do some Belgian wheat beers. The seed is also sometimes used as a thickener. The leaves of the plant, known as cilantro, are also a common flavoring. They are used as a raw garnish in Asian, North African, and Mexican cooking. The root is also edible and may be cooked as a vegetable.

Other Uses

Coriander seed is one of the traditional bitter herbs of Passover. The seeds, mixed with cumin and vinegar, have been used to preserve meat. During World War II, coriander seeds were coated with sugar and marketed as sugar drops; they were thrown from carnival wagons, but this became considered wasteful, so little balls of paper were substituted, hence the coining of the word *confetti,* Italian for "sweetmeat." Coriander essential oil is used to flavor tooth-

paste and scent perfumes and soaps. Coriander (the seed and the leaf) can also be made into a breath-freshening mouthwash. The herb is also included in deodorants to deter body odor.

Constituents

Flavonoids, essential oils (borneol, coriandrol, linalool, terpinene, camphor, pinene), tannin, coumarin

Energetic Correspondences

- Flavor: pungent
- Temperature: hot
- Moisture: dry
- Polarity: yang
- Planet: Mars/Venus/Saturn/Moon
- Element: fire

Contraindications

Excessive use of coriander can have a narcotic effect. There have been rare reports of allergic reactions to coriander.

Range and Appearance

Coriander is an annual or biennial, native to the Mediterranean region and Asia, that grows in the wild in disturbed areas but is often cultivated in the home garden. The plant reaches a height of 3 feet. The leaves are pinnate; the lower leaves are ovate with scalloped edges, and they become more finely divided as they progress up the stem. The flowers are white or pink and grow in umbels; the tiny seeds are globular in shape.

CORNSILK

Botanical Name

Zea mays (formerly *Stigmata maidis*)

Family

Poaceae (Grass Family)

Etymology

The genus name, *Zea,* is Latin for "cause of life." The species name, *mays,* derives from *mahiz,* "mother," the name given the plant by the Taino people of the northern Antilles. The common name *corn* derives from the Old English *kurnam,* "small seed."

Also Known As

English: Indian corn, jugnog, maize, sea mays, turkey corn
French: blé de Turquie, fromment des Indes, gaude, maís,
German: indianisches korn, kukurutz, mais
Italian: granoturco, mais
Japanese: gyokumaishu
Korean: okmisu
Mandarin: yù mi xù
Russian: kukuruza, maize
Sanskrit: yavanala
Spanish: barba de elote, barba de maíz, cabelo de elote, estilos de maíz
Turkish: misir bugdayi

Parts Used

Stigma (from female flower), style (collected when plant sheds pollen)

Physiological Effects

Alterative, anodyne, anti-inflammatory, antiseptic, cholagogue, demulcent, diuretic, galactagogue, lithotriptic, stimulant (mild), tonic, vulnerary

Medicinal Uses

Corn silk, or the silky styles found on an ear of corn, has a soothing effect upon the urinary tract and helps restore tissue tone. It clears heat and excess uric acid and dries dampness. It is used for a wide range of genitourinary complaints but is often combined with herbs that have more antiseptic qualities. Even though it is diuretic, it can also be used to treat too-frequent urination due to bladder irritation. Research from China indicates that cornsilk can lower blood pressure in cases of hypertension and reduce blood clotting time. Corn-silk tea is used to treat bedwetting, benign prostatic hypertrophy, bladder inflammation, bladder stones, cystitis, dropsy, edema, gallstones, gonorrhea, gout, hypertension, incontinence, jaundice, kidney stones, prostatitis, rheumatism, urethritis, and urinary infection.

Corn-silk tea can be used to make a soothing enema. Powdered corn silk can be applied topically to heal wounds.

Edible Uses

Corn silk is not generally considered edible, aside from as tea. The grain of corn, however, was such an important food to the early Native Americans that ceremonies were held to honor the Corn Mother as a deity. Some tribes referred to corn as "giver of life." Today corn is still a popular grain; it is eaten on its own and is used to make corn oil, cornmeal, polenta, popcorn, corn syrup, and a multitude of other food products.

Other Uses

Corn silk can be added to smoking mixtures for its mildly sweet flavor.

Constituents

Ascorbic acid, panothenic acid, vitamin K, flavonoids (anthocyanins), calcium, potassium, silica, malic acid, maizenic acid, alkaloid (hordenine), cryptoxanthin, mucilage, saponins, sterols (sitosterol, stigmasterol), allantoin, resin, tannin

Energetic Correspondences

- Flavor: sweet
- Temperature: cool
- Moisture: moist
- Polarity: yin
- Planet: Sun/Mercury/Venus/Saturn/Pluto
- Element: earth

Contraindications

Generally considered very safe.

Range and Appearance

Corn is an annual cereal grass native to South and Central America. Its tall stalks, bearing large ears of grains protected by husks and corn silk, are easily recognized by most people.

CORYDALIS

Botanical Name

Corydalis ambigua, C. aurea, C. bulbosa, C. cava, C. formosa, C. turtschaninovii, C. yanhusuo (syn. *C. solida*)

Family

Papaveraceae (Poppy Family)

Etymology

The genus and common name, *Corydalis,* derive from the Greek *korudallis,* "crested lark," in reference to the birdlike shape of the flowers.

Also Known As

Cantonese: yin wu, yin wu sok, yun wu
English: dicentra, Dutchman's breeches, golden smoke, squirrel corn, turkey corn
French: corydale
German: lerchensporn
Japanese: engosaku
Korean: yônhosaek
Mandarin: xuan hu, yan hu, yán hú sûo

Part Used

Rhizome

Physiological Effects

Alterative, analgesic, anesthetic, antispasmodic, bitter, deobstruent, diuretic, emmenagogue, hemostatic, hypnotic, muscle relaxant, sedative, tonic

Medicinal Uses

Corydalis relaxes stagnant chi, promotes circulation to all parts of the body, slows the breakdown of choline, and helps relieve pain by binding with opium receptors in the body. Although corydalis has only one one-hundredth the strength of morphine, it is an effective, nonaddictive pain reliever. Its tetrahydropalmatine alkaloid seems to block the nervous system's dopamine receptors. Corydalis is used to treat aches and pains, anxiety, arthritic pain, ataxia, bruises, dysmenorrhea, hernia pain, lumbago, migraine, nervous hysteria, palsy, Parkinson's disease, rheumatism pain, pain from traumatic injury, tics, tremors, and twitching.

Topically, corydalis can be used as a poultice or compress to relieve pain, including toothache.

Edible Uses

Not generally considered edible, aside from as tea.

Other Uses

None known

Constituents

Alkaloids (bulbocapnine, corydaline, leonticine, protopine, tetrahydropalmatine)

Energetic Correspondences

- Flavor: pungent, bitter
- Temperature: warm
- Moisture: dry
- Polarity: yang
- Planet: Mars/Neptune/Moon
- Element: air

Contraindications

Use corydalis only as needed, and do not take more than is needed. Large amounts can be toxic. Avoid during pregnancy. Overdose can cause twitching and tics, rather than remedy them. Do not combine with other remedies that affect the central nervous system or with alcohol. Avoid using *Corydalis* species that are not regarded as medicinal, as they can have dangerous effects.

Range and Appearance

Corydalis, a perennial native to Siberia, Japan, and northern China, grows in hedges and open woods, reaching a height of about 12 inches. The dissected leaves are soft and bluish green. The plant bears racemes of pealike pale magenta, pink, purple, yellow, or white flowers.

COUCH GRASS

Botanical Name

Elytrigia repens (syn. *Agropyron repens;* formerly *Triticum repens*)

Family

Poaceae (Grass Family)

Etymology

The genus name, *Elytrigia,* derives from the Greek *elymos,* "millet," another grass in the same family. The species name, *repens,* is Latin for "creeping." The plant is sometimes called dog grass because dogs (and also cats) will eat it as an emetic when they are sick.

Also Known As

English: dog grass, quack grass, quickens, quick grass, quitch grass, triticum, twitchgrass, wheatgrass, witch grass

French: chiendent commun, chiendent rampant, pied de poule

German: echte quecke, gemeine quecke, grasquecken, kriechende quecke, quickengrass, rebel, rechgrass, schiliessgrass

Italian: caprinella, dente caprino, gramigna, granaccino

Russian: pirey polzutchy

Parts Used

Rhizome, root

Physiological Effects

Antiseptic, aperient, demulcent, diuretic, tonic

Medicinal Uses

Couch grass's high mucilage content makes it soothing to mucous membranes. It helps the body excrete excess sodium, reduces inflammation, and clears heat. The Cherokee peoples have used it to treat bedwetting, incontinence, and urinary stones. The plant can also be used to treat bladder stones, bronchitis, cough, cystitis, dysuria, eczema, enlarged prostate, fever, gallstones, gout, high cholesterol, irritable bladder, jaundice, kidney stones, laryngitis, lumbago, lymphatic congestion, nephritis, prostatitis, rheumatism, urethritis, and venereal disease.

Topically, a decoction of couch grass can be used as a soothing wash for inflamed legs.

Edible Uses

The roots can be ground into a flour or chewed whole as a sweet. They also can be roasted and used as a coffee substitute.

Other Uses

The rhizomes are sometimes used as cattle fodder. Couch grass contains a rubberlike compound that has been used to cover golf balls.

Constituents

Beta-carotene, vitamin B, vitamin C, iron, silica, potassium, zinc, triticin, glucose, levulose, mannitol, inositol, inulin, mucilage, essential oil, vanillin

Energetic Correspondences

- Flavor: sweet
- Temperature: cool
- Moisture: moist
- Polarity: yin
- Planet: Jupiter/Venus
- Element: water

Contraindications

Generally regarded as safe.

Range and Appearance

Couch grass is a perennial grass native to Europe and North America. It grows to a height of 2 to 4 feet and produces spikes of green flowers that are 3 to 4 inches long. The leaves are drooping, flat, and rough and clasp the stem. It is found in cultivated areas and along roadsides with rich soil. Though it is considered an invasive weed, couch grass has its uses: it helps prevent soil erosion and is drought resistant.

CUBEB

Botanical Name

Piper cubeba

Family

Piperaceae (Pepper Family)

Etymology

The genus name, *Piper*, derives from the Greek *peperi*, "pepper." The species name, *cubeba*, and the common name *cubeb* derive from the Indonesian *cabe*, "pepper."

Also Known As

Arabic: kabaaba
Bulgarian: kubebe
Cantonese: dou sai geun
Czech: cubéba
English: Java pepper, tailed pepper
French: cubèbe
German: kubebe, kubenpfeffer
Hindi: kabab-chini
Hungarian: jávai bors
Indonesian: tjabé djawa
Italian: cubebe
Japanese: kubeba
Korean: chaba huchu
Mandarin: bi cheng qie
Polish: kubeba
Portuguese: cubeba
Russian: dikij perets, kubeba
Sanskrit: kankola
Thai: prik hang
Turkish: hint biberi tohumu
Vietnamese: tiêu thâ't
Yiddish: kebebe

Part Used

Fruit (unripe)

Physiological Effects

Analgesic, antiemetic, antiseptic, aphrodisiac, carminative, expectorant, digestive, diuretic, stimulant, stomachic, yang tonic

Medicinal Uses

In traditional Asian medicine, cubeb is said to warm the middle burner and help rebellious chi to descend. It also loosens phlegm and improves energy circulation. It is used to treat belching, bronchitis, catarrh, cystitis, dysentery, flatulence, gonorrhea, hemorrhoids, hernia, hiccups, nausea, obesity, prostatits, rheumatoid arthritis, spermatorrhea, urethritis, urinary tract infection, and vomiting.

Cubeb berries are often included in toothpastes and mouthwashes for their ability to curb dental diseases.

Cubeb is sometimes smoked as an aphrodisiac or to relieve symptoms of asthma and bronchitis. Edgar Rice Burroughs enjoyed smoking cubeb cigarettes and often joked that if it had not been for this diversion, Tarzan may never have been brought to life.

Edible Uses

Cubeb is a close relative of black pepper and began being imported into Europe in the thirteenth century; it soon became a common culinary herb there. A king of Portugal later forbade it in trade in order to promote the sale of black pepper.

Cubeb is used to flavor many dishes in Asian, Indonesian, and North African cookery. It is used much like pepper or allspice. It is a component of ras el hanout, a popular Moroccan spice mixture, and is one of the flavoring agents used in Bombay Sapphire gin and Pertsovaka gin.

Other Uses

The essential oil is used in massage oil, anti-aging cosmetics, throat lozenges, and perfumes. In magical traditions, cubeb berries are thought to attract love.

Constituents

Cubebic acid, bitter principle (cubebin), fatty acids (lauric, oleic, capric), essential oils (citral, cineole, citronellal, furfurol, methylpeptenone), sesquiterpenes, piperidine

Energetic Correspondences

- Flavor: pungent
- Temperature: warm

- Moisture: dry
- Polarity: yang
- Planet: Mercury/Mars
- Element: fire

Contraindications

Avoid in cases of inflammation of the digestive tract or nephritis.

Range and Appearance

Cubeb is a perennial climbing vine that is native to Indonesia, and mainly Java. It can grow to 20 feet in length. The leaves are oval to oblong, and the white dioecious flowers grow in spikes. The reddish brown fruits grow in clusters; they resemble black peppers with stalks attached. Cubeb is often grown on coffee plantations to provide shade for the coffee plants.

CUMIN

Botanical Name

Cuminum cyminum

Family

Apiaceae (Parsley Family)

Etymology

The genus name, *Cuminum,* and common name *cumin* derive from the Greek name for the plant, *kyminon,* which in turn derives from previous Arabic and Semitic names, perhaps going all the way back to ancient Sumeria, where the spice was known as *gamun.*

Also Known As

Arabic: qimnoni, qimron
Cantonese: siu wuih heung
Czech: rímsky' kmín
Danish: spidskommen
Dutch: komjin
Esperanto: kumino
Estonian: vürtsköömen
Finnish: juustokumina
German: kümmel
Greek: kimino

Hebrew: kamon
Hindi: jeera
Icelandic: kummin
Indonesian: jinten
Italian: cumino
Japanese: umazeri
Korean: keomin
Mandarin: kuming, xiao hui xiang
Norwegian: spisskummen
Polish: kmin rzymski
Portuguese: cominho
Romanian: chimion amar
Russian: kmin
Sanskrit: jiraka
Spanish: comino
Swahili: jamda, jira
Swedish: spiskummin
Thai: thian-khao
Turkish: kimyon
Vietnamese: thì là ai câp
Yiddish: kminik

Part Used

Seed

Physiological Effects

Antioxidant, antiseptic, antispasmodic, aphrodisiac, carminative, galactagogue, stimulant

Medicinal Uses

Cumin was an important medicine in ancient Egypt. The seeds calm digestive distress and increase peripheral circulation. They are used in the treatment of bloating, colic, coughs, diarrhea, digestive distress, flatulence, headache, indigestion, morning sickness, and nausea.

Topically, cumin seed can be applied as a poultice to reduce swelling in the breasts or testicles or as a liniment to speed the healing of bruises and sprains. The essential oil of the seeds is sometimes included in massage oils to get rid of cellulite.

Edible Uses

Cumin has long been a popular culinary spice. Early Romans used ground cumin much like we use black pepper today. Today it is a popular seasoning in

North African, Latin, Chinese, Vietnamese, Arabic, Indian, and Cajun cuisine.

Other Uses

Cumin is mentioned in the Bible as a currency with which to tithe priests. In ancient Egypt it was used in the mummification process. In magical traditions it is burned as incense to attract love and encourage fidelity.

Constituents

Beta-carotene, calcium, iron, manganese, fats, carbohydrates, essential oils (aldehydes, phellandrene, pinene, thymol), flavonoids

Energetic Correspondences

- Flavor: slightly bitter
- Temperature: warm
- Moisture: neutral
- Polarity: yang
- Planet: Mars
- Element: fire

Contraindications

Generally regarded as safe.

Range and Appearance

Cumin, native to Eurasia and northern Africa, is believed to have been one of the first herbs to be cultivated. This annual grows to about 6 to 12 inches in height. The leaves can be pinnate or bipinnate. The flowers are white, pink, or purple and grow in small compound umbels. The plant thrives with full sun, rich soil, and moderate water.

DAMIANA

Botanical Name

Turnera aphrodisiaca, T. diffusa (syn. *T. microphylla*)

Family

Turneraceae (Turnera Family)

Etymology

The genus name, *Turnera,* was given in honor of Giorgio della Turra, an Italian botanist (1607–1688).

Also Known As

English: turnera
French: thé bourrique
German: grossblä
Spanish: aguita de damiana, pasrorcita, yerba del pastor

Part Used

Aboveground plant

Physiological Effects

Antidepressant, alterative, anti-inflammatory, aperient, aphrodisiac, astringent, carminative, cholagogue, diuretic, emmenagogue, hormone regulator, laxative (mild), nervine, stimulant, stomachic, urinary antiseptic, yang tonic

Medicinal Uses

Damiana nourishes yang, invigorates the brain and nerves, regulates the pituitary gland, and promotes physical endurance. The bitter principle, damianin, stimulates the nervous system and genitals and allows nerve messages to more readily spread through the body. Damiana was used by the Mayans and Aztecs as a sexual stimulant and to treat respiratory disorders. It was listed in the U.S. National Formulary from 1888 to 1947. Today, damiana is used to treat anxiety, asthma, bedwetting, catarrh, constipation, coughs, debility, depression, dysentery, dyspepsia, emphysema, erectile dysfunction, exhaustion, hangover, headache, hot flashes, infertility, low libido, Lou Gehrig's disease, malaria, menstrual cramps, Parkinson's disease, prostatitis, urinary tract infection, venereal disease, and vertigo. It has been used as a tea to help teenagers overcome the shyness and self-consciousness that sometimes accompanies puberty, and it can also be used to help adults overcome sexual "performance anxiety."

As a flower essence, damiana diminishes feelings of inadequacy and restores feelings of sensuality and energy.

Edible Uses

Damiana is not generally considered edible, aside from as tea. It is sometimes prepared as a therapeutic liqueur and added to margaritas.

Other Uses

Damiana's aphrodisiac properties are well known. Livestock breeders of the 1930s were known to use the herb to encourage animals to breed. Couples sometimes smoke the herb in a waterpipe as a prelude to lovemaking and to induce visions. Damiana is also sometimes burned as an incense to inspire visions.

Constituents

Vitamin C, phosphorous, selenium, silicon, sulfur, flavonoids, essential oils (cineol, cymol, pinene, thymol), glycosides (gonzalitosin), damianin, beta-sitosterol, arbutin, tannin

Energetic Correspondences

- Flavor: bitter, pungent
- Temperature: warm
- Moisture: dry
- Polarity: yang
- Planet: Mars/Pluto
- Element: fire/water

Contraindications

Damiana is generally considered safe, but avoid using it in cases of urinary tract disease or during pregnancy. Long-term use may interfere with the body's assimilation of iron. Large doses may be somewhat laxative.

Range and Appearance

Damiana is a small deciduous shrub native to the American Southwest, Mexico, and the West Indies. The leaves are smooth and pale green on top and ovolanceolate in shape, with three to six teeth and a few hairs on the ribs. The small, yellow, aromatic flowers each have five petals, are hermaphroditic, are borne singularly, and rise from the leaf axils.

DANDELION

Botanical Name

Taraxacum officinale

Family

Asteraceae (Daisy Family)

Etymology

Opinions differ on the origin of dandelion's genus name, *Taraxacum*. Some believe that it derives from the Persian *talkh chakok,* "bitter herb." Others propose that it derives from the Greek *taraxos,* "disorder," and *akos,* "remedy." Still others believe it could be derived from the Greek *taraxia,* "eye disorder," and *akeomai,* "to cure," as the plant was traditionally used as a remedy for eyes.

The common name *dandelion* derives from the French *dent de lion,* "tooth of the lion," in reference to the jagged shape of the leaves.

Also Known As

English: amarga, bitterwort, blowball, cankerwort, chicoria, clockflower, consuelda, devil's milkpail, doonhead clock, fairy clock, fortune-teller, heart-fever grass, Irish daisy, lion's tooth, milk gowan, milk witch, monk's head, peasant's cloak, puffball, priest's crown, sun-in-the-grass, swine's snout, tell time, tramp with the golden head, piddly bed, yellow gowan, wet-a-bed, wild endive

French: dent-de-lion

German: kihblume, löwenzahn

Greek: radiki

Hindi: dudhal

Italian: diente di lieone, tarasso

Japanese: hokoei

Korean: p'ogongyông

Mandarin: pú gong ying

Persian: trakhasnkun

Russian: oduvanchik, pushki

Sanskrit: dughdapheni

Spanish: chiccoria, diente de leon

Turkish: kara hindiba ootu, yabani

Welsh: dant y llew

Parts Used

All (leaf, flower, root, sap)

Physiological Effects

Leaf: alterative, anodyne, antacid, antioxidant, aperient, astringent, bitter, decongestant, depurative, digestive, diuretic, febrifuge, galactagogue, hypotensive, immune stimulant, laxative, lithotriptic, nutritive, restorative, stomachic, tonic, vulnerary

Root: alterative, anodyne, antibacterial, antifungal, anti-inflammatory, antirheumatic, aperient, astringent, bitter, cholagogue, choleretic, decongestant, deobstruent, depurative, digestive, discutient, diuretic, galactagogue, hepatic, hypnotic, immune stimulant, laxative, lithotriptic, nutritive, purgative, sedative, stomachic, tonic

Flower: anodyne, cardiotonic, emollient, hepatic, vulnerary

Sap: anodyne, antifungal, discutient

Medicinal Uses

Dandelion is one of the planet's most famous and useful weeds. This wonderful plant is a blood purifier that aids in the process of filtering and straining wastes from the bloodstream. It cools heat and clears infection from the body. It is especially useful in treating obstructions of the gallbladder, liver, pancreas, and spleen. Dandelion is also used to help clear the body of old emotions such as anger and fear that can be stored in the liver and kidneys. Women who are pregnant will find it useful in preventing edema and hypertension.

The leaf aids in the elimination of uric acid and is used primarily for liver, kidney, and bladder concerns. It can be used to treat amenorrhea, anemia, anorexia, appetite loss, arthritis, bedwetting, breast cancer, breast tenderness, bronchitis, candida, colitis, congestive heart failure, cysts, debility, diabetes, dropsy, dyspepsia, edema, endometriosis, fatigue, flatulence, gallstones, hangover, high cholesterol, hypertension, hypochondria, insomnia, kidney stones, mastitis, mononucleosis, muscular rheumatism, nervousness, obesity, poison oak and ivy, prostatitis, rashes, rheumatism, scrofula, scurvy, sinusitis, spleen enlargement, stomachache, tonsillitis, ulcers, urinary tract infection, and uterine fibroids.

The root is used primarily for problems related to the liver, spleen, stomach, and kidneys. It is used to treat abscess, acne, age spots, alcoholism, allergies, anorexia, appetite loss, arthritis, boils, breast cancer, breast tenderness, bronchitis, candida, chickenpox, cirrhosis, colitis, congestive heart failure, constipation, cysts, depression, diabetes, dizziness, dyspepsia, eczema, endometriosis, fatigue, flatulence, gallstones, gout, hangover, hayfever, headache, heartburn, hemorrhoids, hepatitis, herpes, high cholesterol, hypertension, hypochondria, hypoglycemia, jaundice, kidney stones, mastitis, measles, mononucleosis, morning sickness, mumps, obesity, osteoarthritis, ovarian cysts, poison oak and ivy, premenstrual syndrome, prostatitis, psoriasis, rashes, rheumatism, sinusitis, spleen enlargement, tonsillitis, tuberculosis, tumors, ulcers, uterine fibroids, varicose veins, and venereal warts.

Dandelion flowers are used to treat backache, depression, headache, menstrual cramps, and night blindness.

Topically, the flowers can be used as a healing poultice for wounds. The sap from the fresh stem can be applied to warts to get rid of them. The leaf can be made into a wash to treat fungal infections.

As a flower essence dandelion reduces tension, especially muscular tension in the neck, back, and shoulders. It fosters spiritual openness and encourages the letting go of fear and trust in one's own ability to cope with life. It is beneficial for those who love life but overextend themselves.

Edible Uses

Dandelion is considered one of the five most nutritious vegetables on Earth. The young leaves, gathered before the flower stalk achieves full height and the flowers have not yet formed, may be eaten raw, used as a potherb, or juiced. The young flowers, with the green sepals removed, have a sweet, honeylike flavor and can be eaten raw. The root can be cleaned and prepared like carrots or pickled. The roots are sometimes roasted and used as a coffee substitute. Dandelion wine and beer are most enjoyable.

Other Uses

Dandelion is one of the bitter herbs of the Passover tradition. It is an excellent herb for weight loss as the leaves are diuretic and the root improves fat metabolism.

Constituents

Leaf: beta-carotene, vitamins B_1 and B_2, choline, inositol, folic acid, vitamin C, calcium, iron, manganese, phosphorous, potassium, taraxacin, bitter glycosides, terpenoids
Root: calcium, iron, phosphorous, zinc, choline, flavonoids (lutein, luteolin flavoxanthin, violaxanthin), pectin, inulin, taraxacin, taraxacerin, triterpenes (taraxol, taraxerol, taraxasterol, amyrin), coumestrol, levulin, mucilage, tannin, essential oil, asparagin, lactupicrine, phenolic acids (quinic acid, chlorogenic acid), caffeic acid, gallic acid, fatty acids (myristic, palmitic, stearic, lauric)
Flower: flavonoids (luteolin)
Sap: sesquiterpene lactone (taraxinic acid)

Energetic Correspondences

- Flavor: bitter, sweet, slightly salty
- Temperature: cold
- Moisture: moist
- Polarity: yang
- Planet: Sun/Mercury/Jupiter/Mars
- Element: air

Contraindications

Dandelion is generally regarded as safe, even in large amounts and even during pregnancy. However, as is the case with any plant, there is always a possibility of an allergic reaction. There have been a very few cases reported of abdominal discomfort, loose stools, nausea, and heartburn associated with dandelion. The fresh latex of the plant can cause contact dermatitis in some sensitive individuals. Consult with a qualified health-care practitioner prior to using dandelion in cases of obstructed bile duct or gallstones. Some individuals that have gastric hyperacidity may find that excessive use of dandelion leaf aggravates the condition.

Range and Appearance

Dandelion is a native of Eurasia but is now naturalized in many regions around the world. Growing from 2 to 18 inches high, the plant has a hollow, unbranching stem with a basal rosette of shiny, hairless, coarsely toothed green leaves that are broader toward the top. The teeth are usually downward directed. A plant bears a single yellow flower, which is actually composed of many tiny bisexual florets. Each floret has five tiny teeth on its edge. Dandelion has one of the longest flowering seasons of any plant, and when a warm spell occurs in an off-season, it is not unusual to see dandelion in flower. Beneath the flower is a green calyx with downward-curving outer bracts. The seeds develop as achenes bearing a feathery pappus; they are dispersed by the wind, often as many as five miles from their origin.

In addition to *Taraxacum officinale*, there are more than one hundred and fifty useful species, including *T. magellanicum, T. erythrosperum* (red-seeded dandelion), *T. autumnalis* (fall dandelion or hawkbit), *T. ceratophorum* (horned dandelion), *T. eriophorum* and *T. scopulorum* (both known as Rocky Mountain dandelion), *T. ceratophyllum* (tundra dandelion), and *T. lyratum* (dwarf alpine dandelion).

DEVIL'S CLAW

Botanical Name

Harpagophytum procumbens

Family

Pedeliaceae (Sesame Family)

Etymology

The genus name, *Harpagophytum,* is Greek for "grapple plant." The species name, *procumbens,* is Latin for "lying down" or "prostrate." The common name *devil's claw* refers to the hooklike seed capsules.

Also Known As

Afrikaans: bobbejaandubbeltjie, duiwelsklou, kloudoring, veldspinnakop
English: grapple plant, wood spider

French: tête de mort
German: teufelskralle, trampelklette
Setswana: kanako, lekgagamare, sengaparile

Parts Used

Secondary tubers

Physiological Effects

Alterative, analgesic, anodyne, antiarthritic, antibacterial, anti-inflammatory, bitter, diuretic, febrifuge, hypotensive, laxative, lithotriptic, liver tonic, sedative, smooth muscle relaxant, stimulant

Medicinal Uses

Devil's claw has been used for over two hundred and fifty years by many cultures in South Africa, including the Bantu and Khoikhoi (Hottentot). The herb stimulates the detoxifying and protective mechanisms of the body, helps potentiate the body's natural antirheumatic agents, aids in the elimination of uric acid, and relaxes the muscles.

Devil's claw is used to treat acne, allergies, arthritis, asthma, bursitis, coughs, diabetes, dyspepsia, fever, gout, hay fever, headache, high cholesterol, indigestion, lumbago, neuralgia, osteoarthritis, pain, and rheumatism. It is considered more effective for the treatment of osteoarthritis than for rheumatoid arthritis.

Topically, devil's claw can be applied as a healing poultice to boils, lesions, and wounds.

As a flower essence, devil's claw is helpful for those who manipulate others with their looks and charm, encouraging them to be responsible for their charisma.

Edible Uses

Not generally considered edible, aside from as tea.

Other Uses

None known

Constituents

Luteolin, procumbine, harpagia, iridoid glycosides (harpagoside, aceteoside, procumbide), phytosterols (beta-sitosterols)

Energetic Correspondences

- Flavor: bitter
- Temperature: cool
- Moisture: dry
- Polarity: yin
- Planet: Saturn
- Element: earth

Contraindications

There are no known harmful side effects from long-term use of devil's claw, though there have been some reports of allergic reactions to the plant. It may take a couple of weeks to notice results. Use devil's claw in combination with demulcent herbs to avoid irritating the digestive tract, and avoid it during pregnancy.

Range and Appearance

Native to the sandy soils of the Kalahari Desert and Nubian steppes of Africa, devil's claw is a prostrate evergreen perennial. Its gray-green leaves are opposite and irregularly divided into several lobes. The trumpet-shaped flowers have reddish orange or red to purple petals with yellow, white, or purple centers. The flowers bloom for only three or four days. The plant bears sharp, hooklike seeds that look like claws and cling to passersby.

DEVIL'S CLUB

Botanical Name

Oplopanax horridus (formerly *Echinopanax horridus*)

Family

Araliaceae (Ginseng Family)

Etymology

Devil's club's former botanical name, *Echinopanax horridus,* translates from the Latin as "prickly porcupine ginseng." The genus name, *Oplopanax,* derives in part from the Greek *panakes,* "panacea." The species name, *horridus,* is Latin for "prickly."

Also Known As

Dakelh: hoolhgulh
English: Alaskan ginseng, Pacific ginseng, prickly porcupine ginseng
Finnish: pirunnuija
French: aralie épineuse, bois piquant
German: teufelskeule
Halkomelem: qwa'pulhp
Japanese: haribuki
Russian: zamanikha
Swedish: djävulsklubba

Parts Used

Root, bark, first foot of stem

Physiological Effects

Adaptogen, alterative, analgesic, antiarthritic, antibacterial, antifungal, antirheumatic, antiviral, aromatic, cathartic, diaphoretic, emetic, expectorant, hypoglycemic, immune stimulant, purgative, rejuvenative, respiratory stimulant, stomachic, tonic

Medicinal Uses

Devil's club helps the body and mind adapt to both physical and emotional stresses. It fights infection, helps make coughs more productive, and helps stabilize blood sugar levels. It was used by Native Americans of northern North America as a preventive and treatment for cancer, and it is still used for that purpose today. It is also used to treat adrenal exhaustion, arthritis, autoimmune diseases, broken bones, bronchitis, colds, constipation, cough, diabetes (adult onset and insulin resistant), exhaustion, fever, gallstones, gonorrhea, hangover, irregular menses after childbirth, measles, osteoarthritis, rheumatism, stress, sugar cravings, swollen glands, tuberculosis, and ulcers. It also can be used to encourage weight loss.

Topically, devil's club can be used as a poultice to treat burns, insect bites and stings, toothache, and wounds. It can be added to the bath to relieve sore muscles or prepared as a tea and poured on the hot rocks of a sweat lodge to relieve rheumatism. The berries can be prepared as a hair rinse or poultice to treat lice and dandruff.

Edible Uses

In very early spring, the very young, tender green stalk may be peeled and eaten as a vegetable, and the leaves can be added to dishes such as omelets, soups, or stir-fries. Once the plant's spines stiffen, it is no longer edible.

Other Uses

Shamans of the Tlingit tribe in Alaska fast and take devil's club as part of their initiation. The herb is traditionally hung over doorways and on fishing boats or worn in a medicine pouch as a protective amulet. It is also sometimes burned as incense or prepared as a bath herb for spiritual purification. The powdered root can be used as a deodorant.

Constituents

Essential oils (busnesol, cadenene, cedrol, dodecenol, nerolidol, torreyol), araliasides, panaxosides

Energetic Correspondences

- Flavor: pungent, bitter
- Temperature: cool
- Moisture: dry
- Polarity: yang
- Planet: Mars/Saturn
- Element: air

Contraindications

Diabetics should consult with a qualified health-care practitioner before using this herb, as it may affect the amount of insulin they need. Large amounts can be intoxicating and potentially, if large enough, toxic.

Range and Appearance

Devil's club, a close relative of Eleuthero, also known as Siberian ginseng (*Eleutherococcus senticosus*), is a highly aromatic shrub that is densely covered in yellowish spines. It can stand up to 9 feet tall. It has large, alternate, palmate, three- to seven-lobed leaves that are shaped somewhat like maple leaves and bear yellowish spines on their veins and petioles. The greenish white flowers grow on long, terminal, oblong clusters. Bright red fruits, each holding two seeds, follow the flowers. Devil's club is found growing in wooded areas and along streams in Canada and the northern United States.

Wear gloves when harvesting devil's club, as the spines can embed in the skin.

DILL

Botanical Name

Anethum graveolens, A. sowa

Family

Apiaceae (Parsley Family)

Etymology

The Latin name *Anethum graveolens* means "heavy scented." The common name *dill* is a corruption of an old Norse word, *dylla,* meaning "to soothe or lull," in reference to the herb's use in soothing colicky babies.

Also Known As

Arabic: shibith
Armenian: samit
Bulgarian: kopur
Cantonese: ngau jau sih loh, sih loh
Croatian: kopar
Czech: kopr
Danish: dild
Dutch: dille
English: aneto, dilly
Esperanto: aneto
Estonian: aedtill
Finnish: ryytitilli, tilli
French: aneth odorant
German: gurkenkraut
Greek: anitho
Hebrew: shamir, shevet rehani
Hindi: anithi, sowa
Hungarian: kapor
Icelandic: sólselja
Indonesian: adas manis
Italian: aneto

Japanese: diru
Korean: inondu, tir
Lithuanian: krapas
Mandarin: shih lo
Polish: koper ogrodowy
Portuguese: aneto, endro
Romanian: mãrar
Russian: ukrop
Sanskrit: mishreya
Serbian: kopar
Spanish: eneldo, hinojo
Swedish: dill
Thai: dil, pak chee lao
Turkish: dereotu
Ukrainian: koper, kpin, krip
Vietnamese: tiêu h'ôi hu'o'ng
Yiddish: koper

Part Used

Seed

Physiological Effects

Antibacterial, antioxidant, antispasmodic, aromatic, calmative, carminative, cholagogue, diaphoretic, digestive, emmenagogue, galactagogue, stimulant, stomachic

Medicinal Uses

Dill increases circulation, moves stagnation, and helps regulate metabolism. It is an excellent children's remedy. It is used to treat colic, diarrhea (in infants), dyspepsia, flatulence, halitosis, heartburn, hiccups, indigestion, insomnia, muscle spasms, and nightmares.

Topically, dill seed can be prepared as a wash to treat head lice or hemorrhoids or as a handbath to nourish weak fingernails.

As a flower essence, dill is helpful for children who have too much expected of them. It can help one to digest and process experiences that seem overwhelming and is useful for those who feel oversensitive to their environments. It also facilitates clear thinking and the release of feelings of victimization. It can be used to encourage situations to "come to a head" so that change may occur.

Edible Uses

Dill seed is a popular spice that is widely used in Russian, Polish, and Scandinavian cuisine. The seeds can also be sprouted and eaten like alfalfa sprouts. The flowers are also edible, as are the leaves; both are rich in vitamin C, calcium, iron, and potassium.

Other Uses

Among early American settlers, dill seeds were referred to as "meetin' seeds" and given to small children to chew to keep them calm during long church sermons and to adults to keep their stomachs from rumbling.

The essential oil is used to scent soaps and perfumes. The seeds can be sewn into a sachet and placed in a bed pillow to help lull a person to sleep. The seeds are sometimes included in mouthwashes as a breath freshener.

In magical traditions, dill seed is a component of love potions, prosperity spells, and sachets placed in cradles to protect children.

Constituents

Essential oils (limonene, phellandrene, carvone), flavonoids, linoleic acid

Energetic Correspondences

- Flavor: pungent, bitter
- Temperature: warm
- Moisture: neutral
- Polarity: yang
- Planet: Sun/Mercury/Moon
- Element: fire/air

Contraindications

Avoid therapeutic doses during pregnancy.

Range and Appearance

Dill is native to southern Asia but is cultivated worldwide. It is an annual or biennial growing from 2 to 5 feet tall, with large, finely dissected, bluish green leaves that clasp the grooved stem. The yellow flowers are borne on umbels.

DIVINING SAGE

Botanical Name

Salvia divinorum, S. pipizintzintli

Family

Lamiaceae (Mint Family)

Etymology

The genus name *Salvia* derives from the Latin *salvus*, "healthy." The species name *divinorum* derives from the Latin *divinare*, "to divine."

Also Known As

English: diviner's mint, diviner's sage, leaves of the shepherdess, magic mint, María pastora, sage of the seers

Mazatec: ska pastora, ska Maria pastora

Spanish: hojas de la pastora, la hembra, la Maria, yierba de Maria

Part Used

Leaf

Physiological Effects

Hallucinogen, psychoactive, refrigerant

Medicinal Uses

Research suggests that divining sage has compounds that lock into the opioid receptors in the brain, thus causing an altered state of consciousness, like opiates. The herb can be used to treat anemia, headache, and rheumatism.

Edible Uses

Though the leaves are eaten, it is more for their psychoactive effects than as a food.

Other Uses

Divining sage was a traditional hallucinogen used by the Indians of Central America before the Spanish conquest. Recall of childhood experiences, futuristic divinations, and short-term visual hallucinations are common side effects.

Constituents

Diterpenoids (salvinorin A and C, divinatorins, salvinicins)

Energetic Correspondences

- Flavor: pungent
- Temperature: cold
- Moisture: neutral
- Polarity: yin
- Planet: Mars/Pluto
- Element: earth

Contraindications

Feelings of coldness are a common side effect. Nausea, vertigo, and muscle uncoordination are rare side effects. Should not be used without supervision.

Range and Appearance

This perennial, native to only a few square miles in southern Mexico, grows to about 3 feet in height. It has a hollow square stem and large green leaves. The seeds are largely sterile and rarely set roots; instead, the plant must be grown from cuttings. It seldom flowers, but when it does, they are white with purple calyces.

DONG QUAI

Botanical Name

Angelica polymorpha, A. sinensis

Family

Apiaceae (Parsley Family)

Etymology

The genus name, *Angelica,* derives from the Greek *angelos,* "messenger," which is also the root of the English word *angel.* The English spelling of the Chinese name appears variously as *dong quai, tang kuei,* and *tang kwei.* The Chinese name translates as "state of return," in reference to the belief that the herb helps blood return to where it belongs, rather than stagnating.

Also Known As

Cantonese: dong gwai
English: female ginseng, honeywort, mountain celery, tang kuei, tang kwei
Japanese: toki
Mandarin: dang gui

Part Used

Root

Physiological Effects

Alterative, analgesic, antibacterial, antifungal, anti-inflammatory, antispasmodic, antitumor, aperient, aphrodisiac, aromatic, blood tonic, chi tonic, circulatory stimulant, digestive, diuretic, emmenagogue, hepatoprotective, hypotensive, immune stimulant, laxative, sedative (mild), postpartum tonic, uterine relaxant, stimulant and tonic, yin tonic

Medicinal Uses

Record of dong quai's use first appeared in the *Shen Nong Ben Cao Jing* (Divine Husbandman's Classic of the Materia Medica), compiled during the Han Dynasty (A.D. 25–220). It is still one of the most frequently used herbs in Asia.

Dong quai helps stabilize blood sugar levels, thereby helping to support feelings of calm. It builds the blood, relaxes the uterus, improves circulation, and disperses congestion in the pelvic region; women who are going off birth control pills can use dong quai to help reestablish regular menstrual cycles. Dong quai also helps nourish dry, thin vaginal tissues and beautifies the skin. Though it is not estrogenic, its effects are similar in that it binds to estrogen receptor sites.

In vitro studies have shown dong quai to have activity against strep, shigella, dysentery, and various fungi. It speeds up wound healing and stimulates the production of white blood cells, including B-lymphocytes and T-lymphocytes. Dong quai may help those with environmental allergies by inhibiting production of allergenic antibodies.

Dong quai is used to treat amenorrhea, anemia, arthritis, blood deficiency, blood stagnation, blurry vision, boils, cancer, candida, chills, chronic bronchitis, cirrhosis, constipation (due to dryness), dry skin, dysmenorrhea, endometriosis, exhaustion, hair loss, headache, hypertension, infertility (female), insomnia, irregular menses, menopause symptoms (hot flashes, vaginal dryness, and heart palpitations), muscle spasms, pain, restless leg syndrome, PMS, restlessness in a fetus, sciatica, stroke, tinnitus, and traumatic injury.

Edible Uses

Dong quai root is edible and is often added to poultry or grain dishes or soups. In fact, in some parts of Asia it is traditional for new mothers to eat dong quai chicken soup for a month following childbirth.

Other Uses

None known

Constituents

Vitamin B$_2$, niacin, folic acid, vitamin B$_{12}$, chromium, iron, magnesium, phosphorous, potassium, flavonoids, coumarins, polysaccharides, essential oils (carvacrol, safrole, isosafrole), butylidene phthalide, n-valerophenone-o-carboxylic acid, beta-sitosterol, angelic acid, angelicone

Energetic Correspondences

- Flavor: sweet, pungent, bitter (but extremely bitter roots are of poor quality)
- Temperature: warm
- Moisture: moist
- Polarity: yin
- Planet: Venus/Mars/Jupiter/Moon
- Element: water

Contraindications

Avoid dong quai during pregnancy, except under the supervision of a qualified health-care practitioner. Avoid in cases of diarrhea, poor digestion, abdominal distention, heavy menstrual flow, or high fever with a strong fast pulse, or when using blood-thinning medications. Use of dong quai can increase photosensitivity.

Range and Appearance

Dong quai is a 2- to 3-foot-tall perennial native to the mountain forests of China. Its root consists of a whitish or yellowish gray main section with longer branches, both of which are used medicinally. The stem is purplish, glabrous, and slightly striated. The inferior and often the superior leaves are pinnate. The fragrant, five-petaled, white flowers grow in umbels of twelve to thirty-six blossoms.

A plant must be two to three years old before the root is considered mature enough to harvest.

ECHINACEA

Botanical Name

Echinacea angustifolia, E. pallida, E. purpurea

Family

Asteraceae (Daisy Family)

Etymology

The genus name and common name, *Echinacea*, derives from the Greek *echinops*, "hedgehog," in reference to the stiff, bristly flower head. The species names derive from Latin, with *angustifolia* meaning "narrow leaved," *pallida* meaning "pale" (in reference to the color of the flowers), and *purpurea* meaning "purple" (in reference to the color of the flowers).

Also Known As

Danish: smalbladet, solhat
Dutch: kogelbloem
English: black Sampson (*E. angustifolia*), coneflower, rudbeckia, snakeroot
French: rudbeckie à feuilles étroites
German: igelkopf, kegelblume, kupferblume, stachelkopf
Icelandic: sólhattur
Norwegian: smalbladet, solhatt
Polish: jezowka
Spanish: equinácea
Swedish: liten läkerudbeckia

Parts Used

Root, rhizome, leaf, flower, seed

Physiological Effects

Alterative, anodyne, antibacterial, anticatarrhal, antifungal, anti-inflammatory (mild), antioxidant, antiseptic, antitumor, antiviral, astringent, carminative, depurative, diaphoretic, digestive, febrifuge, immune stimulant, sialogogue, stimulant, vulnerary

Medicinal Uses

Echinacea is an excellent anti-infection agent. It is most effective when taken at the onset of symptoms. The herb stimulates the formation of leukocytes and enhances phagocytosis. It inhibits the enzyme hyaluronidase, which aids the infection process by thinning cellular matrix, thereby making cells more permeable to infection. Echinacea also stimulates wound healing and has cortisone-like activity. One of its constituents, echinacin, exhibits interferon-like activity. Another constituent, properdin, helps neutralize bacterial and viral blood toxins and increases the total number of immune cells developing in the bone marrow. Echinacea also exhibits some antitumor activity.

In addition to its ability to ward off or mitigate illness, echinacea is used in the treatment of abcess, acne, allergy, blood poisoning, boils, bronchitis, cancer, candida, chicken pox, chronic fatigue, colds, diphtheria, ear infection, eczema, fever, flu, gangrene, herpes, laryngitis, Lyme disease, lymphatic congestion, mastitis, measles, mumps, pneumonia, prostatitis, scarlet fever, sinusitis, smallpox, snakebite, sore throat, tonsillitis, tuberculosis, typhoid, and urinary tract infection. It also can lessen the side effects of vaccinations.

Applied topically, echinacea stimulates the reticulo-epithelial layers of skin, increases the formation of antibodies, and speeds tissue repair. It is excellent in salves, compresses, and washes to treat cuts, boils, burns, carbuncles, gangrenous tissue, hives, infected wounds, sties, tendonitis, and venomous bites such as those from scorpions and spiders. It can be used in mouthwashes to treat canker sores, gingivitis, or pyorrhea.

Edible Uses

The leaves are the only plant part considered edible, but they are rarely used as a food, as they are prickly and bitter. Echinacea has an aromatic, earthy flavor when prepared as a tea.

Other Uses

Echinacea was used in Native American sweat lodges to help the participants endure extreme temperature; its effectiveness could perhaps be attributed to its cooling properties.

Constituents

Beta-carotene, vitamin C, vitamin E, calcium, chromium, polysaccharides (inulin), glycosaminoglycans, echinacoside, echinaceine, isobutylmines, caffeic acid, chicoric acid, linoleic acid, palmetic acid, essential oils, glycosides, inulin, polyacetylenes, sesquiterpenes, betaine, tannin

Energetic Correspondences

- Flavor: pungent, bitter
- Temperature: cool
- Moisture: dry
- Polarity: yin
- Planet: Jupiter/Mars/Saturn
- Element: air

Contraindications

Excessive use of echinacea can cause throat irritation, nausea, dizziness, and excessive salivation. Rare cases of allergic reactions have been reported. Those with a compromised immune system, such as might result from lupus, should use echinacea only under the advice of a qualified health-care professional. Echinacea can be taken frequently (every couple of hours) during acute infection, but this sort of dosing should be undertaken only for a few days. Herbalists disagree about the effectiveness of the herb's long-term use; many recommend taking it for cycles of ten days to three weeks, with breaks in between, while others recommend it for continuous long-term use.

Although echinacea can often be used in place of antibiotics, it does not strongly affect the genito-urinary system, so don't rely on it to treat infections for that part of the body.

Echinacea commonly produces a slightly tingly sensation on the tongue, which is a harmless reaction.

Range and Appearance

This perennial herb, native to the prairies of North America, usually attains a height of about 3 feet. The stiff, hairy flower is a cone-shaped disc surrounded by spreading rays from white to pale to deep purple. *E. angustifolia* has narrow, lance-shaped leaves. *E. pallida* can grow up to 4 feet tall, and its flower has strongly drooping rays. *E. purpurea* has oval leaves that are coarsely toothed, and the inner bristly disc of its flower is more orange than that of other species.

Echinacea prefers full sun, has low water requirements, and will grow in a wide variety of soil conditions.

Overharvesting from the wild, especially of *E. angustifolia,* is leading to endangerment of this genus. When you purchase this herb, please make sure it has been organically cultivated rather than wildcrafted.

ECLIPTA

Botanical Name

Eclipta alba (syn. *E. prostrata, Verbesina alba, Verbesina prostrata*)

Family

Asteraceae (Daisy Family)

Etymology

The genus name and common name, *Eclipta,* derive from the Greek *ekleipo,* "deficient," referring to the plant lacking a pappus. The species name, *alba,* is Latin for "white."

Also Known As

Arabic: kadim-el-bint
Cantonese: lien-tzo ts'ao ("lotus herb"),
　shui han-lien
English: bhringaraj, false daisy, swamp daisy
French: éclipta blanche
Hindi: babri, bhangra
Mandarin: hàn lían cao
Japanese: kanrenso
Korean: hannyônch'o
Sanskrit: bringaraj, kesharaja
Spanish: hierba de tajo
Zulu: ungcolozi

Parts Used

Entire plant

Physiological Effects

Alterative, anodyne, antibacterial, anti-inflammatory, antiviral, astringent, carminative, cholagogue, demulcent, deobstruent, depurative, febrifuge, hemostatic, hepatic, hypotensive, laxative, nervine, purgative, refrigerant, rejuvenative, styptic, vulnerary, yin tonic

Medicinal Uses

Eclipta is widely used in Asian medicine; *E. alba* is more common in Ayurvedic medicine and *E. prostrata* in Chinese treatments. Eclipta tonifies and nourishes liver and kidney yin, cools the blood, stops bleeding, and promotes beautiful skin. It is used to treat abscess, alopecia, anemia, balding, blurred vision, boils, cirrhosis, diphtheria, dizziness, dysentery, hepatitis, insomnia, jaundice, liver enlargement, loose teeth, nosebleed, premature gray hair, restlessness, spleen enlargement, stress, tinnitus, and tuberculosis.

Topically, eclipta can be prepared as an oil and applied to the scalp to curb hair loss, to reduce graying, and to promote luster. The oil also can be rubbed on the forehead to relieve headaches. Eclipta can be prepared as a compress to reduce inflammation, including from hemorrhoids, or as a salve, liniment, or poultice to remedy dermatitis, eczema, and wounds. The leaves can be prepared as a poultice to treat scorpion sting and snakebite. In Nepal, the juice from the leaf is diluted in sesame oil and used as drops in the ears, nose, and eyes to treat sinusitis, migraines, and eye, ear, and nose inflammation.

Edible Uses

Eclipta can be eaten as a potherb or vegetable.

Other Uses

A black dye obtained from the plant is used to color hair and as a tattooing agent.

Constituents

Saponins, lactones, nicotine, tannin, beta-carotene, ecliptine

Energetic Correspondences

- Flavor: bitter, sweet, sour
- Temperature: cool
- Moisture: moist
- Polarity: yin
- Planet: Mercury
- Element: air

Contraindications

Avoid eclipta in cases of severe chills, diarrhea, or poor digestion.

Range and Appearance

There are three varieties of eclipta, all growing throughout the Himalayan foothills and wet areas of India: a white-flowering variety, a yellow-flowering variety, and a black-fruiting variety. Eclipta is an annual herb with a soft stem and numerous branches. The leaves are opposite and covered on both sides with fuzzy hairs. When bruised the stems ooze a milky white fluid that soon turns black.

ELDER

Botanical Name

Sambucus canadensis, S. nigra

Family

Caprifoliaceae (Honeysuckle Family)

Etymology

The genus name, *Sambucus*, is from the Greek *sackbut*, the name of a musical instrument made of elder. The species name *nigra* refers to the black berries of this species, and *canadensis* means "originating in Canada." The common name *elder* comes from the Anglo-Saxon *aeld*, "fire," in reference to the young hollow stems of this shrub having been used to blow into a fire to get it burning.

Also Known As

Czech: bozinka
Danish: hyld
Dutch: vlier
English: blood elder, bour tree, danewort, ellanwood, ellhorn, fever tree, hylder, pan pipes, pipe tree, sambu, tree of medicine, tree of music, Viking elder, walewort
French: sureau noir
German: flieder, holunder, schwiztee
Hungarian: bodzafa
Italian: sambreo, sambuco nero
Mandarin: chieh-ku mu
Norwegian: hyll
Polish: bez czarny
Portuguese: sabuguiero
Russian: busine
Spanish: sauco
Swedish: fläder
Welsh: eirin ysgaw

Parts Used

Flower, berry

Physiological Effects

Flower: alterative, anticatarrhal, anti-inflammatory, antirheumatic, antiseptic, antispasmodic, antitumor, astringent, carminative, decongestant, depurative, diaphoretic, digestive, discutient, diuretic, emollient, expectorant, febrifuge, galactagogue, laxative, nervine, purgative, rejuvenative, restorative, stimulant (gentle), tonic, vasodilator, vulnerary
Berry: alterative, anticatarrhal, anti-inflammatory, antirheumatic, antiseptic, antispasmodic, antiviral, decongestant, depurative, diaphoretic, digestive, discutient, diuretic, expectorant, laxative, nervine, rejuvenative, restorative, tonic

Medicinal Uses

Elder flower and berry encourage the body to release toxins through their diaphoretic and diuretic action.

They also dry dampness, relieve congestion, and help clear the heat of infection. The flavonoids in the berry help bind and disarm hemagglutinins, tiny viral spikes covered with the enzyme neuraminidase, which allows the virus to penetrate cellular membranes.

Elderberry juice and syrup have been used for more than two thousand years in the treatment of colds, flu, and coughs. Elder flowers and berries prepared as a tea are used to remedy acne, asthma, boils, catarrh, chicken pox, chills, colds, colic, cough, eczema, eye twitches, fever, flu, gout, hayfever, headache, measles, neuralgia, respiratory infection, rheumatism, sore throat, and tonsillitis.

Topically, elder flowers can be prepared as an anti-inflammatory wash, salve, eyewash, or gargle. A headache may be relieved by a cool elderflower compress.

Edible Uses

The berries and flowers of elder are edible. Elderberries are both delicious and healthful; in fact, in the early 1900s hospitals served elderberry jam because of its high vitamin and mineral content and ability to improve appetite and digestion and promote regular elimination. Today elderberries are commonly used to make fruit soups, pies, cobblers, jams, ice cream, and syrups.

When elder flowers are used in food, they are referred to as "elder blow." The flowers can simply be added to preparations such as fruit salads, jellies, vinegars, muffins, or punches. Try elderflower fritters with elderberry syrup!

Other Uses

Ancient Celts considered elder a sacred tree, symbolic of birth and death. In many ancient cultures elder was held to be so sacred that it was neither burned as firewood nor used in woodworking lest it bring bad luck to the household, and it was planted by homes and worn in amulets to encourage prosperity, happy marriage, healthy children, and protection from both lightning and evil forces.

The leaves can be bruised and then rubbed on the body or worn in a hat to keep away pestering insects. A tea prepared from the leaves, cooled and strained, can be applied to other plants to prevent aphid infestation.

Elder flowers are sometimes used in cosmetic preparations such as skin washes, toners, lotions, and hair rinses. The berries were once used in hair dye to rejuvenate fading color.

Constituents

Flower: flavonoids (rutin, quercitin, kaempferol), essential oils, phytosterols (sitosterol, stigmasterol, campestrol), viburnic acid, phenolic compounds (chlorogenic acid, caffeic acid, p-coumaric acid), triterpenes (ursolic acid, 30-b-hydroxyursolic acid, oleanolic acid, a-amyrin, b-amyrin, free esterified solids, fixed oil), tannins
Berry: beta-carotene, vitamin C, iron, potassium, tyrosine, alkaloids (sambucine, hydrocyanic acid)

Energetic Correspondences

• Flavor: flower—bitter; berry—sweet, bitter
• Temperature: cool
• Moisture: dry
• Polarity: yin
• Planet: Mercury/Venus/Mars/Jupiter
• Element: water

Contraindications

Avoid elder in cases of fluid depletion, as elder is a diuretic. Cook or dry the ripe berries before consuming large quantities of them, as excess quantities of the fresh berries can have a laxative effect. Avoid elder bark and root, except under the guidance of a qualified health-care practitioner; although they have medicinal benefits, they are strongly purgative and emetic. Know your species and avoid using red-berried elders, as many of them are poisonous.

Range and Appearance

There are over 30 species of elder. *Sambucus nigra* is native to Europe, western Asia, and northern Africa, while *S. canadensis* is native to North and Central America. These small deciduous trees have soft wood and grow to a height of between 5 and 25 feet, depending on the species and climate. Elder grows in clumps, with ten to thirty canes (stems) together. The leaves are divided into five to eleven slender glabrous leaflets, each about 3½ inches long, that grow in opposite pairs, often with an extra leaf; they are shiny green above and duller light green beneath. The small white flowers form a flat-topped cluster. The berries are usually purplish black, although they sometimes appear to be blue, which is the result of a powdery blush upon them. They contain ovate greenish brown seeds. Many songbirds and wild animals, including moose and elk, depend upon elderberries for sustenance.

ELECAMPANE

Botanical Name

Inula conyzae, I. helenium

Family

Asteraceae (Daisy Family)

Etymology

The species name, *helenium,* is said to be a reference to Helen of Troy, who was supposedly collecting elecampane when Paris captured her. The common name *elecampane* is derived from the Latin *campana,* "of the field."

Also Known As

Dutch: griekse alant
English: elfdock, elfwort, horse elder, horseheal,
   scabwort, velvet dock, wild sunflower
Finnish: isohirvenjuuri
French: grande aunée, heleniaire, herbe d'Hélène,
   inule aunee, oeil de cheval
German: beinerwell, echter alant, lionne,
   lugenwurz, odenkopf, stickwurz
Italian: enula elemie, inula campana
Japanese: senpukuku
Korean: sônbokhwa
Mandarin: xúan fù hua
Portuguese: enula-campana
Russian: devial sil, de-via-sil, inula
Sanskrit: pushkaramula

Spanish: enula campana, helopia, raíz del moro
Swedish: alant, elinsrot
Welsh: marchalan

Parts Used

Root, leaf, flower

Physiological Effects

Alterative, analgesic, anthelmintic, antibacterial, antifungal, anti-inflammatory, antiparasitic, antiseptic, antispasmodic, antiscorbutic, antitussive, antivenomous, aromatic, astringent, bitter, bronchial dilator, cardiotonic, carminative, cholagogue, diaphoretic, digestive, diuretic, emollient, emmenagogue, expectorant, hemostatic, hepatic, immune stimulant, lung tonic, rejuvenative, stimulant, stomachic, vulnerary

Medicinal Uses

Asian medicine uses primarily the flower of elecampane, while Western medicine employs mainly the root. The root is known to loosen phlegm, stimulate its expulsion, inhibit its production, relieve irritation in the respiratory passages, and deter a wide range of pathogens. It is used to treat asthma, auto-immune disorders, bronchitis, candida, catarrh, chest colds, cough, cystitis, diphtheria, dyspepsia, emphysema, exhaustion, fever, hay fever, laryngitis, nose bleed, parasites, pleurisy, pneumonia, shortness of breath, sinusitis, tuberculosis, ulcers, wheezing, whooping cough, and worms. The root can also be chewed to prevent tooth decay.

Topically, a wash can be made of the roots and leaves to cleanse the skin and to treat blemishes and other skin eruptions, facial neuralgia, and sciatica. The leaf can be applied as a poultice to treat nettle sting. The root is sometimes prepared for use as an enema.

Edible Uses

The roots, leaves, and seeds are edible. The roots can be cooked like other root vegetables; they also can be candied, made into lozenges, used to flavor sweet dishes, or used in the making of wines and liqueurs. The leaves and seeds can be eaten raw.

Other Uses

Elecampane flowers are sometimes included in potpourris, and the root can be burned as incense. In magical traditions, elecampane has long been used in amulets for protection against negative energy, to enhance psychic power, and in love charms.

Constituents

Calcium, magnesium, carbohydrate (inulin), mucilage, essential oils (azulene, camphor, helenin), lactones (helenine), sterols (sitosterol, stigmasterol), sesquiterpenes

Energetic Correspondences

- Flavor: bitter, pungent, sweet
- Temperature: warm
- Moisture: dry
- Polarity: yang
- Planet: Sun/Mercury/Uranus
- Element: air

Contraindications

Do not use during pregnancy. Large doses may cause diarrhea, vomiting, gastric spasms, allergic hypersensitivity, or even symptoms of paralysis.

Range and Appearance

Elecampane is a perennial native to Europe and northern Asia; it can be found growing in ditches and other waste places and reaches a height of between 3 and 8 feet. The upper leaves are large, toothed, and ovate and clasp the stem. The lower leaves are stalked. The entire plant has a downy quality. The ray flowers are solitary, large, and golden yellow.

EPHEDRA

Botanical Name

Ephedra distachya (syn. *E. vulgaris*), *E. equisetina*, *E. sinica*

Family

Ephedraceae (Joint Fir Family)

Etymology

The genus name, *Ephedra,* derives from the Greek *ephedros,* "sitting upon." The common name *ma huang* is an Anglicized spelling of the Chinese name. *Ma* translates as "astringent" or possibly "hemp" (in reference to the starlike stems of the plant), while *huang* translates as "yellow," in reference to the plant's color.

Also Known As

Cantonese: ma wong
English: Chinese joint fir, ma huang
Finnish: efedra
French: ephèdre du valais
German: meertäubl
Japanese: mao
Korean: mahwang
Mandarin: má húang
Sanskrit: somalata
Spanish: canutillo, popotillo
Swedish: efedra

Parts Used

Stem, branch

Physiological Effects

Antiallergenic, anti-inflammatory, antispasmodic, antitussive, aphrodisiac, astringent, bronchial dilator, circulatory stimulant, decongestant, diaphoretic, diuretic, expectorant, metabolic stimulant

Medicinal Uses

Humans have been using ephedra since the inception of our species. In fact, ephedra was found in the grave of a Neanderthal skeleton discovered in Shanidar Cave, in northeastern Iraq, and dating to some sixty thousand years ago.

Ephedra relaxes the muscles of the lung region, dilates the blood vessels of the coronary system and on the skin's surface, stimulates the sympathetic nervous system, and stimulates metabolism. It is used to treat allergies, arthritis, asthma, bronchitis, cocaine withdrawal symptoms, colds with chills, congestion, cough, dropsy, dyspnea, edema, emphysema, excessive appetite, fainting, fever with chills and no perspiration, hay fever, obesity, and wheezing. The milder American varieties (*E. nevadensis, E. viridis*) are more suitable for the treatment of allergies and asthma in children.

When combined with caffeine, ephedra has a thermogenic effect that helps metabolize fat and promote weight loss. However, use of ephedra can have many potential side effects (see "Contraindications," below), and there are many safer ways to lose weight.

In 1926 the German firm Merck synthesized ephedra's alkaloid, ephedrine, a chemical that is related to the endogenous brain hormone adrenaline. Synthetic ephedrine and pseudoephedrine are currently found in pharmaceuticals including Contac, Sinutab, Sudafed, Actifed, and Robitussin PE.

Topically, the resin from the ephedra shrub can be applied to cuts to promote healing.

Edible Uses

The red berries on the plant are the only parts considered edible.

Other Uses

Guards of Genghis Khan's army used ephedra to help them stay awake (they would be beheaded if caught dozing!). Taoist monks use ephedra to sharpen awareness. The herb also has been smoked as an aphrodisiac.

Constituents

Ascorbic acid, chromium, catechin, ephedrine, pseudoephredine, N-methyl-ephedrine, n-methyl-pseudoephedrine, norephedrine, norpseudoephedrine

Energetic Correspondences

• Flavor: sweet, pungent
• Temperature: warm
• Moisture: dry
• Polarity: yang
• Planet: Saturn/Uranus/Mars
• Element: earth

Contraindications

Ephedra has had a lot of negative press in recent years because of its potential side effects. Much of

the reason for this is that companies have concentrated the ephedrine alkaloids in products intended to promote energy and weight loss; this unnaturally strong concentration of ephedrine alkaloids has caused serious health problems and even death in users. Nevertheless, with proper precautions, as described below, ephedra can be a medicinal ally.

Ephedra can cause dizziness, manic episodes, nervousness, hypertension, rapid heartbeat, tingling, nausea, sweating, insomnia, or in rare cases a rash. Concentrated extracts of ephedra are more likely than a simple infusion to cause these side effects; a tea made from the dried plant is the safest method of use.

Do not use ephedra while pregnant, while nursing, or in children under the age of eighteen. Avoid in cases of weakness and debilitation, high blood pressure, adrenal weakness, anorexia, bulimia, kidney disease, heart disease, thyroid disorder, diabetes, prostatitis or enlarged prostate, ulcer, hepatitis, weak digestion, glaucoma, Raynaud's disease, insomnia, excessive sweating, or yin deficiency. Do not use ephedra in conjunction with monoamine oxidase inhibitors, steroids, beta-blockers, or antidepressants. Avoid ephedra at least three days before surgery to prevent blood pressure elevation concerns.

Never exceed the recommended dosage. Avoid using ephedra for extended periods. For safest use, ephedra is best taken under the guidance of a qualified health-care practitioner.

Ephedra brings internal energy to the surface of the body, which can leave one depleted at the core. To minimize this effect, ephedra can be combined with licorice root, which provides moisture to counteract ephedra's drying effect.

Range and Appearance

There are about forty species of ephedra, native to Asia, the Mediterranean, and North and Central America. This small shrub grows to a height of about 3 feet and has broomlike stems. The opposite branches are short, erect, and notched by reddish brown nodelike joints. The leaves are actually tiny scales on the branches. The shrub's small yellow flowers are followed by red berries.

E. nevadensis (also known as Mormon tea or Brigham tea) and *E. viridis* (also known as green ephedra) are closely related herbs that grow in the American West and have a much milder effect than the ephedra species described here, containing little to no ephedrine alkaloids.

EPIMEDIUM

Botanical Name

Epimedium spp., including *E. aceranthus, E. acuminatum, E. brevicornum, E. grandiflorum, E. koreanum, E. macranthum, E. pubescens, E. sagittatum*

Family

Berberidaceae (Barberry Family)

Etymology

The genus name, *Epimedium,* derives from the Greek *epi,* "upon," and *media,* in reference to the ancient country of Media, southwest of the Caspian Sea. The Mandarin name *yín yáng hùo* translates as "licentious goat wort," in reference to the fact that goats that graze upon this herb have increased seminal emissions and are more sexually active.

Also Known As

Cantonese: gan yeng fuk, seun líng pei
English: barrenwort, bishop's hat, horny goat weed
Japanese: inyokaku
Korean: ûmyanggwak
Mandarin: xian ling pi, yín yáng hùo

Parts Used

Aboveground plant

Physiological Effects

Anti-inflammatory, antispasmodic, antiviral, aphrodisiac, circulatory stimulant, endocrine tonic, hormone regulator, hypotensive, hypothyroidism, immune stimulant, kidney yang tonic, neuromuscular stimulant, restorative, tonic, vasodilator

Medicinal Uses

Epimedium warms the kidneys, tonifies yang, and removes excess moisture from the body. It stimulates the pituitary gland and thus the gonads and increases sperm production and motility. It also dilates capillaries and larger blood vessels, strengthens bones, improves metabolism, and exhibits a mild androgenic effect. Epimedium is used to treat atherosclerosis, bronchitis, depression, drug and chemical withdrawal symptoms, erectile dysfunction, exhaustion, forgetfulness, hay fever, herpes, infertility, low libido, lumbago, memory loss, menopause symptoms, numbness, osteoporosis, pain, polyuria, poor circulation, premature ejaculation, prostatitis, and rheumatism.

Edible Uses

The leaf is edible; it is used as a potherb in Asia and is a common additive to spring wines.

Other Uses

None known

Constituents

Vitamin E, manganese, flavonoids (quercetin, luteolin, kaempferol), icariin epimedin, methylicariin, anhydrocaritin), linolenic acid, palmitic acid, polysaccharides, alkaloids (magnoflorine, berberine, coptisine), sterols, tannin

Energetic Correspondences

- Flavor: pungent, sweet
- Temperature: warm
- Moisture: dry
- Polarity: yang
- Planet: Jupiter
- Element: fire

Contraindications

Epimedium is not recommended for those who have an excessive sex drive, experience wet dreams, or are overly hot or irritable. Excess use can cause vertigo, vomiting, dry mouth, decreased thyroid activity, or nosebleed. Use for short periods of time only.

Range and Appearance

Epimedium is a perennial evergreen herb native to the subtropics of Asia. It grows on hillsides, in cliff crevices, or in shady bamboo groves, reaching about 6 to 15 inches in height. It has somewhat heart-shaped basal leaves, compounded into two or three parts, that are green with sometimes purple or reddish tinges. The central leaflet is ovate-lanceolate with a cordate base. Pale yellow terminal flowers appear in panicles or racemes.

EUCALYPTUS

Botanical Name

Eucalyptus spp., including *E. globulus*

Family

Myrtaceae (Eucalyptus Family)

Etymology

The genus and common name are derived from the Greek *eucalyptos,* "well covered," in reference to the cuplike membranes that surround the flower.

Also Known As

English: blue gum tree, blue malee (*E. polybractea*), fever tree, gum tree, iron bark (*E. staigeriana*), stringy bark tree
Finnish: eukalyptuspuu, kuumepuu
French: arbre à la fievre, gommier bleu
German: blauer eucalyptusbaum, blauer gummibaum, fieberbaum
Italian: eucalipto
Mandarin: ta-hsieh an (*E. robusta*)
Sanskrit: tailaparni
Spanish: dolár, eucalipto
Swedish: feberträd

Parts Used

Young leaf

Physiological Effects

Antibacterial, antifungal, anti-inflammatory, antiseptic, antispasmodic, antiviral, aromatic, astringent, bronchial dilator, circulatory stimulant, decongestant, diaphoretic, expectorant, febrifuge

Medicinal Uses

In traditional Aboriginal medicine, eucalyptus leaf is used to treat wounds and infections. It stimulates mucus secretions, remoistening the mucous membranes while inhibiting infectious microorganisms from growing on them. It also relieves pain and clears the head, soothes and stimulates the lungs, deters infection, and stimulates immunity.

Eucalyptus leaves are used in the treatment of arthritis, asthma, bronchitis, catarrh, chicken pox, cholera, colds, croup, diabetes, diarrhea, diphtheria, dysentery, emphysema, encephalitis, flu, herpes, leukemia, malaria, measles, pneumonia, rheumatism, scarlet fever, sinusitis, sore throat, typhoid, typhus, tuberculosis, whooping cough, and worms. The dried leaves are included in smoking mixtures used for the treatment of asthma and bronchitis. Eucalyptus honey (honey infused with eucalyptus leaf) in particular is excellent for clearing catarrh and respiratory ailments.

Eucalyptus can be prepared as a tea that can be gargled to treat throat infection. It also makes an excellent bath herb to relieve muscle and joint soreness and respiratory congestion.

Eucalyptus yields one of the most antiseptic of essential oils. The essential oil is diluted and applied topically to treat blisters, boils, burns, gangrene, herpes sores, and wounds. It is included in salves and massage oils to relieve chest and sinus congestion, headache, painful arthritic joints, and stiff joints. The oil can also be used in steam baths, saunas, and vapor inhalations as a decongestant.

Edible Uses

Not generally considered edible, except as tea. However, koala bears feed on leaves that are between 12 and 18 months old.

Other Uses

Eucalyptus is a natural insect repellent; the pods are sometimes made into dog collars and the leaves are stuffed into dog beds to deter fleas and other pests, and the essential oil is often an ingredient in insect repellent preparations. The tree is planted in hot, swampy parts of the world to dry swampland and to discourage the proliferation of malaria-carrying mosquitoes. Aborigines use the leaves to catch fish, as when the leaves are soaked, they release a mild tranquilizer that temporarily stuns fish in the area, allowing them to be easily scooped up.

Tea made from the leaves can be used as a breath-freshening mouthwash. The leaves are sometimes included in potpourris, and the wood of the tree is used in construction, as firewood, and in the crafting of digeridoo instruments. Eucalyptus is also a dye plant, yielding shades of green, brown, and orange.

Constituents

Vitamin C, flavonoids (rutin, quercitin, hyperoside), essential oils (cineol, pinene, citronellal), polyphenolic acids, tannins, aldehydes, resin

Energetic Correspondences

- Flavor: pungent, bitter
- Temperature: cool
- Moisture: moist
- Polarity: yin
- Planet: Saturn/Moon/Pluto
- Element: water

Contraindications

Large doses can cause headache, vertigo, convulsions, and even death. The essential oil may cause irritation or burning; avoid contact of the essential oil with mucous membranes.

Range and Appearance

Eucalyptus is an evergreen tree native to Australia and the Malay Archipelago; more than 700 species exist. It ranks among the world's tallest trees; *E. globulus,* for example, the most common species, grows to a height of about 200 feet. The bark is grayish brown and peels off annually. The blue-green leaves are leathery, sickle shaped, and from 6 to 12 inches long. The white flowers grow in umbellate clusters. The fruit is enclosed in a hardened calyx composed of three or four cells, with two or three fruits per cell.

EUCOMMIA

Botanical Name

Eucommia ulmoides

Family

Eucommiaceae (Eucommia Family)

Etymology

The genus name, *Eucommia,* is derived from the Greek *eu* and *kommi,* meaning "true gum," in reference for the tree's ability to produce rubber. The Chinese names and Anglicized *du zhong* are taken from the name of a legendary Taoist sage, Du Zhong, who apparently attained enlightenment after using this herb.

Also Known As

Cantonese: dou jung
English: gutta-percha tree, hardy rubber tree, wood cotton
German: guttaperchabaum
Japanese: tochu
Mandarin: dù zhòng

Part Used

Bark

Physiological Effects

Analgesic, anti-inflammatory, antispasmodic, aphrodisiac, aromatic, astringent, blood tonic, chi tonic, depurative, diuretic, hepatic, hypotensive, immune stimulant, kidney tonic, liver tonic, restorative, sedative, yang tonic, vasodilator

Medicinal Uses

In Chinese medicine eucommia has been used for more than three thousand years and ranks second only to ginseng. In recent years there has been extensive research into its ability to lower high blood pressure without negative side effects. Eucommia is also known to stimulate the production of interferon, strengthen the bones and muscles, and aid in the smooth movement of chi and blood. It is used in the treatment of broken bones, chronic fatigue, dizziness, erectile dysfunction, fatigue, fetal restlessness, headache, high cholesterol, hypertension, infertility (female), kidney deficiency, knee pain, lumbago during pregnancy, osteoporosis, polyuria, premature aging, prostate weakness, and threat of miscarriage.

Edible Uses

The bark is not generally considered edible, except as tea, but the young leaves can be eaten as a vegetable.

Other Uses

Eucommia produces a latex that can be used to make a type of rubber. The leaves contain a nonelastic rubber, called gutta-percha, that is used as an insulating material for electric wires. The bark is peeled from the tree in early spring and then folded so the inner surfaces meet. This setup is left to age for several weeks, until the inner surface blackens. Then the bark is untied and dried in the sun. When dried, the bark is cracked to reveal the white threads of latex, which can then be harvested.

Constituents

Potassium, vitamin C, flavonoids, latex (gutta-percha), alkaloids, lignan glycosides, pinoresinol, iridoids (acubin), geniposide, reptoside

Energetic Correspondences

- Flavor: sweet, mildly pungent
- Temperature: warm
- Moisture: dry
- Polarity: yang
- Planet: Jupiter
- Element: fire

Contraindications

Avoid eucommia in cases of excessive heat or yin deficiency. Large doses can be sedative but are not considered dangerous.

Range and Appearance

Eucommia is native to central China, where it grows in mountainous regions at sunny woodland edges. This deciduous tree resembles an elm and has oval leaves and pale green or reddish flowers. The tree is

dioecious, meaning that male and female flowers grow on different trees.

Because China limits the sale of eucommia overseas, it has become rather expensive.

EYEBRIGHT

Botanical Name

Euphrasia nemorosa (syn. *E. americana, E. canadensis*), *E. rostkoviana* (syn. *E. officinalis*)

Family

Scrophulariaceae (Figwort Family)

Etymology

The genus name, *Euphrasia,* derives from the name of Euphrosyne, one of the Three Graces or Charites; she was the goddess of joy. The name refers to the joy a person would feel when his or her vision was improved from using eyebright.

Also Known As

English: euphrasia, euphrosyne, ocularia
Finnish: ahosilmäruoho
French: brise-lunettes, casse-lunettes, euphraise
German: augentröst, augstenzeiger, hirnkraut, schabab, weisses ruhrkraut, wiesenaugentrost, zwangkraut
Italian: eufrasia di rostkov
Spanish: eufrasia
Swedish: stor ögontröst

Part Used

Aboveground plant

Physiological Effects

Alterative, antibacterial, anticatarrhal, anti-inflammatory, antiseptic, astringent, digestive, decongestant, expectorant, febrifuge, hepatic, ophthalmic, tonic, vulnerary

Medicinal Uses

The flower of eyebright somewhat resembles a bloodshot eye, which may have been part of the reason ancient peoples valued this plant for treating eye ailments. Appearances aside, eyebright is beneficial for the treatment of many ailments of the eye. It stimulates the liver to clean the blood, dries dampness, curbs discharge, and reduces inflammation, thereby clearing the eyes and head and relieving conditions that congest visual clarity. It has an antihistamine-like effect and is a specific for mucus discharge from the eyes, ears, and nasal passages.

Eyebright is used to treat allergies, blepharitis, cataracts, catarrh, conjunctivitis, cough, earaches, eye inflammation, eye irritation (itchiness and watering), eyestrain, hay fever, headache with congestion, head cold, hoarseness, jaundice, leukorrhoea, memory loss, ophthalmia, photophobia, rhinitis, sinusitis, sore eyes, sore throat, styes, vertigo, and weak vision.

Topically, a tea or the fresh-pressed juice of eyebright can be used as an eyewash, compress, or nasal wash to relieve irritation in the eyes and nose. It also can be used as a poultice to encourage the healing of wounds.

Edible Uses

Eyebright leaves, though slightly bitter, can be eaten raw.

Other Uses

The dried leaves of the plant are sometimes included in smoking mixtures. In magical traditions, eyebright is said to enhance psychic ability.

Constituents

Beta-carotene, vitamin C, flavonoids, choline, tannins (acubin), glycosides (aucubine, aucuboside, aneobin, rhynanthin), phenolic acids, euphrastanic acid, essential oil, glucose, mannose

Energetic Correspondences

- Flavor: bitter, pungent
- Temperature: cool
- Moisture: dry
- Polarity: yang
- Planet: Sun
- Element: air

Contraindications

Eyebright is generally regarded as safe. In cases of serious eye disorders, however, eyebright is best used under the guidance of a qualified health-care professional. Avoid eyebright in cases of extreme congestion, as it may be worsened by eyebright's astringent properties. Avoid during pregnancy.

Range and Appearance

Native to Europe, eyebright is a small annual herb, reaching a height of only 2 to 8 inches. The leaves are deeply toothed, oval, and pubescent and the stems are square. The small hermaphroditic plants are white with yellow and purple spots. Eyebright is semiparasitic, in that its roots attach to those of grasses. It does best in open areas, such as pastures.

FENNEL

Botanical Name

Foeniculum officinale, F. vulgare

Family

Umbelliferae (Parsley Family)

Etymology

The genus name, *Foeniculum*, and common name *fennel* derive from the Latin *foenum*, "hay," in reference to the finely divided leaves of the plant.

Also Known As

Afrikaans: vinkel
Arabic: shamaar
Armenian: samit
Bulgarian: rezene
Cantonese: wuih heung
Czech: fenykl
Croatian: koromac
Danish: fennikel
Dutch: venkel
English: sweet cumin
Esperanto: fenkolo
Estonian: harilik apteegitill
Finnish: fenkoli

French: fenouil
German: fenchel
Greek: finkokio
Hebrew: shumar
Hindi: saunf
Hungarian: édeskömény
Icelandic: fennika
Indonesian: jinten manis
Italian: finocchio
Japanese: shouikyo, uikyo
Korean: hoehyang
Lithuanian: paprastasis pankolis
Mandarin: hui xiang
Nepali: saunf
Norwegian: fennikel
Polish: fenkul
Portuguese: funcho
Romanian: anason dulce, fenicul
Russian: aptechnyj ukrop
Sanskrit: madhurika
Serbian: komorac
Slovak: fenikel
Spanish: hinojo
Swahili: shamari
Swedish: fänkål
Thai: thian-kaupeluengk
Turkish: rezene
Ukrainian: fenkhel zvychajniy
Vietnamese: cây thì làà
Zulu: imboziso

Part Used

Seed

Physiological Effects

Anesthetic, antibacterial, antiemetic, antifungal, anti-inflammatory, antispasmodic, antitussive, aperient, aromatic, calmative, carminative, digestive, diuretic, expectorant, galactagogue, laxative (mild), mucolytic, phytoestrogenic, stimulant, stomachic

Medicinal Uses

Fennel seed improves the body's energy by enhancing the digestion and assimilation of food. It clears phlegm, stimulates interferon production, relaxes the bronchi, loosens bronchial secretions, decongests the liver, and clears stagnation. It aids in the digestion of fatty foods and is often added to laxative blends to ease gripe. It also helps stabilize blood sugar levels, thus curbing appetite. It is considered an excellent herb for children.

Fennel is used in the treatment of amenorrhea, asthma, bloating, bronchitis, colic, cough, diabetes, dyspepsia, endometriosis, fatigue, fever, flatulence, gout, halitosis, hangover, heartburn, hernia, hiccups, hypertension, indigestion, jaundice, kidney stones, laryngitis, low libido, malabsorption, menstrual cramps, nausea, obesity, premenstrual syndrome, rheumatism, stomachache, teething, weak vision (including floaters), and vomiting.

Topically, fennel seed tea can be used as a soothing anti-inflammatory eyewash.

Edible Uses

Fennel seed makes for sweet breath, with a flavor similar to that of aniseed and licorice; it is a popular culinary seasoning. The leaves of the plant are also edible raw or cooked.

Other Uses

Fennel seed can be prepared as a compress, bath herb, or facial steam to moisten dry skin or as a mouthwash to freshen the breath. In magical traditions, fennel is hung over doorways to offer protection against evil.

Constituents

Beta-carotene, vitamin C, calcium, iron, magnesium, potassium, phosphorous, silicon, zinc, essential oils (anethole, fenchone, pinene, limonene, safrole), phenolic ether, flavonoids, coumarins, stigmasterol

Energetic Correspondences

- Flavor: pungent, sweet
- Temperature: warm
- Moisture: moist
- Polarity: yang
- Planet: Mercury
- Element: fire

Contraindications

Excess use of fennel seed can overstimulate the nervous system. Avoid therapeutic dosages during pregnancy.

Range and Appearance

Fennel, native to the Middle East and Mediterranean, is a perennial that can grow from 5 to 6 feet in height. The plant has a bluish green hue and grows in colonies in waste places, on roadsides, along fence lines, and in vacant lots. When crushed, it gives off a distinct licorice-like aroma. It has clustered basal leaves and alternate stem leaves. Both the basal and stem leaves are pinnate, look fernlike, and are compounded three or four times. The yellow flowers grow in flat-topped umbels.

Fennel prefers full sun and low to moderate amounts of water, and it does best in well-worked, well-drained soil.

FENUGREEK

Botanical Name

Trigonella foenum-graecum

Family

Fabaceae (Legume Family)

Etymology

The genus name, *Trigonella,* derives from the Greek *trigonon,* "triangle," in reference to the three-sided corolla of the flower. The species name, *foenum-graecum,* is Latin for "Greek hay," in reference to the fact that fenugreek was once used to scent inferior grades of hay.

Also Known As

Arabic: hilbeh, hulba
Armenian: chaiman
Bulgarian: sminduh
Cantonese: wuh louh ba
Croatian: piskavica
Czech: pískavice recké, senenka
Danish: bukkehornskløver
Dutch: fenegriek
English: bird's foot, Greek hay
Esperanto: fenugreko
Estonian: kreeko lambalääts
Finnish: sarviapila
French: fenugrec, trigonelle
German: bockshornklee, griechisch heu
Greek: trigonella
Hebrew: hilbeh
Hindi: methi (seed), sag methi (leaf)
Hungarian: görögszéna
Indonesian: kelabet
Italian: fieno greco
Japanese: henu-guriku, koruha
Korean: horopa
Lithuanian: vaistine ozrage
Mandarin: hú lú ba
Nepali: methi
Norwegian: bukkehornklover
Polish: kozieradka pospolita
Portuguese: feno-grego
Romanian: molotru
Russian: pazhitinik grecheski
Sanskrit: methika
Serbian: piskavica
Spanish: alholva
Swahili: uwatu
Thai: luk sat
Tibetan: meeti
Turkish: çemen
Ukrainian: hunba sinna
Vietnamese: h'ô lo ba
Yiddish: fenigrekum, khilbe

Parts Used

Seed (but in Ayurvedic medicine, the entire plant)

Physiological Effects

Alterative, anthelmintic, anti-inflammatory, antiseptic, aphrodisiac, aromatic, carminative, demulcent, digestive, diuretic, emmenagogue, emollient, expectorant, febrifuge, galactagogue, hypoglycemic, mucolytic, nutritive, phytoestrogenic, restorative, stimulant, vulnerary, yang tonic

Medicinal Uses

Fenugreek has long been used in Egyptian, Ayurvedic, and Chinese medicine. It contains six compounds that help stabilize blood sugar levels. It increases levels of the "good" cholesterol HDL (high-density lipoprotein), reduces blood glucose levels, warms the kidneys, lubricates the intestines, nourishes the glands, and stimulates the production of digestive secretions. It is used in the treatment of anorexia, bronchitis, catarrh, constipation, cough, diarrhea, dyspepsia, erectile dysfunction, fever, flatulence, debility, diabetes, gout, hernia, high cholesterol, kidney chi deficiency, menopause symptoms, menstrual cramps, neuralgia, pain, premature ejaculation, sciatica, scrofula, sore throat, swollen glands, tuberculosis, and vaginal dryness.

Topically, fenugreek can be used as a compress to treat abscesses, boils, burns, cellulitis, and swollen glands. It makes a fine gargle for sore throat, douche for leukorrhea, eyewash for inflamed eyes, and compress for chapped hands, and it also can be used as a facial wash.

Edible Uses

Fenugreek seeds can be sprouted as a salad green. They have a flavor somewhere between that of bitter celery, burnt sugar, and maple syrup, and they combine well in tea with a bit of cinnamon bark or a spoonful of honey. The roasted seeds can be brewed as a coffee substitute. The fresh leaves of the plant are edible and can be eaten raw or cooked.

Other Uses

None known

Constituents

Beta-carotene, B-complex vitamins (especially niacin and choline), vitamin C, vitamin E, calcium, iron, lysine, tryptophan, glutamic acid, aspartic acid, lecithin, carbohydrates (galactomannans), steroidal saponins (diosgenin, yamogenin), alkaloids (trigonelline, carpaine, gentianine), glycosides, flavonoids (apigenin, quercitin, luteolin), coumarin, mucilage, protein, fatty acids (linoleic, linolenic, oleic)

Energetic Correspondences

- Flavor: bitter
- Temperature: warm
- Moisture: moist
- Polarity: yang
- Planet: Mercury
- Element: air

Contraindications

Avoid fenugreek seed during pregnancy, as it can be a uterine stimulant. Although fenugreek can be used to lower blood sugar levels, diabetics should use it for this purpose only with guidance from a qualified health-care practitioner.

Range and Appearance

Fenugreek, an annual native to western Asia and the Middle East, grows to about 1 to 2 feet in height and resembles a large clover. The flowers are trifoliate and toothed; the flowers, which grow in the leaf axils, have a yellow-violet corolla. The brownish seeds are contained in long, narrow, sickle-shaped pods. Each seed is oblong, with a deep furrow dividing it into two unequal lobes.

Fenugreek thrives in dry, fertile soil. To grow, sow the seeds thickly in the spring in an area that receives full sun. Avoid cold, wet soil or the seeds will rot before germinating.

Green Manures: Both fenugreek and licorice make good green manures. Cultivating these plants and then turning under the crop will help fix nitrogen in the soil.

FEVERFEW

Botanical Name

Tanacetum parthenium (formerly *Chrysanthemum parthenium*)

Family

Asteraceae (Daisy Family)

Etymology

The genus name, *Tanacetum,* derives from the Latin *anthanasis,* "immortal," referring to the long life of the flowers. The species name, *parthenium,* derives from the Greek *parthenonos,* "virgin," in reference to the famous temple dedicated to the goddess Athena; legend tells that feverfew was used to save the life of a worker who fell from the walls of the temple. The common name *feverfew* derives from the Latin *febrifuga,* "to chase away fevers," in reference to the plant's medicinal use.

Also Known As

English: altamisa, bachelor's buttons, featherfew, featherfoil, featherfowl, feather-full pyrethrum, flirtwort, mayweed, midsummer daisy, mother herb, nosebleed, vetter-voo, whitewort, wild chamomile,

Finnish: reunuspäivänkakkara

French: espargoutte, grande camomille

German: bertram, metram, mutterkraut

Italian: camomilla grande, erba madre, matricale, partenio

Sanskrit: atasi

Spanish: altamisa mexicana, santa maria, yerba de santa maria

Swedish: mattram

Parts Used

Flower, leaf

Physiological Effects

Alterative, anti-inflammatory, antimicrobial, antiseptic, antispasmodic, aperient, aromatic, bitter, carminative, diaphoretic, diuretic, emmenagogue, febrifuge, nervine, purgative, stimulant, tonic, vasodilator, vermifuge

Medicinal Uses

Feverfew prevents blood platelet aggregation and inhibits the release of inflammatory substances from cells, including leukotriene and thromboxane prostaglandins. It also inhibits the release of histamine and serotonin. It is used in the treatment of allergies, amenorrhea, arthritis, colds, dysmenorrhea, fever, flu, headache, indigestion, migraine, pain, placenta retention, rheumatism, stomachache, toothache, and worms. It may take several weeks to get results from using feverfew. Eating a few leaves every day can help prevent migraines.

Topically, feverfew can be applied as a compress to the head to relieve headache, to the gums to reduce swelling after a tooth extraction, or to bruises to facilitate healing. It also can be used in a sitz bath to relieve menstrual cramps or in an enema to get rid of worms. The fresh flowers can be rubbed onto the skin to soothe insect bites.

Edible Uses

Feverfew is edible, though it is not generally considered a food source. It has been used to flavor pastries and wine.

Other Uses

The flowers deter bugs and moths and are sometimes added to sachets kept with clothing. They also can be rubbed fresh onto the skin as an insect repellent. The essential oil is used in perfumery. In magical traditions, feverfew is burned as incense for spiritual cleansing.

Constituents

Sesquiterpene lactones (parthenolide), essential oils (borneol, camphor, terpene), camphor, pyrethirin, tannins

Energetic Correspondences

• Flavor: bitter

• Temperature: warm

• Moisture: dry

• Polarity: yin

• Planet: Sun/Venus

• Element: water

Contraindications

Avoid during pregnancy and while nursing. Because it can diminish blood-clotting ability, feverfew should not be used in conjunction with blood-thinning medications and should be avoided for at least a week prior to surgery. In rare cases feverfew can cause irritation of the gastrointestinal tract, mouth, or tongue; taking it with food can minimize this possibility. In cases of severe allergy to ragweed, a close relative of feverfew, use feverfew under the guidance of a qualified health-care practitioner. In rare cases topical use of feverfew can cause contact dermatitis.

Range and Appearance

Feverfew is a perennial native to southeastern Europe. The plant reaches a height of 6 to 18 inches. The leaves are strongly scented, feathery, greenish yellow, and bipinnate. The flowers are daisylike, with white petals and yellow centers.

FLAX

Botanical Name

Linum lewisii, L. perenne, L. usitatissimum

Family

Linaceae (Flax Family)

Etymology

The genus name, *Linum,* is the Latin name for this plant. The common name *flax* derives from the Old English word for cloth made from this plant, *fleax.*

Also Known As

English: linseed
Finnish: pellava
French: lin
German: flaches
Italian: lino
Sanskrit: uma
Spanish: lino
Swedish: lin

Part Used

Seed

Physiological Effects

Analgesic, anti-inflammatory, antitussive, demulcent, emollient, expectorant, laxative

Medicinal Uses

Flaxseed moistens the body and soothes irritation and inflammation, due to its demulcent and oily qualities. It is used in the treatment of arthritis, asthma, breast cysts, bronchitis, colitis, constipation, coughs, cystitis, eczema, gastritis, hemorrhoids, and sore throat. For a laxative effect, eat 1 to 2 tablespoons of the seeds, along with plenty of fluits.

Topically, flaxseed can be used as a healing poultice for boils, burns, carbuncles, inflammation, pleurisy, psoriasis, and shingles.

Edible Uses

This truly useful plant has been cultivated as a food source for more than seven thousand years. In the eighth century, Charlemagne passed a law requiring French citizens to consume flaxseeds so that they would be healthy subjects. Centuries later, Mahatma Ghandi said that when flaxseed became a regular food, all people would have better health. The seeds may be eaten raw or cooked.

Other Uses

The seeds are often included in lotions and gels for its holding effect. They can be used in soothing pillows for eye soreness and headaches. In magical traditions, flaxseed is used to attract prosperity.

The fibers of the plant are used to make paper, linen, and twine. The oil from the seeds was used to make linoleum.

Constituents

Omega-3 fatty acids, omega-6 fatty acids, cyanogenic glycosides (linamarin), mucilage, protein, betacarotene, vitamin B, vitamin E

Energetic Correspondences

- Flavor: sweet
- Temperature: warm
- Moisture: moist
- Polarity: yang
- Planet: Mercury/Saturn/Uranus
- Element: fire

Contraindications

Avoid the immature (unripe) seeds, which may be toxic. Once the seeds have been ground or processed into oil, they should be used soon, as they can quickly go rancid.

Range and Appearance

Linum perenne is native to Europe and eastern Asia, while *L. lewesii* is native to North America and *L. usitassimum* is cultivated only. The plant grows in dry, well-drained soil in full to partial sun. Its leaves are narrow and stems slender. The flowers are bright blue and have five stamens. The seeds are oval, flattened, and brown or black.

FRANKINCENSE

Botanical Name

Boswellia sacra (syn. *B. carteri*), *B. thurifera*

Family

Burseraceae (Frankincense or Balsam Family)

Etymology

The genus name *Boswellia* was given in honor of Scottish botanist John Boswell (1719–1780). The common name *frankincense* is believed to be a rephrasing of "incense of the Franks," as the herb was introduced into Europe by Frankish crusaders.

Also Known As

Arabic: al lubán, mogar, sheehaz
English: galibanum, olibanum
French: arbre à encens, oliban, salai tree
German: weihrauchzbaum
Hebrew: laban
Italian: olibano
Sanskrit: dhup, salai guggul
Spanish: olibano

Part Used

Resin

Physiological Effects

Alterative, anticatarrh, antidepressant, anti-inflam-matory, antioxidant, antiseptic, antispasmodic, aromatic, diuretic, emmenagogue, expectorant, immune stimulant, nervine, rejuvenative

Medicinal Uses

Frankincense improves circulation, of both blood and chi, and clears obstructions. It helps the sinews to be more flexible, shrinks inflamed tissue, and helps relieve pain. It also helps prevent free-radical damage. It is used in the treatment of arthritis, asthma, bronchitis, cancer, colitis, delayed menses, dysmenorrhea, and hypertension.

Topically, frankincense can be prepared as a liniment to relieve the pain of rheumatism or injury. It also can be used as a salve to help heal wounds and prevent scarring. It can be prepared as a mouthwash to treat ulcers or as a steam inhalation to treat respiratory problems such as asthma, bronchitis, and emphysema.

Edible Uses

Not generally considered edible.

Other Uses

Frankincense, along with gold and myrrh, is renowned as one of the gifts of the Magi to the infant Christ. It is often burned as incense, a practice dating back to the Egyptians, who burned it at sunrise to honor Ra, the sun god. Its smell is said to calm and clear the mind. Its essential oil is used in perfumery. It is included in skin-care products such as creams and lotions to prevent wrinkling of the skin.

Constituents

Boswellic acids, olibanoresene, arabic acid, essential oils (pinene, d-borneol), bassorin

Energetic Correspondences

- Flavor: pungent, bitter
- Temperature: warm
- Moisture: dry
- Polarity: yang
- Planet: Sun
- Element: fire

Contraindications

When using frankincense internally, use it only in small amounts and only for a short period of time. Overdose can cause nausea and vomiting. Avoid during pregnancy.

Range and Appearance

Native to the northern Africa and the Arabian peninsula, the frankincense tree is small, deciduous, and usually found growing in full sun in hot, dry conditions. When the tree's bark is damaged or scored, a white emulsion exudes that hardens into "tears" when dry; this is the part used medicinally. The star-shaped flowers are white and sometimes tipped with green or pink. The compound, glossy leaves grow in seven to nine serrate leaflets.

GALANGAL

Botanical Name

Alpinia galanga

Family

Zingerberaceae (Ginger Family)

Etymology

The genus name, *Alpinia,* was given to honor the Italian botanist Prospero Alpini (1533–1617). The common name *galangal* is derived from the Persian/Arabic *qulanan,* which most likely comes from the Chinese *liang-jiang,* meaning "mild ginger" or "excellent ginger."

Also Known As

Arabic: khalanjan
Bosnian: kulinjan
Cantonese: daaih gou leuhng geung
Croatian: galanga
Czech: galgán obecny'
Danish: stor galanga
Dutch: grote galanga
English: chewing John, China root, East Indian
    catarrh root, galingale, languas, Laos root,
    Siamese ginger, spice ginger
Estonian: suur kalganirohi

French: galanga de l'Inde
German: galant, siamesische ingwerlilie
Greek: galanki
Hebrew: galangal
Hindi: kulinjan
Hungarian: galanga
Indonesian: laos
Italian: galanga maggiore
Japanese: garanga, koryokyo
Korean: kallengal
Laotian: kha ta deng
Lithuanian: alpinija
Mandarin: da gao liang jiang
Persian: xuz rishe
Polish: galanga
Portuguese: gengibre do laos
Russian: al'piniia galanga
Sanskrit: kulanja, rasna
Serbian: galanga
Spanish: calanga, galang, garengal
Thai: kha
Turkish: galanga
Vietnamese: ríêng â'm
Yiddish: galgan

Part Used

Rhizome

Physiological Effects

Antibacterial, antifungal, antitumor, aromatic, carminative, digestive, stimulant

Medicinal Uses

The mystic and herbalist Hildegard de Bingen called galangal "the spice of life" and believed it was a gift from God to keep sickness away. The herb is known to improve circulation, clear energy blockages, and increase digestive secretions. It is used in the treatment of bronchitis, candida, catarrh, cholera, flatulence, hiccups, indigestion, leukemia, malaria, measles, nausea, rheumatoid arthritis, and ulcers. The powdered dried rhizome is used as a snuff to relieve the congestion of colds.

Edible Uses

Galangal is a popular seasoning in Thai and other

South Asian cuisines. The rhizomes are edible and are often included in curries, meat dishes, and soups. The young shoots and flowers can be eaten raw, boiled, or pickled.

Other Uses

Galangal is sometimes used in perfumery. In magical traditions it is burned as an incense to attract good luck and prosperity, as well as for psychic protection and good health.

Constituents

Essential oils (pinene, cineole, eugenol, eucalyptol), sesquiterpene lactones (alpinin, galangin, galangol, kaempferride), starch

Energetic Correspondences

- Flavor: pungent, sweet
- Temperature: hot
- Moisture: dry
- Polarity: yang
- Planet: Mars
- Element: fire

Contraindications

Avoid using large amounts on a continuous basis.

Range and Appearance

The plant is native to China, India, and Indonesia and thrives in moist, fertile, well-drained soils in partial shade. It grows in clumps of stiff stalks up to 7 feet in height with abundant, long, bladelike leaves. The orchidlike flowers are greenish white with a red-veined tip. The berries are red.

GARCINIA

Botanical Name

Garcinia atroviridis, G. gummi-gutta (syn. *G. cambogia*), *G. indica*

Family

Clusiaceae, also known as Guttiferaceae (Saint John's Wort Family)

Etymology

The genus name, *Garcinia*, was given in honor of the French botanist Laurent Garcin, who first described this plant in 1734.

Also Known As

English: brindal berry, gutta, Malabar tamarind
Danish: gummiguttræ
Dutch: geelhars
French: gamboge, gomme-gutte
German: gummiguttbaum, gutti
Italian: gommagutta
Japanese: garushinia kanbogia
Russian: gartsiniia
Sanskrit: kankusta, vrikshamla
Thai: som khaek
Ukrainian: gartsiniia kambodzhiiskaia

Part Used

Rind of fruit (pericarp)

Physiological Effects

Antiseptic, appetite suppressant, astringent, digestive, diuretic, thermogenic, vermifuge

Medicinal Uses

Garcinia appears to inhibit the body's conversion of calories into fats, to improve the body's ability to burn calories, and to lower the body's production of low-density lipoproteins (LDL), or "bad" cholesterol. It is used in the treatment of high cholesterol, indigestion, obesity, and rheumatism.

Topically, garcinia can be used as a gargle and mouthwash to treat spongy gums.

Edible Uses

The rind of the garcinia fruit is used primarily as a culinary seasoning. The fruit is very acidic and is not usually eaten raw.

Other Uses

The dried rind is used to polish gold and silver. It is also used to coagulate rubber latex.

Constituents

Hydroxycitric acid, gum, resin, essential oil

Energetic Correspondences

- Flavor: sour
- Temperature: warm
- Moisture: dry
- Polarity: yin
- Planet: Saturn
- Element: earth

Contraindications

Avoid during pregnancy and while nursing. Large doses may be cathartic. Those who are allergic to citric acid may be sensitive to garcinia as well.

Range and Appearance

The garcinia tree is native to India, Burma, Thailand, and Malaysia. It features orange-brown bark and long, laurel-like leaves. The tree is dioecious; the flowers are small and yellow. The fruits are about the size of crab apples, smooth, and orangish green. Each fruit bears a single seed.

GARLIC

Botanical Name

Allium sativum

Family

Lilliaceae (Lily Family)

Etymology

The genus name, *Allium,* is the Latin word for this plant. The species name, *sativum,* is Latin for "cultivated." The common name *garlic* derives from the Anglo-Saxon *gae,* "lance," in reference to the shape of the leaf, and *lic,* "leek."

Also Known As

Arabic: fum, thoum
Armenian: skhdor
Bulgarian: chesan, chesnov luk
Cantonese: syun tauh
Croatian: bijeli luk
Czech: cesnek
Danish: hvidlog
Dutch: knofloock
English: stinking rose
Esperanto: ajlo
Estonian: küüslauk
Finnish: valkosipuli
German: knoblauch
Greek: skordo
Hebrew: shum
Hindi: lasan
Icelandic: hvítlauker
Indonesian: bawang putih, kesuna
Italian: aglio
Japanese: garikku, ninniku, taisan
Korean: kallik
Laotian: van mahakan
Latvian: kiploki
Mandarin: da suan
Nepali: lasun
Norwegian: hvitlok
Polish: czosnek pospolity
Romanian: usturoi
Russian: chesnok
Sanskrit: lashuna
Serbian: beli luk
Spanish: ajo
Swahili: kitunguu sauma
Swedish: vitlök
Thai: gratiem
Tibetan: gogpa, sgog pa
Turkish: sarmisak
Ukrainian: chasnyk
Vietnamese: cây toi
Yiddish: knobl

Part Used

Bulb

Physiological Effects

Alterative, antibiotic, antifungal, aphrodisiac, carminative, diaphoretic, diuretic, expectorant, hypoglycemic, hypotensive, parasitacide, vasodilator, yang tonic

Medicinal Uses

Garlic shows activity against many types of infectious diseases, including staphylococcus, streptococcus, and salmonella bacteria. It also helps prevent blood platelet aggregation, which makes it of use in addressing problems of the circulatory system. It is used in the treatment of arterosclerosis, asthma, candida, catarrh, diabetes, high cholesterol, hypertension, obesity, tuberculosis, whooping cough, and worms.

Topically, garlic can be prepared as a bolus to treat yeast infection or an enema to treat dysentary. An uncut clove can be used as a suppository to treat hemorrhoids. Garlic-infused oil can be used as ear drops to treat ear infection or as a wash to treat gangrenous wounds and snakebite.

Edible Uses

The garlic rhizome is edible and has been used as a seasoning since ancient times. However, it loses its medicinal properties when heated.

Getting Rid of Garlic Breath

Garlic breath can result from garlic consumption, lasting for as long as ten hours. It can be overcome by chewing some anise, caraway, cardamom, cumin, or fennel seeds; chewing pieces of cinnamon or sprigs of parsley; or taking one drop of pure peppermint oil in a cup of water.

Other Uses

Eating garlic is said to repel mosquitoes and ticks (and vampires). Planting garlic in the garden helps repel pests.

Constituents

Allicine, essential oils (diallyl bisulphide, diallyl trisulphide, ajone), sulfur, germanium, selenium

Energetic Correspondences

- Flavor: pungent
- Temperature: hot
- Moisture: dry
- Polarity: yang
- Planet: Mars
- Element: fire

Contraindications

Excess amounts of garlic can be irritating to the stomach and kidneys; some people find that even small amounts of raw garlic can cause heartburn. Avoid large doses during pregnancy and while nursing, as it may cause digestive distress in the mother and baby. Some people may be allergic to garlic. Excessive use can provoke anger and emotional irritability.

Do not apply cut garlic directly to the skin for more than a few minutes, as it can burn the skin.

Range and Appearance

Garlic is believed to be native to central Asia but is widely cultivated. The leaves are long and flat, reaching up to 3 feet in length. The white, star-shaped flowers grow in umbels. Garlic, a perennial, is a popular garden plant and does well in fertile, moist soils in full sun.

GENTIAN

Botanical Name

Gentiana andrewsii (closed gentian), *G. lutea* (yellow gentian), *G. macrophylla*, *G. officinalis*, *G. scabra*, *G. villosa*

Family

Gentianaceae (Gentian Family)

Etymology

The genus name, *Gentiana*, and common name *gentian* derive from that of the second-century Illyrian king Gentius, who is said to have introduced this herb as a medicine.

Also Known As

Arabic: jintiyania
English: bitter root, longdan, Sampson's snakeroot
Finnish: keltakatkero
French: gentiane
German: bitterwurzel, enzianworzel, schnapswurzel
Italian: genziana
Japanese: jingyo, ryutan

Korean: chin'gyo
Mandarin: qín jiao
Sanskrit: trayamana
Swedish: gullentiana
Turkish: güsad

Parts Used

Root, rhizome

Physiological Effects

Alterative, anthelmintic, antiseptic, bitter, cholagogue, emmenagogue, febrifuge, ophthalmic, refrigerant, siliagogue, stomach tonic

Medicinal Uses

Gentian has been used as a digestive aid for centuries; it improves the assimilation of nutrients such as iron and vitamin B_{12} and aids in the breakdown of proteins and fats. Gentian is used in the treatment of amenorrhea, anorexia, appetite loss, arthritis, dog bite, dyspepsia, flatulence, gout, hepatitis, jaundice, joint inflammation, and malaria. It is also used as a poison antidote. For greatest effectiveness as a digestive aid, take tincture of gentian 10 to 30 minutes before mealtime.

Topically, a wash of gentian can be used to clean wounds and to treat snakebite.

As a flower essence, gentian is helpful for pessimists, helping them to have a more positive attitude.

Edible Uses

Gentian is so bitter that even when it is diluted to 1 part bitter to 12,000 parts other fluids; the bitterness can still be tasted. It is not generally considered edible, aside from therapeutic use, though it is used to flavor beverages such as vermouth and bitters.

Other Uses

Veterinarians use gentian to stimulate the appetite of animals. Folk wisdom of Appalachia holds that carrying a piece of gentian root in your pocket will increase your physical strength.

Constituents

Bitter principles (amarogentian, gentiopricin), quinic acid, inulin, pectin, galacton, iron, phosphorous, resin

Energetic Correspondences

- Flavor: bitter
- Temperature: cold
- Moisture: dry
- Polarity: yin
- Planet: Saturn/Mercury/Mars
- Element: earth

Contraindications

Gentian can aggravate hyperacidic conditions and ulcers. Large doses can cause nausea and vomiting.

Range and Appearance

Gentian is an annual or perennial native to North America and Eurasia. It produces long, branched, opposite whorls or pairs of simple leaves and four to seven hermaphroditic, lobed, bell- or funnel-shaped flowers that are white, yellowish green, or blue-violet to purple. The seeds are long and winged. The fleshy rhizome is yellowish brown and wrinkled. The plant prefers moist soil in full sun to partial shade.

GINGER

Botanical Name

Zingiber officinale

Family

Zingiberaceae (Ginger Family)

Etymology

The genus name, *Zingiber,* and common name *ginger* derive from the ancient Greek word for the plant, *zingiberi,* which is itself thought to be of Indo-Aryan origin and possibly to mean "shaped like a horn."

Also Known As

Arabic: zanjabeel
Armenian: gojanghbegh
Bulgarian: dzhindzhifil
Cantonese: geung

Croatian: dumbir, ingver

Danish: ingefær

Dutch: gember

Esperanto: zingibro

Estonian: harilik ingver

Finnish: inkivääri

French: gingembre

German: ingwer

Greek: dzinder, piperoriza

Hebrew: sangvil

Hindi: adi

Hmong: kai

Hungarian: gyömbér

Icelandic: engifer

Indonesian: jahé, lia

Italian: zenzero

Japanese: jinja, shoga

Korean: jinjeo, kon-gang

Loatian: khing

Mandarin: jiang

Nepali: aduwa

Norwegian: ingefær

Polish: imbir

Portuguese: gengibre

Romanian: ghimbir

Sanskrit: adraka, nagara, shunthi

Serbian: ingver

Slovenian: ingver

Spanish: jengibre

Swahili: tangawizi

Swedish: ingefära

Thai: kinkh

Tibetan: gamag, sga smug

Turkish: zencefil

Ukranian: imbyr

Vietnamese: can khuong, gùng

Yiddish: imber, ingber

Part Used

Rhizome

Physiological Effects

Analgesic, antibacterial, antiemetic, antifungal, anti-inflammatory, antioxidant, antiparasitic, antiseptic, antispasmodic, antitussive, antiviral, aperient, aphro-disiac, aromatic, cardiotonic, carminative, choleretic, circulatory stimulant, diaphoretic, emmenagogue, expectorant, febrifuge, hepatoprotective, rubefacient, sialogogue, stimulant, stomachic, vermifuge, yang tonic

Medicinal Uses

Ginger has been found to be even more effective than Dramamine in curbing motion sickness, without causing drowsiness. As a digestive aid, it warms the digestive organs, stimulates digestive secretions, increases the amylase concentration in saliva, and facilitates the digestion of starches and fatty foods. It also strengthens the tissues of the heart, activates the immune system, prevents blood platelet aggregation and leukotriene formation, and inhibits prostaglandin production, thus reducing inflammation and pain. Ginger is often included in other herbal formulas, especially those that contain laxative herbs to reduce gripe.

The dried root is hotter than the fresh root and is more effective in relieving nausea and warming the body. Fresh ginger is considered best for respiratory problems and dried ginger for digestive ailments.

Ginger root is used in the treatment of amenorrhea, angina, ankylosing spondylitis, anxiety, arthritis, asthma, atherosclerosis, bloating, bronchitis, cancer, catarrh, chemotherapy side effects, chills, claudication (intermittent), colds, colic, cough (with white phlegm), cramps, delayed menses, depression, dyspepsia, erectile dysfunction, fatigue, flatulence, flu, food poisoning, gastritis, headache, high cholesterol, hypertension, hypothyroidism, indigestion, irritable bowel, laryngitis, low libido, lumbago, menstrual cramps, migraines, morning sickness, nausea, obesity, pain, poor circulation, post-anesthesia nausea, Raynaud's disease, low sperm count and motility, stomachache, vertigo, wheezing, and worms. It is also used to prevent blood clots, stroke, and heart attack.

Topically, ginger can be prepared as a compress and applied over arthritic joints, bunions, sore muscles, and toothaches to relieve pain; over the kidneys to relieve the pain and assist in the passage of stones; over the chest or back to relieve asthma symptoms;

or over the temples to relieve headache. Ginger is wonderful in the bath in cases of chills, muscle soreness, sciatica, and poor circulation. It can be used in foot soaks to treat athlete's foot or to relieve the head congestion associated with colds and flu. It also can be brewed as a tea and gargled to relieve a sore throat.

Edible Uses

Ginger root is a popular spice that adds a pungent, warming quality to dishes. Slices of pickled ginger are often served with sushi, while candied ginger is a popular snack that also calms nausea. The leaves are also sometimes used as a flavoring agent.

As a tea ginger root is aromatic with a pleasant zesty bite. The flowers can also be made into a tea with a similarly spicy but milder flavor.

Other Uses

In magical traditions, ginger is said to attract love, prosperity, and success.

Constituents

Sulfur, protein, proteolytic enzyme (zingibain), bisabolenel, oleoresins, starch, essential oils (zingiberene, zingiberole, gingerols, shogoal, camphene, cineol, borneol, citral), acetic acid, mucilage

Energetic Correspondences

- Flavor: pungent, sweet, bitter
- Temperature: warm
- Moisture: dry
- Polarity: yang
- Planet: Mars
- Element: fire

Contraindications

Although ginger can relieve morning sickness, pregnant women should not ingest more than 1 gram daily. Avoid in cases of peptic ulcers, hyperacidity, or other hot, inflammatory conditions. Avoid excessive amounts of ginger in cases of acne, eczema, or herpes. Ginger may cause adverse reactions when used in combination with anticoagulant drugs such as Coumadin or aspirin; if you are using such medica-

tions, seek the advice of a qualified health-care practitioner before commencing use of ginger.

Range and Appearance

Ginger, native to tropical eastern Asia, is a perennial with long green stalks that can grow to 4 feet in height and long, narrow, alternate leaves. The greenish, yellow, or white flowers are streaked with purple and are borne on short, dense spikes. The root is a creeping tuber with several fingerlike protrusions and a pale skin that turns brownish upon drying; it is commonly sold in grocery stores.

The plant thrives in partial shade in fertile, moist, well-drained soils. In gardens in temperate climates, the plant will need to be brought indoors when the cold weather begins.

Do not confuse ginger with wild ginger (*Asarum canadensis*), which is unrelated.

GINKGO

Botanical Name

Ginkgo biloba

Family

Ginkgoaceae (Ginkgo Family)

Etymology

The genus name, *Ginkgo*, derives from the Japanese *ginkyō*, meaning "silver apricot." The species name, *biloba*, derives from the Latin *bis*, "double," and *loba*, "lobes," in reference to the two-lobed leaves.

Also Known As

Cantonese: baak gwat yip, gan hang yip
Czech: jinan dvoulalocny'
Danish: tempeltræ
Dutch: tempelboom
English: Buddha's fingernails, fossil tree,
    grandfather and grandson tree, maidenhair tree
Finnish: neidonhiuspuu, temppelipuu
French: noyer du japon
Icelandic: musteristré
German: ginkgobaum
Hindi: balkuwari

Hungarian: páfrányfenyõ
Italian: ginco
Japanese: ginkyō
Korean: hangjamok, unhaeng
Mandarin: bai guo ye (leaf), yin guo (seed), yin xing ye (leaf)
Portuguese: nogueira-do-japão
Spanish: arbol de las pagodas, arbol sagrado
Swedish: tempelträd
Turkish: mabet agaci
Vietnamese: cây lá quat

Parts Used

Leaf (harvested when starting to yellow, then dried), seed (nut)

Physiological Effects

Leaf: antibacterial, anticoagulant, antifungal, anti-inflammatory, antioxidant, brain tonic, cardiotonic, circulatory stimulant, decongestant, kidney tonic, neuroprotective, rejuvenative, vasodilator
Seed: anthelmintic, antibacterial, antifungal, antitussive, astringent, cardiotonic, digestive, expectorant, sedative

Medicinal Uses

Ginkgo is the oldest tree species on the planet, having been common even when dinosaurs roamed the earth. It has a high resistance to disease, insects, and pollution.

Ginkgo leaf helps relax blood vessels, improving circulation and the delivery of nutrients, including oxygen and glucose, throughout the body, including the brain. It strengthens fragile capillaries and interferes with platelet-activating factor, a protein that can trigger spasms in the lungs. Concentrated ginkgo leaf increases the synthesis of dopamine, norepinephrine, and other neurotransmitters. Ginkgo leaf is used in the treatment of allergies, altitude sickness, Alzheimer's disease, angina, anxiety, arteriosclerosis, asthma, bronchitis, cataracts, claudication (intermittent), cough, dementia, depression, dizziness, dysentery, eczema, erectile dysfunction, fatigue, hearing loss, hemorrhoids, high cholesterol, leg cramps, leukorrhea, macular degeneration, memory loss, nerve-related deafness, optic neuropathy, pain in the extremities, poor circulation, Raynaud's disease, senility, shortness of breath, tinnitus, tuberculosis, varicose veins, vertigo, and vision loss. It is also used to prevent and speed recovery from stroke and in the prevention and treatment of blood clots.

Ginkgo seed (nut) inhibits the production of phlegm and shows activity against a variety of pathogens. It is used in the treatment of alcohol toxicity, asthma, bladder irritation, bronchitis, cancer, catarrh, cough, diphtheria, dysentery, gonorrhea, hangover, incontinence, kidney weakness, leukorrhea, polyuria, spermatorrhea, typhoid, tuberculosis, vaginal infection, and wheezing.

Topically, ginkgo seed can be used as a poultice to rid the body of scabies, ringworm, and sores.

Edible Uses

The inner seeds are edible if boiled or roasted. The leaves are not generally considered edible, aside from as tea.

Other Uses

Ginkgo leaves can be placed in books to prevent insects from eating the pages.

Constituents

Leaf: beta-carotene, vitamin C, superoxide dismutase, flavonoids (ginkgolide, quercitin, rutin, kaempferol), ginkgolic acid, terpene lactones ginkgolides, bilobalide, bilobetin, ginkgolides, proanthocyanidins
Seed: calcium, iron, phosphorous, gibberellin, essential oil, ginkgolic acid, fatty acid, tannin, resin

Energetic Correspondences

- Flavor: sweet, bitter
- Temperature: leaf—neutral; seed—warm
- Moisture: dry
- Polarity: yin
- Planet: Sun/Mercury/Venus/Mars
- Element: air

Contraindications

Side effects from using unstandardized ginkgo leaves are rare. However, large amounts or concentrations have been reported to cause gastrointestinal disturbance, irritability, restlessness, and headache. Ginkgo leaf can negatively affect the blood's ability to clot, so avoid ginkgo for at least a week before surgery; in cases of hemophilia; or in concurrence with anticoagulant drugs such as Coumadin, aspirin, or monoamine-oxidase inhibitors.

Fruit from the female trees may cause contact dermatitis or mouth lesions. Do not eat the pulp of the fruit. (It smells like dog poop, so who would want to?) Even standing over roasting seeds can cause eye irritation and dermatitis.

Avoid long-term use of the seed, and do not take more than ten seeds at a time. Excess use may cause fever, headache, irritation of the mucous membranes and skin, or emotional irritability.

Range and Appearance

Ginkgo is a large deciduous tree that is native to China. It reaches a height of about 130 feet and has an erect trunk with cracked gray bark. The leaves are broad and fan shaped, with two lobes and numerous parallel veins. The tree is dioecious, meaning female and male flowers are produced on separate trees. The male flowers grow on catkins; female flowers grow in pairs on 12-inch stalks. The fruits are yellow-orange and plum shaped.

GINSENG

Botanical Name

Panax ginseng (Asian ginseng), *P. quinquefolium* (American ginseng)

Family

Araliaceae (Ginseng Family)

Etymology

The common name *ginseng* derives from the Mandarin name for the plant, *ren shen,* which translates roughly as "essence of the earth in the form of a man," a reference to the humanlike shape of some ginseng roots. The genus name, *Panax,* derives from

the Greek *panakes,* "panacea," and *seng,* the term for a fleshy root that is used as a tonic.

Also Known As

Cantonese: sei yang sam (*P. quinquefolium*)
English: divine herb, essence of man, five fingers, human root, pannag, red berry, sang, spirit herb, tartar root
French: panax
German: gensang
Italian: ginseng
Japanese: ninjin (*P. ginseng*), siyojin (*P. quinquefolium*)
Korean: insam (*P. ginseng*)
Spanish: ginsen
Mandarin: hua qi shen (*P. quinquefolium*), ren shen (*P. ginseng*), xi shen (*P. quinquefolium*), xi yang shen (*P. quinquefolium*)
Sanskrit: lakshmana
Turkish: sinseng

Part Used

Root

Physiological Effects

Adaptogen, analgesic, antiallergenic, anti-inflammatory, antioxidant, antispasmodic, antiviral, aphrodisiac, cardiotonic, carminative, chi tonic, demulcent, digestive, endocrine tonic, febrifuge (*P. quinquefolium*), hepatoprotective, hypoglycemic, hypotensive, immune tonic, nervine, nutritive, phytoandrogenic, rejuvenative, restorative, sialagogue, stimulant, tonic

Medicinal Uses

Asian ginseng has an incredibly long history of use in Chinese medicine, dating back some six thousand years. It is valued especially for its restorative and energizing properties. In the 1700s French missionaries discovered that a plant growing near the Great Lakes and being used by native peoples in love potions and as a tonic was a New World relative of the Asian species. Due to overharvesting of wild ginseng in China, there was a ripe market for this American commodity, which of course led to the overharvesting on this continent as well. Even Daniel

Boone was a ginseng harvester. American ginseng has properties similar to those of Asian gingeng, but it is considered to be milder, and it is more likely to be prescribed for younger people.

Ginseng, of either variety, helps the body better utilize oxygen, spares glycogen utilization, increases cerebral circulation, helps the adrenal glands to better conserve their stores of vitamin C, aids in stabilizing blood sugar levels, helps balance hormone levels in men and women, reduces LDL ("bad" cholesterol) levels while elevating HDL ("good" cholesterol) levels, and aids in the production of DNA, RNA, interferon, and red and white blood cells. It can improve stamina, reaction time, and concentration, which make it useful for such pursuits as studying, taking tests, long-distance driving, and meditating. It also speeds recovery time from sickness, surgery, childbirth, athletic performance, and other stressors to the body.

Ginseng is used in the treatment of adrenal deficiency, AIDS, Alzheimer's disease, anemia, appetite loss, atherosclerosis, chemotherapy side effects, chronic fatigue, depression, diabetes, diarrhea (chronic), drug addiction and withdrawal symptoms, erectile dysfunction, fatigue, heart palpitations, infertility (male and female), insomnia, low libido, low sperm count, malabsorption, memory loss, menopause symptoms, night sweats, organ prolapse, post-traumatic stress (physical and emotional), radiation exposure, shortness of breath, stress, stroke, and tuberculosis.

American ginseng is white; the root is simply harvested and cleaned. Asian ginseng, on the other hand, is often steamed with herbs and wine, which gives it a reddish color and a more warming quality. Thus American ginseng is more often used during the warmer times of the year, while Asian ginseng is best used during cooler seasons.

Ginseng's effects are cumulative, and most benefit occurs after a period of use, although some users will notice immediate effects. Many athletes use it for a week prior to a competition.

Although the root is the primary medicinal component of the plant, the leaves of both varieties can be used to treat hangover and fever.

When to Take Ginseng

For best effect, take ginseng between meals rather than with food. It is best not to take ginseng at night, as it could impair sleep.

Edible Uses

The root is edible when soaked or cooked if dried; it is commonly added to soups and grain dishes. The root also makes a delicious and therapeutic candy. It also can be infused in liqueur or wine.

Other Uses

Ginseng is often included in anti-wrinkle facial products as it helps heal and soften the skin.

Constituents

B vitamins, acetylcholine, copper, germanium, manganese, phosphorous, selenium, saponins (ginsenosides, also known as panaxosides), triterpene glycosides, phytosterols (beta-sitosterol, stigmasterol, campesterol), essential oils (farnesene, hexadecane, gurjunene)

Energetic Correspondences

- Flavor: sweet, slightly bitter
- Temperature: *P. ginseng*—warm; *P. quinquefolium*—warm
- Moisture: *P. ginseng*—dry; *P. quinquefolium*—moist
- Polarity: yang
- Planet: Sun
- Element: fire

Contraindications

Avoid ginseng in cases of heat and inflammation, such as fever, flu, pneumonia, hypertension, or constipation. Do not give to children for prolonged periods, as it may cause early sexual maturation. Avoid during pregnancy and while nursing. Do not take ginseng in conjunction with cardiac glycosides except under the guidance of a qualified health-care professional.

The neck of ginseng root is mildly emetic and not used as a tonic.

Range and Appearance

Ginseng is a perennial that grows in shady hardwood forests of North America (*P. quinquefolius*) and temperate regions of Asia (*P. ginseng*). The stalk reaches a height of 1 to 2 feet. The leaves are palmate and divided into three to seven (usually five) sharply toothed leaflets. The hermaphroditic flowers are white to yellowish and grow in round umbels. Red berries follow the flowers.

Ginseng is not a quick cash crop, as the roots must be five to seven years old before they become ready for harvesting.

GOJI

Botanical Name

Lycium barbarum, L. chinense

Family

Solanaceae (Nightshade Family)

Etymology

Lycium, the genus name, is believed to derive from the name of the mid-Asian region Lydia, from which this plant may have originated. The common name *goji* derives from the Chinese names for this plant.

Also Known As

Cantonese: gei ji
English: boxthorn, desert thorn, happy berry, lycii, matrimony vine, wolfberry
German: bocksdorn
Italian: licio
Japanese: jikoppi, kuko, kukoshi
Korean: kugicha
Mandarin: gou ji zi, gou qi zi, zhou qi
Thai: gao gèe

Parts Used

Berry (primarily), root bark (rarely), leaf (rarely)

Physiological Effects

Alterative, antibacterial, antimutagenic, antioxidant, aphrodisiac, blood tonic, decongestant, demulcent, diuretic, febrifuge, hemostatic, hepatoprotective, hypoglycemic, hypotensive, immune stimulant, kidney tonic, liver tonic, nutritive, rejuvenative, restorative, vasodilator, yin tonic

Medicinal Uses

In Asia goji berry is traditionally used as a longevity tonic that nourishes the kidneys and liver. It is known to stimulate the production of hormones, interferon, white blood cells, enzymes, and blood. It also increases levels of the antioxidant superoxide dismutase and hemoglobin while decreasing levels of lipid peroxides, and it nourishes bone marrow and helps remove toxins from the blood by strengthening the kidneys and liver.

Goji berries are used to treat anemia, asthma, bronchitis, cancer, chemotherapy and radiation side effects, colds, complexion problems, cough, diabetes, dizziness, erectile dysfunction, exhaustion, eye problems (cataracts, dry eye syndrome, macular degeneration, night blindness, photosensitivity, retinitis, blurred vision, and poor vision due to malnutrition), fatigue, fever, hair loss, hiccups, high cholesterol, hypoglycemia, infertility, knee weakness, leukorrhea, low libido, low testosterone levels, lumbago, menopause symptoms, night sweats, pneumonia, premature aging, prematurely gray hair, seminal and nocturnal emissions, senility, thirst, tinnitus, tuberculosis, and vertigo.

The root bark calms coughs, lowers fever, and reduces blood pressure.

Goji leaves appear to increase collagen synthesis. They are used topically as a poultice to treat bedsores, burns, frostbite, furuncles, and insect bites.

Edible Uses

Goji berries are edible fresh or dried (like raisins). They are often an ingredient in medicinal wines. The young leaves and shoots are also edible; they can be eaten raw. The root is edible but should be cooked.

Other Uses

Asian folklore claims that goji berries enhance beauty and cheerfulness when taken for long periods. The plants have an extensive root system and are sometimes used to stabilize soil in sandy areas in an effort to combat soil erosion.

Constituents

Carotenoids (physalin, zeaxanthin, beta-carotene), vitamin C, vitamins B_1 and B_2, niacin, iron, selenium, zinc, linoleic acid, amino acids (tryptophan, arginine, leucine, isoleucine), polysaccharides, phenols, betaine, beta-sitosterol

Energetic Correspondences

- Flavor: sweet, slightly sour
- Temperature: neutral
- Moisture: moist
- Polarity: neutral (yin/yang)
- Planet: Mars/Venus
- Element: water

Contraindications

Avoid in cases of acute fever or dampness, such as diarrhea and bloating. Otherwise goji is considered very safe, even for daily consumption.

Range and Appearance

Goji, native to eastern Asia, is an evergreen, thorny plant with spine-tipped stems that can grow to 6 feet in height. The leaves are narrow, succulent, and covered with a whitish film. The hermaphroditic flowers are tubular and purple hued. The berries are a vibrant red. Goji grows well in poor, well-drained soils in full sun.

Although the berries are bright red when on the bush, they lose some color when dried. When purchasing goji berries, avoid those that remain bright red; they probably have been treated with sulfite preservatives.

GOLDENROD

Botanical Name

Solidago spp.

Family

Asteraceae (Daisy Family)

Etymology

The genus name, *Solidago,* comes from the Latin *solidus* and *agere,* meaning "to make whole" or "to bring together." The common name *goldenrod* refers to the long panicle of golden blossoms.

Also Known As

English: Aaron's rod, blue mountain tea, fastening herb, golden wings, pagan wound herb, Saint Peter's staff, sun medicine, wound weed, yellow weed

Finnish: isopiisku, kanadanpiisku

French: herbe aux juifs, herbe des juifs, verge d'or

German: goldrute, heidnisch wundkraut

Italian: erba giudaica, pioggia d'oro, verga aurea, verga d'oro

Mandarin: hsiao pai-lung

Russian: zolotarnik obiknovenny

Spanish: oreja de libre

Swedish: höstgullris, kanadensiskt gullris

Part Used

Aboveground plant

Physiological Effects

Analgesic, anthelmintic, anticatarrhal, antifungal, anti-inflammatory, antioxidant, antiseptic, antitumor, aromatic, astringent, carminative, cordial, diaphoretic, diuretic, expectorant, febrifuge, hemostatic, hepatic, hypotensive, kidney cleanser, mucolytic, stimulant, styptic, tonic, vulnerary

Medicinal Uses

Goldenrod was a prominent wound-healing remedy during the Middle Ages. Goldenrod was an official herb in the United States Pharmacopoeia from 1820 till 1882. It is known to cleanse the kidneys, promote tissue healing, dry dampness, help thin mucus secretions, and reduce inflammation. Goldenrod is used to treat amenorrhea, arthritis, asthma, bedwetting, bladder stones, bladder weakness or injury, Bright's disease, bronchitis, candida, catarrh, cholera, colds, coughs, cystitis, diarrhea, diphtheria, dropsy, dysentery, dysuria, eczema, exhaustion, fever, flu, gallstones, gout, hay fever, intestinal ulceration, jaundice, kidney stones, kidney chi and yin deficiency, kidney inflammation, lung hemorrhage, malaria, measles, menorrhagia, menstrual cramps, nausea, nephritis, prostate enlargement, rheumatism, scrofula, sore throat (the Zuni chewed the fresh flower for this purpose), stomachache, tuberculosis, urethritis, urinary infection (chronic), worms, and yeast infection.

Topically, a wash, compress, liniment, or poultice of goldenrod can be used to treat arthritis, boils, burns, eczema, headache, rheumatism, snakebite, swelling, or wounds. The plant can be prepared as a poultice to treat insect bites and burns; as a gargle to treat sore throat, laryngitis, or thrush; as a mouthwash to treat toothache; as a douche to treat yeast infection; or as a hair rinse to prevent hair loss. Goldenrod is also traditionally prepared as a wash for women to use after giving birth.

Edible Uses

Young goldenrod leaves and flowers can be eaten raw or added to cooked dishes. The seeds are also edible and sometimes are used to thicken soup. The flowers are sometimes infused in wine.

Other Uses

Goldenrod is sometimes added to smoking mixtures. It can be hung in the home as a natural air freshener. The leaves and flowers yield a yellow, green, or gold dye. The plant was once used to make sneezing powder, which was sold as a gag. Thomas Edison developed a rubberlike substance from goldenrod, but it proved too expensive to market commercially.

Constituents

Flavonoids (quercitin, rutin, isoquercitrin, astragalin), saponins, diterpenes, phenolic glycosides, inulin, leiocarposide, salicylic acid, essential oil, tannins

Energetic Correspondences

- Flavor: bitter, pungent
- Temperature: warm
- Moisture: dry
- Polarity: yin
- Planet: Sun/Venus
- Element: air

Contraindications

In cases of chronic kidney disorder, consult with a qualified health-care practitioner before using goldenrod. Avoid in cases of edema resulting from heart failure or kidney failure.

Goldenrod is often accused of causing hay fever. However, its pollen is actually quite heavy and falls to the earth rather than becoming airborne. It is more likely ragweed, which blooms at the same time as goldenrod that is culprit.

Range and Appearance

Goldenrod is native to all temperate regions on the earth. Nearly one hundred species grow in North America alone. It is found growing in clearings, fields, woodlands, roadsides, and just about any spot that gets a good amount of sunshine, whether in dry or moist conditions. The stalk of the plant reaches about 5 feet in height. The leaves are alternate, lanceolate, oblong, and slightly dentate. The hermaphroditic flowers (both ray and discs) are bright golden yellow and arranged in panicles. Bees, butterflies, and flies all drink goldenrod nectar.

In the garden, goldenrod provides food for butterflies, bees, and many valuable insects, including lacewings and ladybugs.

GOLDENSEAL

Botanical Name

Hydrastis canadensis

Family

Ranunculaceae (Buttercup Family)

Etymology

The genus name, *Hydrastis,* is from the Greek *hydrastina,* "water acting," in reference to the drying effect goldenseal has upon the body's mucous membranes. It is called goldenseal because of the appearance of seals (like those used with sealing wax) on the root, which are the result of the stalk dying down.

Also Known As

English: eye balm root, ground raspberry, Indian dye, Indian paint, jaundice root, Ohio curcuma, orange root, turmeric root, yellow puccoon, yellow root, wild curcuma

Finnish: hydrastis

French: racine d'or, racine orange, sceau d'or

German: gelbwurzel, hydrastisrhizom, wasserblatt, wasserkraut

Italian: idraste

Spanish: hidrastide del Canada

Part Used

Rhizome

Physiological Effects

Alterative, antibacterial, antibiotic, anticatarrhal, antifungal, anti-inflammatory, antiseptic, antispasmodic, antiviral, astringent, bitter, cholagogue, decongestant, digestive, diuretic, endocrine tonic, febrifuge, glandular deobstruent, hemostatic, hypertensive, laxative, mucous-membrane tonic, oxytocic, restorative, spleen tonic, stomachic, stomach tonic, styptic, vasoconstrictor

Medicinal Uses

Goldenseal was widely used by Native Americans, especially the Cherokee, Comanche, Crow, and Iroquois. It was an official herb in the United States Pharmacopoeia from 1831 to 1841 and again from 1863 to 1936, and it was included in the National Formulary from 1936 to 1960. Goldenseal clears heat, breaks up congestion, arrests bleeding, dries mucus and dampness, and fights infection. Berberine, one of goldenseal's alkaloids, has activity against amoebas, cholera, *E. coli,* giardia, staph, strep, yeast, and protozoas.

Goldenseal is used to treat appetite loss, bladder infection, bronchitis, cancer, catarrh, cholera, colds, colitis, cystitis, diabetes, diarrhea, dysentery, ear infection, fever, flu, gallstones, gastritis, gastrointestinal infection, giardia, gonorrhea, hemorrhage, hepatitis, herpes, indigestion, infection, jaundice, malaria, measles, menorrhagia, parasites, pelvic inflammatory disease, pharyngitis, pneumonia, postpartum bleeding (excessive), scarlet fever, small pox, sinusitis, sore throat, tonsillitis, typhoid, tuberculosis, ulcers, and urinary tract infection.

Topically, goldenseal can be used as a compress, wash, or poultice to treat acne, athlete's foot, eczema, herpes, impetigo, poison ivy, ringworm, and wounds. It makes an excellent gargle to treat gum infection, mouth sores, sore throat, pyorrhea, and thrush and can be used as a powder to treat tooth and gum infection. It can be used as an eyewash to treat conjunctivitis, corneal inflammation, and sties or as eardrops (mixed with olive oil) to treat ear infection. A goldenseal douche helps curb leukorrhea, candida, chlamydia, pelvic inflammatory disease, trichomonas, and vaginitis. Goldenseal is also a traditional snuff to treat nasal congestion, nose polyps, and sinus infection.

Edible Uses

Goldenseal is extremely bitter and so is not considered an edible plant.

Other Uses

Many Native American tribes used goldenseal as an ingredient in face paint, to dye clothing, and to repel insects.

Constituents

Calcium, chromium, manganese, potassium, silicon, sulfur, unsaturated fatty acids, alkaloids (berberine, hydrastine, canadine, berberastine, canadaline, hydrastinine), flavonoids, resin, albumin, starch, chlorogenic acid

Energetic Correspondences

• Flavor: bitter

• Temperature: cold

- Moisture: dry
- Polarity: yin
- Planet: Sun/Saturn
- Element: earth

Contraindications

Avoid during pregnancy, in cases of high blood pressure, or in the week preceding surgery, as it may increase blood pressure. It also can elevate blood sugar levels and blood pressure in one who is already so inclined; use only under the guidance of a qualified health-care professional in such cases. Use only for short periods (three weeks or less), as long-term use can kill off friendly intestinal flora and reduce assimilation of B vitamins. Follow a course of goldenseal with probiotics such as acidophilus. Large amounts may cause diarrhea and over stimulate the nervous system. The fresh plant can be irritating to mucous membranes.

Range and Appearance

Goldenseal, native to Canada and the eastern United States, is a perennial that grows from 6 to 12 inches tall in the rich soil of moist, shady woods. It usually has two leaves, each with five to seven lobes, doubly toothed, with one leaf larger than the other. The flowers are single, small, and greenish white, with rose-colored sepals. A raspberry-looking fruit, containing ten to thirty black seeds, appears after the flower (note that it is not edible).

Goldenseal is endangered in the wild; overharvesting is contributing to its demise. To protect the few remaining wild populations, buy only cultivated goldenseal.

GOTU KOLA

Botanical Name

Centella asiatica (formerly *Hydrocotyle asiatica*)

Family

Apiaceae (Parsley Family)

Etymology

The origin of the genus name, *Centella,* is uncertain; it may derive from the Greek *kentron,* "sharp point." The former genus name, *Hydrocotyle,* derives from two Greek words, *hydro,* "water," and *kotyle,* "plant." The species name, *asiatica,* denotes that the plant is native to Asia. The leaves resemble Chinese coins, hence the folk name *pennywort.*

Also Known As

Afrikaans: varkoortjies
Arabic: arrtaniyal-hindi
Cantonese: gam hok chou
English: elixir of life, gagan-gagan, ground ivy, marsh pennywort, pennywort, white rot
Finnish: intiansammakonputki, makonputk, rohtosammakonputki
French: ecueille d'eau, hydrocotyle asiatique
German: wassernabel, wasswenabel
Hindu: brahmamanduki
Italian: idrpcotile, scodella d'acque
Mandarin: han ke cao
Sanskrit: manduka parn, brahmi
Turkish: su tasi

Part Used

Aboveground plant

Physiological Effects

Adaptogen, alterative, analgesic, antibacterial, anti-inflammatory, antioxidant, antirheumatic, antiseptic, antispasmodic, astringent, brain tonic, circulatory stimulant, decongestant, demulcent, depurative, diuretic, endocrine tonic, febrifuge, hypotensive, immune tonic, laxative, nervine, rejuvenative, tonic, vasodilator, vulnerary

Medicinal Uses

In Asia gotu kola has long been considered to be a longevity tonic. An old Singhalese proverb says of gotu kola, "Two leaves a day will keep old age away." And there are reports of a Chinese herbalist, Li Ching Yun, who supposedly lived to be 256 years old and was a regular consumer of gotu kola.

Gotu kola is known to strengthen the body's membranes, help restore strength to the venous walls and connective tissue, calm the mind, improve neural transport, and help the body detoxify. It is believed to improve the movement of energy from the left and right brain hemispheres. It is used to treat age spots, AIDS, amnesia, appetite loss, asthma, attention deficit disorder, boils, cellulite, cirrhosis, convulsions, depression, dermatitis, drug addiction, eczema, encephalitis, epilepsy, fatigue, fever, hair loss, hay fever, hemorrhoids, hepatitis, insanity, jaundice, keloid scars, leprosy, lupus, malaria, memory loss, mental confusion, mental retardation, nervous breakdown, neuralgia, neurosis, phlebitis, poisoning, premature aging, scleroderma, schizophrenia, scrofula, senility, sinusitis, syphilis, tuberculosis, tumors, varicose veins, venereal disease, vision weakness, and wound healing. It is also used to encourage convalescence after surgery or accident.

Both when taken internally and when applied topically in the form of an oil or salve, gotu kola can help stimulate collagen production, improve cutaneous microcirculation, and stimulate cellular mitosis. It can prevent scar formation and improve wound healing time and is used in the treatment of burns, eczema, gangrene, hemorrhoids, leprosy, lupus, and psoriasis. It also can encourage the healing of skin grafts.

Edible Uses

The fresh leaves can be eaten raw or cooked. In Asia you can find a variety of gotu-kola-based sodas.

Other Uses

Gotu kola is often taken as a brain tonic. On the first day of spring in Nepal, for example, gotu kola leaves are given to schoolchildren to improve their concentration and memory skills. The herb is sometimes used in cosmetics for its regenerative and skin-firming properties.

Constituents

Beta-carotene, B vitamins, vitamin C, calcium, iron, magnesium, glutamate, serine, lysine, histidine, Asiatic acid, madecassic acid, triterpene glycosides (asiaticoside, brahmoside, thankuniside), alkaloid (hydrocotyline), sterols (stigmasterol, sitosterol) tannin, vallarin, essential oil

Energetic Correspondences

- Flavor: bitter, sweet
- Temperature: cool
- Moisture: moist
- Polarity: yin
- Planet: Moon/Neptune
- Element: water

Contraindications

Large doses can cause headache, itching, stupor, and vertigo. Avoid during pregnancy, except under the guidance of a qualified health-care practitioner. Avoid in cases of overactive thyroid.

Range and Appearance

Gout kola is native to eastern Asia, Australia, and the South Pacific. It is a spreading, low-growing annual that thrives in swampy conditions such as marches and riverbanks. Its flexible stalks run close to the ground. The leaves are bright green, kidney shaped or round, and alternate. The white or pinkish flowers grow from the leaf axils in umbellate florescences.

GRAVEL ROOT

Botanical Name

Eupatorium maculatum, E. purpureum, E. ternifolium, E. verticullatum

Family

Asteraceae (Daisy Family)

Etymology

The genus name, *Eupatorium,* honors an ancient Persian king, Mithrades Eupator, who was a renowned herbalist. The common name *gravel root* refers to the plant's long history of use in helping the body rid itself of stones. The common names *joe-pye weed* and *jopi weed* derive from that of Joe Pye (or Jopi), who, according to folklore, was a Native American medicine man in New England who used the plant to treat typhus. The common name *queen* _of the meadow_ is a reference to the plant's beautiful and stately purple or pink flowers.

Also Known As

English: feverweed, hempweed, joe-pye weed, jopi weed, kidney root, marsh milkweed, purple boneset, queen of the meadow, tall boneset, thoroughwort, trumpetweed

Finnish: punalatva

French: eupatoire

German: purpur-wasseredost

Italian: canapa

Swedish: rosenflockel

Parts Used

Root (primarily), entire plant (rarely)

Physiological Effects

Antirheumatic, astringent, carminative, diaphoretic, diuretic, emmenagogue, immune stimulant, lithotriptic, nervine, stimulant, tonic

Medicinal Uses

Ojibwa Indians would wash their children, up until about the age of six, with a solution of gravel root tea to strengthen them. The plant was widely used by Native American tribes in treating kidney problems. It is known to balance the genitourinary system, cleanse the kidneys, clear heat, calm inflammation, and help the body eliminate uric acid. It is used to treat arthritis, asthma, bedwetting, bladder irritation, bladder stones, cough, cystitis, difficult labor, dropsy, enlarged prostate, erectile dysfunction, fever, flu, gallstones, gout, hematuria, incontinence, kidney stones, lumbago, polyuria, prostatitis, rheumatism, threatened miscarriage, typhus, urethritis, and uterine prolapse.

Edible Uses

Gravel root is not generally considered edible. The roots were at one time burned and powdered for use as a salt substitute.

Other Uses

A red dye can be made from the seeds.

Constituents

Protein, carbohydrates (polysaccharides), flavonoids (quercitin, euparin), oleoresin (eupatorin), sesqiuterpene lactones, essential oil, resin, tannin

Energetic Correspondences

- Flavor: bitter, pungent
- Temperature: cool
- Moisture: dry
- Polarity: yin
- Planet: Saturn
- Element: earth

Contraindications

Large doses may cause vomiting. Avoid during pregnancy. Gravel root contains some pyrrolizidine alkaloids (see page 100 [comfrey]), and it is not recommended for use for periods of more than six weeks.

Range and Appearance

Gravel root is a perennial native to the meadows, woodlands, and lowlands of Europe and eastern North America. It usually reaches a height of about 6 feet but on occasion 12 feet. The stems are green, with a purplish hue at the leaf nodes. The leaves are broad, rough, and jagged and grow three to five at a joint. The hermaphroditic flowers are tubular and white or pale pink to purple and grow in rounded clusters.

GRINDELIA

Botanical Name

Grindelia camporum (syn. _G. robusta_), _G. rigida_, _G. squarrosa_

Family

Asteraceae (Daisy Family)

Etymology

Grindelia is named after the German botanist David H. Grindel. The common name _gumweed_ refers to the sticky resin that covers the plant.

Also Known As

English: gumweed, rosin weed, Spanish gold, tarweed
German: harzkraut, sperriges gummikraut
Spanish: boton de oro

Parts Used

Top (flower, bud, upper leaves), resin

Physiological Effects

Alterative, antispasmodic, aromatic, demulcent, diuretic, expectorant, hypotensive, sedative, stomachic

Medicinal Uses

Grindelia helps the body expel mucus. It also helps calm the heart and relax the spasms associated with asthma and bronchitis. It is used in the treatment of asthma, bronchitis, catarrh, colds, cough, emphysema, hay fever, malaria, measles, small pox, tuberculosis, and whooping cough. The leaves are reputed to calm asthma attacks when smoked.

Topically, grindelia can be used as a bath herb to treat paralysis and rheumatism. It also can be prepared as a liniment to treat eczema, herpes lesions, impetigo, poison ivy and oak, and varicose veins; as a massage oil to relieve arthritis and bed sores; and as a poultice to soothe insect bites and to speed the healing of burns.

Edible Uses

Grindelia leaves are edible raw or cooked, though strong tasting. The buds and flowers are sometimes made into lozenges.

Other Uses

Sucking on a grindelia bud when at high altitudes helps increase lung capacity. Green and yellow dyes can be made from the flowers and pods.

Constituents

Flavonoids (quercitin), saponins (grindelin), laevoglucose, diterpene (grindelic acid), essential oils, resin, tannins, alkaloid (grindeline)

Energetic Correspondences

- Flavor: pungent, bitter
- Temperature: warm
- Moisture: dry
- Polarity: yang
- Planet: Sun
- Element: fire

Contraindications

Do not use in cases of heart problems, as it can lower blood pressure. Because of the herb's high resin and potentially high selenium content (it absorbs selenium from the soil), large dosages can irritate the kidneys.

Range and Appearance

Grindelia is a biennial or perennial native to western North America. It has a smooth, round stem that reaches about 3 feet in height; its leathery leaves extend about an inch in length. The buds are covered with bracts; the hermaphroditic, yellow ray flowers are sticky and resinous. Grindelia prefers full sun and will tolerate drought and poor soil.

GUARANA

Botanical Name

Paullinia cupana (syn. *P. sorbilis,* formerly *Cupania americana*)

Family

Sapindaceae (Lychee Family)

Etymology

The genus name *Paullinia* was given in honor of C. F. Paullini, a German botanist who discovered the Guarani tribe of South America in the eighteenth century. The common name *guarana* derives from that of the Guarani, who live where this plant grows.

Also Known As

English: Brazilian cocoa, uabano, uaranazeiro
German: kletterstrauch
Guarani: wara'ná
Tupi: wara'ná

Part Used

Seed

Physiological Effects

Analgesic, antibacterial, antioxidant, aphrodisiac, appetite suppressant, astringent, carminative, diuretic, febrifuge, hyperglycemic, refrigerant, stimulant, thermogenic, vasodilator

Medicinal Uses

Guarana has about two and a half times the caffeine content of coffee; however, it is absorbed more slowly into the gastrointestinal tract, so it has a gentler, longer-lasting effect. It curbs hunger and has been used as an energizer and diet aid. It also has been found to prevent blood platelet aggregation. It is sometimes used in the treatment of attention deficit hyperactivity disorder, cellulite, depression, diarrhea, dysentery, dyspepsia, fatigue, flatulence, hangover, headache, migraine, neuralgia, and obesity.

Topically, guarana can be used in shampoos to treat oily hair and prevent hair loss and in lotions to help diminish cellulite.

Edible Uses

Guarana is prepared much like chocolate: the seeds are pulverized and roasted, mixed with water, formed into bars, and dried. It is sometimes an ingredient in energy sodas, candy bars, and gums.

Other Uses

Woody parts of the vine are used to make carved figurines.

Constituents

Choline, glucose, caffeine, theophylline, theobromine, guaranine, xanthine, allantoin, tannins, saponins, mucilage

Energetic Correspondences

* Flavor: bitter, sweet
* Temperature: warm
* Moisture: dry
* Polarity: yang

* Planet: Mars/Saturn/Uranus
* Element: fire

Contraindications

Guarana is contraindicated for those with heart disease, ulcer, diabetes, or epilepsy. Avoid in cases of high blood pressure, during pregnancy, and while nursing. It can cause nervousness, insomnia, depletion of B vitamins, and caffeine dependency.

Range and Appearance

Guarana is a shrubby climbing vine native to South America, mostly northern Brazil and Venezuela, that can reach up to 20 feet in length. The leaves are finely divided and compound. The yellow flowers grow in clusters, as do the small, pear-shaped, red fruits, each of which contains three capsules. As the fruit ripens, it opens to reveal a black seed that resembles an eye. Guarana thrives in hot, damp environments, such as are found in rain forests.

GUGGULU

Botanical Name

Commiphora africana, C. wightii (syn. *C. mukul*)

Family

Burseaceae (Frankincense Family)

Etymology

The genus name, *Commiphora,* derives from the Greek *kommi,* "gum," and *phoros,* "carrier."

Also Known As

Arabic: mogla, mukulyahuda
Bengali: makal
English: guggul, guggulow, gum guggul, Indian bedelium, mukul tree
Hebrew: bedolach
Hindi: guggul
Nepali: gokuladhoopa
Sanskrit: devadhupa, koushika
Spanish: gugul
Swahili: mbambara

Part Used

Resin

Physiological Effects

Alterative, analgesic, anti-inflammatory, antioxidant, antiseptic, antispasmodic, astringent, carminative, diaphoretic, emmenagogue, expectorant, astringent, nervine, rejuvenative, stimulant, thyroid stimulant

Medicinal Uses

Guggulu lowers levels of low-density lipoproteins (LDL, or "bad" cholesterol) while elevating levels of high-density lipoproteins (HDL, or "good" cholesterol). It also helps prevent blood platelet aggregation and breaks up blood clots. Because it helps activate thyroid function by improving iodine assimilation, it may stimulate weight loss. It stimulates white blood cell production and has an antiseptic effect upon the body's secretions. It also helps stimulate the regeneration of nerve tissue as well as bones and joints. It is used in the treatment of acne, arteriosclerosis, arthritis, bronchitis, cystitis, debility, diabetes, dyspepsia, gout, hemorrhoids, high cholesterol, high triglyceride levels, hypertension, hypothyroidism, lumbago, obesity, osteoarthritis, rheumatism, sciatica, tumors, and whooping cough.

Topically, guggulu can be made into a gargle to treat canker sores and tonsillitis and a salve to treat eczema and leprosy.

Edible Uses

Not generally considered edible, aside from as tea.

Other Uses

Guggulu is sometimes used as a fixative in perfumes. The wood is sometimes burned as incense. In magical traditions, guggulu is associated with strength and triumph.

Constituents

Phytosterols (guggulsterones), terpenes (manusumbionic acid, manusumbinone), essential oil, gum, calcium, magnesium, iron

Energetic Correspondences

- Flavor: bitter, pungent, sweet
- Temperature: warm
- Moisture: dry
- Polarity: yang
- Planet: Mars
- Element: fire

Contraindications

In rare cases guggulu can cause an allergic skin reaction; the reaction will disappear when use of the herb is discontinued. In cases of bowel inflammation, liver disease, or diarrhea, use only under the guidance of a qualifed health-care practitioner. The crude (raw) extract is more likely to have side effects (diarrhea, stomach pain, skin rash) than the dried, purified product.

Range and Appearance

Native to Asia and Africa, guggulu is a small tree reaching only 4 to 6 feet in height. Its stems are covered with thorns. A yellowish resin (known as gum guggul) exudes from the stems. The tree is leafless for much of the year; when leaves appear they occur in groups of one to three leaflets. The flowers are red; the fruit is oval in shape. The bark is ash colored and peels off in rough pieces, exposing a thin, papery underbark.

GYMNEMA

Botanical Name

Gymnema sylvestre (formerly *Asclepias geminata*)

Family

Asclepiadeceae (Milkweed Family)

Etymology

The genus name, *Gymnema,* derives from the Greek *gymnos,* "naked." The species name, *sylvestre,* is Latin for "of the forest." The Hindi common name, *gurmar,* means "sugar destroyer," in reference to the plant's use in blocking the taste of sugar.

Also Known As

Arabic: kharak
English: miracle fruit, periploca of the woods, ram's horn
German: waldschlinge
Hindi: gurmar
Sanskrit: meshashringi, sarpa-darushtrika

Part Used

Leaf

Physiological Effects

Astringent, cough suppressant, diuretic, hypoglycemic, laxative, refrigerant, stomachic, tonic

Medicinal Uses

Gymnema has been used to treat diabetes for more than two thousand years in Ayurvedic medicine. When gymnema is taken before eating, the molecules of one of its constituents, gymnemic acid, fill the sugar-taste receptor sites on the tongue for one to two hours, thus preventing the taste buds from reacting to the sugar molecules in food and blocking the taste of sugar; with the taste of sugar gone, the desire to eat sugar subsides. Gymnema also helps stabilize blood sugar levels, enhances insulin production, promotes the regeneration of beta cells that release insulin into the pancreas, and inhibits adrenaline from stimulating the liver to produce glucose.

Gymnema is used in the treatment of diabetes (types 1 and 2), fever, high cholesterol, hypoglycemia, obesity, and sugar addiction.

Topically, gymnema can be prepared as a poultice with castor oil to reduce swelling in glands. The powdered root has been used in India to treat snakebite.

Edible Uses

The leaf is not generally considered edible, aside from as tea. The fruit is edible and is usually roasted, peeled, and deseeded; it has a potato-like flavor.

Other Uses

None known

Constituents

Gymnemic acid, tartaric acid, calcium oxalate, glucose, stigmasterol, betaine, choline

Energetic Correspondences

- Flavor: sweet
- Temperature: cool
- Moisture: moist
- Polarity: yin
- Planet: Venus
- Element: earth

Contraindications

In cases of insulin dependency, use gymnema only under the guidance of a qualifed health-care practitioner, as use of the herb may necessitate an adjustment in insulin dosage.

Range and Appearance

Gymnema is a woody climbing plant native to the tropical forests of southern and central India, eastern Asia, Australia, and western and southern Africa. It prefers loamy, sandy soil. Its leaves are long, slender, and opposite. The creamy white to beige fruits are roundish and become thinner toward the ends, with one ending in a corkscrew.

HAWTHORN

Botanical Name

Crataegus spp.

Family

Rosaceae (Rose Family)

Etymology

The genus name *Crataegus* derives from the Greek *kratos,* "hard," referring to hardness of the wood. The *haw* in the common name *hawthorn* derives from the Anglo-Saxon *haga,* "hedge" or "enclosure"; indeed, hawthorn, with its long thorns, is sometimes used as a living fence.

Also Known As

English: bread and cheese tree, chastity tree, hagthorn, haw, May blossom, May bush, May Day flower, whitethorn

Finnish: pyöröliuskaorapihlaja

French: épine noble

German: weissdorn, zweigriffeliger

Italian: biancospino

Japanese: sansa

Korean: sanza

Mandarin: shan zha

Sanskrit: ban-sangli (berry)

Spanish: espino

Swedish: hagtorn, rundhagtorn

Parts Used

Leaf, flower, berry

Physiological Effects

Adaptogen, anabolic, anthelmintic, antiabortifacient, antibacterial, antioxidant, antispasmodic, astringent, cardiotonic, carminative, circulatory stimulant, digestive, diuretic, hypotensive, lithotriptic, nervine, nutritive, rejuvenative, sedative, stimulant, vasodilator, yin tonic

Medicinal Uses

In Asian medicine hawthorn is used more as a digestive aid, whereas in Western medicine it is considered more of a heart tonic. In Europe, hawthorn is often prescribed in place of digitalis as a cardiotonic. It normalizes blood pressure, strengthens the heart muscles, dilates the blood vessels, improves circulation, lowers cholesterol, and improves the contractions of the heart muscles. It protects the heart muscle during times of oxygen deprivation, helps soften deposits, reduces blood vessel inflammations, and strengthens connective tissues. It also calms the spirit. The heart is put under a lot of stress during times of serious infection; drinking hawthorn tea during and after these periods helps protect the heart from pathogens. Hawthorn also can be used to strengthen joint lining, collagen, and discs in the back and to help one be better able to retain a chiropractic adjustment.

Hawthorn is used in the treatment of altitude sickness, amenorrhea, anemia, angina, anxiety, arrhythmia, arteriosclerosis, arthritis, Beurger's disease, blood clots, claudication (intermittent), congestive heart failure, coronary insufficiency, diabetes, diarrhea, dropsy, dysentery, dyspepsia, gout, heartache (emotional), heart palpitations, heart weakness, hemorrhoids, hernia, high cholesterol, hypertension, hypotension, indigestion, infertility, insomnia, ligament injury, loose teeth, macular degeneration, obesity, pulse irregularity, shortness of breath, slipped discs, tachycardia, tendonitis, threatened miscarriage, thrombosis, urinary stones, tapeworm, and varicose veins. It is also used in the prevention and recovery from heart attack.

Topically, hawthorn tea is used as a gargle to treat sore throat.

As a flower essence, hawthorn promotes the healing power of hope, love, trust, and forgiveness. It helps relieve negative feelings from the heart and encourages knowledge of the strength and resiliency of the heart.

Edible Uses

Hawthorn fruits can be eaten raw, dried, or cooked; they are a popular jelly or chutney fruit. The berries taste somewhat sour, sweet, and sometimes bitter, yet fruity. When making a tea of the berries, first soak them for about twelve hours, as they will then more easily release their properties.

The flowers are also edible, as are the young leaves. The leaves and flowers have a sweet, pleasant, astringent flavor, similar to that of green tea. In Germany, the leaves are often used in place of green and black tea.

Other Uses

Hawthorn wood is quite hard and resistant to rot; it is valued for use as tool handles and fence posts.

In magical traditions, hawthorn is said to support fertility, chastity, and happiness and to protect homes against lightning and storm damage.

Celtic tradition makes frequent reference to the three sacred trees: oak, ash, and thorn (hawthorn).

Constituents

Vitamin C, choline, acetylcholine, vitamins B_1 and B_2, calcium, tartaric acid, flavonoids (proanthocyanidins, anthocyanidins, hyperoside, vitexin, epicatechin, rutin, quercitin), glycosides (oxycanthine), saponins, triterpenoids (amygdalin, ursolic acid, chlorogenic acid), tannins, pectin, amines, purines (adenosine, adenine, guanine), saponins; the alkaloid crategin is most prevalent in the flowers, then the leaves, then the berries

Energetic Correspondences

- Flavor: sour, sweet, sometimes bitter
- Temperature: warm; the flower is cooler than the berry and leaf
- Moisture: dry
- Polarity: yang
- Planet: Mars
- Element: fire

Contraindications

Using hawthorn may potentate the effects of heart medications such as beta blockers, digoxin, or Lanoxin. If you are using heart medication, consult with a qualified health-care professional before commencing use of hawthorn. Use hawthorn with caution in cases of poor digestion or acid stomach. Hawthorn's effects are slow to manifest; the herb may need to be taken for four to eight weeks before results are observed. It is generally considered extremely safe.

Range and Appearance

Hawthorn, native to northern Asia, Europe, and temperate America, is a family of deciduous shrubs or trees. It hybridizes easily; botanists claim anywhere from one hundred to one thousand species. The shrubs or trees reach 6 to 20 feet in height, with multiple branches and usually has stiff thorns. The leaves can be simple, toothed, lobed or cut and alternate, obovate, or obovate-elliptical. The five-petaled white or pink flowers grow in corymb inflorescences. The reddish fruits, known as haws, resemble rosehips, grow in clusters, and contain one to five hard

seeds. Hawthorn grows by streams and in meadows, forests and open spaces. It prefers full sun to partial shade and moist, well-drained soil, but it will tolerate drought.

HIBISCUS

Botanical Name

Hibiscus spp., including *H. rosa-sinensis,*
  H. sabdariffa, H. syriacus

Family

Malvaceae (Mallow Family)

Etymology

Hibiscus is the Greek name for mallow, the family to which this genus belongs.

Also Known As

Arabic: karkade
English: Guinea sorrel, Jamaica sorrel, mallow,
  rosella, rosemallow, rose of Sharon, sour-sour
Finnish: teehibiskus
French: karkadeh
German: karkade, rosselahanf
Hawaiian: ma'o hau hele
Italian: carcadè
Swedish: rosellhibiskus

Part Used

Flower

Physiological Effects

Alterative, antibacterial (mild), anti-inflammatory, antioxidant, antiparasitic, antiscorbutic, antiseptic, antispasmodic, astringent, cholagogue, demulcent, digestive, diuretic, emmenagogue, emollient, expectorant, febrifuge, hemostatic, ophthalmic, refrigerant, sedative, stomachic, tonic

Medicinal Uses

Hibiscus cools the body, nourishes and soothes the tissues, and helps eliminate excess fluid in the body. It also has mild infection-fighting properties. It is used in the treatment of bladder infection, cancer, constipation, cough, cystitis, debility, diarrhea, dysentery, dysmenorrhea, dyspepsia, fever, hangover, heart ailments, hypertension, leukorrhea, liver disorders, menorrhagia, and neurosis.

Topically, a healing wash made from hibiscus flowers can be used to treat eye infection, itchy skin, and wounds.

As a flower essence, hibiscus helps women who are out of touch with their sexuality and helps relieve psychological sexual blocks resulting from trauma. It comforts women who have suffered abuse and helps reunite the warmth of the soul with the passion of sexuality.

Edible Uses

The flowers are a glorious food and lovely decorations. Their flavor is tart, lemonlike, and refreshing. The leaves, tender stalks, and seeds can also be eaten.

Other Uses

A conditioning shampoo can be made from the leaves. A red dye is made from the flowers. Many hibiscuses have a bark that yields strong fibers; Polynesians use these fibers to make grass skirts.

Constituents

Ascorbic acid, citric acid, tartaric acid, malic acid, flavonoids (anthocyanins), gossypetin, glucoside (hibiscin), phytosterols

Energetic Correspondences

• Flavor: sour, sweet, bitter
• Temperature: cool
• Moisture: moist
• Polarity: yin
• Planet: Venus
• Element: water

Contraindications

Persons who are very chilled should avoid hibiscus, as it is cooling.

Range and Appearance

There are more than two hundred species of deciduous trees and shrubs in the hibiscus genus. The taller

species can grow to about 9 feet in height. The entire plant is covered with fine grayish hairs. The alternate leaves are palmately veined or lobed; they may be simple, ovate, or lanceolate, depending on the species. The hermaphroditic flowers can be white, yellow, pink, red, purple, or multicolored.

Hibiscus is native to Africa but can be cultivated in North America. It will tolerate frost as long as there is adequate moisture, and it prefers full sun and well-drained soil.

HONEYSUCKLE

Botanical Name

Lonicera japonica

Family

Caprifoliaceae (Honeysuckle Family)

Etymology

The genus name, *Lonicera,* is taken from that of Adam Lonicer, a sixteenth-century German physician and naturalist. The common name *honeysuckle* refers to the practice of sucking the sweet nectar from the blossoms.

Also Known As

Cantonese: gam gan tang, yan dong tang
English: gold and silver flower, honey vine, lady's
    fingers, woodbine
French: chèvreféuille
German: geisblatt, heckenkirsche
Italian: capri-foglio
Japanese: kinginka
Korean: kûmûnhwa
Mandarin: jin yin hua

Parts Used

Flower (primarily), stem (rarely)

Physiological Effects

Alterative, antibiotic, antifungal, anti-inflammatory, antiseptic, antispasmodic, antiviral, astringent (mild), depurative, diaphoretic, diuretic, emetic, expectorant, febrifuge, hypotensive, laxative, refrigerant, vulnerary

Medicinal Uses

Honeysuckle clears damp heat and removes toxins. Prolonged use is reputed to prolong life and increase vitality. Research in China is indicating that honeysuckle may be helpful in the treatment of breast cancer.

Honeysuckle flowers are used to treat allergies, appendicitis, asthma, bacterial infection, boils, bronchitis, cancer, carbuncles, colds, cough, Crohn's disease, diarrhea dysentery, ear infection, eczema, eye inflammation (conjunctivitis, uveitis, keratitis), fever, fibrocystic breasts, flu, food poisoning, headache, heavy metal toxicity, hepatitis, high cholesterol, infection due to injury, itchiness, laryngitis, lymphatic swelling, mastitis, pneumonia, poisoning, psoriasis, rheumatism, sinusitis, sore throat, strep throat, tonsillitis, tuberculosis, and ulcers.

The stems are used to treat appendicitis, hepatitis, mumps, pneumonia, and rheumatism.

Topically, honeysuckle can be used as a compress to treat bruises, poison oak or ivy, rash, sore eyes, sunburn, swellings, and tumors or as a gargle to treat sore throat and ulcerations. The flowers are sometimes included in mouthwashes to treat mouth ulcers.

As a flower essence, honeysuckle helps those who are stuck in the past with memories or regrets. It helps one live in the present moment, using the wisdom of past experiences as a foundation and rekindling interest in life. It also helps relieve homesickness.

Edible Uses

Honeysuckle flowers are edible (many remember sucking the raw nectar from honeysuckle flowers); as buds they can be added to stir-fries or other cooked dishes. The tea prepared from the flowers, when iced, makes a refreshing, cooling summer beverage. The leaves also make a delicious tea and are sometimes used as a green tea substitute. Beware the fruits, which are cathartic and emetic.

Other Uses

The stems are placed under bed pillows to facilitate sleep and are also used in basket weaving. The flowers and leaves are sometimes added to potpourri. Honeysuckle is sometimes used in cosmetic creams to soften skin.

In magical traditions, honeysuckle is said to offer psychic protection and to encourage prosperity and intuition.

Constituents

Tannins, glycoside, chlorogenic acid, isochlorogenic acid, flavonoids (luteolin), mucilage, sugars

Energetic Correspondences

- Flavor: sweet, bitter
- Temperature: cold
- Moisture: dry
- Polarity: yang
- Planet: Mercury/Mars/Jupiter/Moon
- Element: earth

Contraindications

Avoid honeysuckle in cases of excessive phlegm, inflammation in the upper respiratory tract, or watery diarrhea due to internal coldness. Do not use for more than seven days in a row. Avoid using honeysuckle berries, which are toxic. The *caprifolium* and *periclymenum* varieties are used only externally.

Range and Appearance

Most varieties of honeysuckle are woody, twining vines, though some are shrubs. The leaves are opposite and oval; the stem is reddish brown. The yellow, white, pink, or red flowers are very fragrant and can attract hummingbirds and butterflies. A reddish orange berry appears after the flowers. Honeysuckle requires only modest amounts of water and will tolerate shade. In warmer climates, however, it is considered an invasive species.

HOPS

Botanical Name

Humulus lupulus (syn. *H. americanus*)

Family

Cannabaceae (Hemp Family)

Etymology

The genus name, *Humulus,* derives from the Latin *humus,* "earth," in reference to the manner in which the plant creeps across the ground. The species name, *lupulus,* comes from the Latin *lupus,* "wolf," in reference to the plant's aggressive growth, which tends to smother other plants around it. The common name *hops* comes from the Latin *hoppan,* "to climb," in reference to the plant being a climbing vine.

Also Known As

English: hop bine
Finnish: humula
French: houblon grimpant
German: hopfen, zaunhapfen
Italian: luppolo
Mandarin: ch-ku-ts'aon
Russian: hmel
Spanish: lupulo
Swedish: humle

Part Used

Strobile (female inflorescence)

Physiological Effects

Anaphrodisiac, anodyne, anthelmintic, antibiotic, anti-inflammatory, antiseptic, antispasmodic, aperient, astringent, cholagogue, diuretic, febrifuge, galactagogue, hypnotic, lithotriptic, muscle relaxant, nervine, sedative, soporific, stomachic

Medicinal Uses

The ancient Hebrews used hops to prevent the plague. Hops clear heat and toxins, nourishes yin, restrains infection, aids digestion, calms the spirit and the nerves, and encourages sleep. It has a strong effect on hormones, a fact that was first noticed when female gatherers of the plants would menstruate earlier in their cycle. It is known to quiet excessive sexual desire, especially in men.

Hops have been used to treat abscesses, acne, attention deficit disorder, attention deficit hyperactivity disorder, anxiety, boils, cancer, chorea, Crohn's disease, cystitis, delirium tremens, eczema, excessive sex drive, headache, hysteria, indigestion, insomnia, irritable bowel, jaundice, mastitis, menstrual cramps, muscle spasms, neuralgia, pain, restlessness, rheumatism, nervous stomach, stress, tuberculosis, urinary stones, and worms. Alcohol extracts of hops have been used successfully to treat dysentery, leprosy, and tuberculosis.

Topically, hops poultices can be used to treat boils, bruises, cysts, earache, eczema, headaches, inflammation, rash, sprains, toothache, tumors, and wounds. Hops can be mixed with eucalyptus and peppermint in a salve to use as a chest rub to quiet a cough. In hair rinses, hops reduce dandruff and highlights brunette; in lotions, it softens the skin. It also makes a relaxing bath herb.

As a flower essence, hops aids in the transition from a playful childlike nature to the sexuality of adolescence. It stimulates physical and spiritual progress and improves group interaction.

Edible Uses

The strobiles are not generally considered edible, except as tea and for flavoring waters and beers. The young leaves (before they have opened) fleshy rhizomes can be eaten, as can the tips of the shoots, which are eaten in spring, like asparagus.

Other Uses

In ancient times hops was used, much like its close relative hemp, to make rope, bedding, cloth, and paper. Some like to smoke hops for their sedative effect. Hops also can be made into sachets and placed in pillowcases as a sleeping aid and to prevent nightmares. Abraham Lincoln and King George III are both said to have slept with hops pillows. However, the most well-known use of hops is in making beer, for which hops have been used since the Middle Ages; it functions as a preservative and also imparts a bitter flavor. A brown dye can be made from the flowers and leaves. The essential oil is used in perfumery.

Constituents

Sulfur, B-complex vitamins, flavonoids (quercitin, rutin), humulone, lupulone, lupulinic acid, bitter principle (lupulin), essential oil, valerianic acid, valeric acid, myrcene, phytoestrogens, methylbutenol

Energetic Correspondences

- Flavor: bitter, pungent
- Temperature: cold
- Moisture: dry
- Polarity: yang
- Planet: Sun/Mars/Saturn/Pluto
- Element: air

Contraindications

Avoid during pregnancy and in cases of depression. Use in conjunction with pharmaceutical sedatives only under the guidance of a qualified health-care professional, as it may exacerbate their effects.

Fresh hops plants may cause contact dermatitis and allergic reactions in some individuals, and tiny hairs from the plant can irritate the eyes if they come in contact with them.

Range and Appearance

Native to Eurasia and North America, hops is a dioecious perennial vine that can grow to 30 feet in length. It is common in damp woodlands and hedgerows. It has prickly stems and opposite, three- or five-lobed leaves. The aromatic fruiting cones, called strobiles, have a yellowish green color. The plant is dioecious, meaning male and female flowers form on different plants. The male flowers form long racemes, while the female flowers form small, round heads, which mature into conelike formations.

HOREHOUND

Botanical Name

Marrubium vulgare

Family

Lamiaceae (Mint Family)

Etymology

The genus name, *Marrubium* is thought to be derived from *marrob*, the Hebrew word for "bitter juice" and others believe it is from *Maria urbs*, a town in ancient Italy. The species name, *vulgare*, is Latin for "common." The common name horehound derives from the Old English *har hune*, "downy plant," in reference to the plant's hoary appearance.

Also Known As

English: bull's blood, eye of the star, hoarhound, houndsbane, seed of Horus, white horehound
Finnish: hurtanminttu
French: herbe vierge, marrube blanc, marrube commun, marrube vulgaire, mont blanc
German: gemeiner, lungenkraut, weisser andorn, weisser dorant
Italian: marrobio
Sanskrit: farasiyun
Spanish: marrubio, marrubium, mastranzo
Swedish: andorn, kransborre

Part Used

Aboveground plant

Physiological Effects

Anthelmintic, antibacterial, antiseptic, antispasmodic, aperient, bitter, cholagogue, choleretic, decongestant, demulcent, diaphoretic, digestive, diuretic, emmenagogue, expectorant, hepatic, laxative, pectoral, resolvent, stimulant, stomachic, tonic

Medicinal Uses

Horehound has been used medicinally since ancient times. Julius Caesar recommended it as an antidote to poisons, while seventeenth-century English herbalists recommended it to help expel the placenta after childbirth. Early European settlers brought the plant to the New World, where it quickly naturalized and found use among Native Americans; the Navajo, for example, used it to ease childbirth.

Horehound mildly stimulates cardiopulmonary activity, encourages the body to expel phlegm, clears heat and toxins, and deters infection. The essential oils in horehound help dilate the arteries and relieve lung congestion. Horehound tea is used to treat anemia, amenorrhea, asthma, bronchitis, catarrh, colds, congestion, coughs, croup, dyspepsia, dyspnea, heart palpitations, hepatitis, hoarseness, jaundice, laryngitis, pharyngitis, placenta retention, pneumonia, rheumatism, sore throat, tuberculosis, typhoid, whooping cough, and worms.

Infused in oil, horehound helps heal wounds. It also can be prepared as a compress to treat dog bites, eczema, shingles, and wounds.

Edible Uses

Horehound, though having a bitter flavor, has long been a popular ingredient in candy, lozenges, syrups, and liqueurs. It is also sometimes an ingredient in beer, where it takes the place of hops.

Other Uses

Horehound is believed to be one of the original bitter herbs of the Jewish Passover tradition. The fresh leaves of the plant can be immersed in milk and set out to kill flies. In magical traditions, horehound is said to offer protection against evil forces.

Constituents

Vitamin C, choline, iron, flavonoids (luteolin), pectin, essential oil (pinene, limonene, campene), diterpene alcohol (marrubiol), sterols, saponins, bitter lactone, alkaloids (betonocine, stachydine) tannin, mucilage, bitter principle (marrubin), and marrubic acid

Energetic Correspondences

- Flavor: bitter, pungent, salty
- Temperature: cool
- Moisture: dry
- Polarity: yang
- Planet: Mercury/Mars
- Element: air

Contraindications

Horehound is considered very safe, even for children. It should be avoided during pregnancy, however. Large doses may be laxative and cathartic. The juice of the fresh plant may cause dermatitis.

Range and Appearance

Horehound is a perennial native to Europe, Asia, and northern Africa. It grows to about 20 inches in height and is covered with downy hairs. The plant has four-sided stems and opposite, ovate, rugose leaves. The small, white, two-lipped flowers occur in dense whorls. Unlike most other mints, it has little aroma.

In the garden, horehound will tolerate poor soil and prefers dry conditions and full sun. It attracts bees and repels flies.

HORSE CHESTNUT

Botanical Name

Aesculus hippocastanum

Family

Hippocastanaceae (Horse Chestnut Family)

Etymology

The genus name, *Aesculus,* is Latin for "acorn." The species name, *hippocastanum,* blends the Greek *hippos,* "horse," and *kastanea,* "chestnut," in reference perhaps to the use of the plant to treat respiratory problems in horses and cattle or perhaps to the horseshoelike markings on the tree's branches.

Also Known As

English: buckeye, conker tree, Spanish chestnut
Finnish: hevoskastanja
German: rosskastanie
Italian: ippocastano
Japanese: toti-no-ki
Swedish: hästkastanj

Part Used

Seed

Physiological Effects

Anti-inflammatory, astringent, circulatory tonic, expectorant, febrifuge, narcotic, nutritive

Medicinal Uses

Horse chestnut helps strengthen the capillaries and decreases their permeability. It also helps move congestion. It is used in the treatment of arthritis, capillary fragility, edema, frostbite, hemorrhoids, phlebitis, and rheumatism.

Topically, horse chestnut can be prepared as a poultice, salve, or compress to treat hemorrhoids, rheumatism, sores, sprains, swelling, and varicose veins.

As a flower essence, horse chestnut helps those who repeat their mistakes over and over, without learning from them, to see themselves more clearly.

Edible Uses

Horse chestnuts are not considered edible unless they have been soaked or boiled in multiple changes of water to leach out the toxins. Some Native Americans prepared a porridge from the nuts using this processing.

Other Uses

Saponins in the seeds can be used to make soap. The wood, though weak, has a nice grain and is used to make household items.

Constituents

Saponins (aescin), glycosides (aesculin, fraxin), hydroquinine, tannins, flavones

Energetic Correspondences

- Flavor: bitter
- Temperature: neutral
- Moisture: dry
- Polarity: yang
- Planet: Jupiter
- Element: fire

Contraindications

The nuts (seeds), as well as the leaves, flowers, and bark, are somewhat toxic unless processed; do not use raw or untreated nuts. The green shell of the nuts can cause digestive distress, drowsiness, and skin flushing and should be peeled off. Use horse chestnut only in small amounts, generally one-fourth that of other herbs. Nausea and gastrointestinal upset are possible side effects; the plant can also thin the blood. Avoid during pregnancy and while nursing.

Range and Appearance

Horse chestnut is a deciduous tree native to Eurasia that can grow 50 to 80 feet tall. It prefers well-drained, moist soil in full sun to partial shade. Its leaves are large, rough, serrated, palmate, and compound. The flowers are hermaphroditic. The nuts are enclosed in prickly green husks.

HORSETAIL

Botanical Name

Equisetum spp., including *E. arvense* (field horsetail)

Family

Equisetaceae (Horsetail Family)

Etymology

The genus name, *Equisetum,* derives from the Latin *equis,* "horse," and *seta,* "bristle," in reference to the plant's resemblance to a horse's tail, with its long stems with cones at their ends. The common name *horsetail* also denotes that resemblance. The species name *arvense* is Latin for "of the fields."

Also Known As

Cantonese: maan chok
Dutch: akkerig paardestaart
English: bottlebrush, bull pipes, devil's guts, Dutch rush, joint grass, paddock pipes, pewterwort, scouring rush, shave brush, shavegrass, tad broom, tin weed, toad pipes, vegetable silica
French: equisette, prêle des champs, prêles, queue-de-chat, queue de cheval

German: ackerschtelhalm, kannenkraut,
   katzenschwanz, schafteu, schlammschachtelhalm
   (*E. limosum*), sumpfschatelhalm (*E. palustre*),
   zinnkraut
Italian: asprella (*E. hyemale*), coda di cavallo
   (*E. arvense*), equiseto palustre (*E. palustre*)
Japanese: mokuzoku, tsukushi
Korean: mokchok
Mandarin: mù zéi
Spanish: cañutillo del llano, carricillo, cola
   de caballo, equiseto
Turkish: at ruyrugi

Part Used

Sterile stem (collected in spring)

Physiological Effects

Alterative, anodyne, antibacterial, antifungal, anti-inflammatory, antiseptic, astringent, diaphoretic, diuretic, hemostatic, kidney tonic, lithotriptic, nutritive, rejuvenative, styptic, tonic, vulnerary

Medicinal Uses

Horsetail has ancient roots, having been predominant during the Carboniferous period, some four hundred million years ago, when dinosaurs roamed the planet. At that time, the plant grew 40 feet or more in height.

Horsetail's high silicon content helps repair bones, cartilage, and connective tissues. It also helps to clear heat, dry dampness, and clear toxins. It was used by Native Americans to help expel the placenta after childbirth and as a treatment for gonorrhea. In Asian and American Indian traditions, shamans throw horsetail into a burning fire to create impressive sounds to drive away illness. Today, horsetail is used to treat acne, arthritis, bedwetting, blood loss, blurred vision, broken bones, bursitis, cancer (fresh juice), catarrh, cystitis, diarrhea, dropsy, dysentery, dysuria, eczema, edema, fractures, gallstones, gout, hair loss, hematuria, hemorrhage, hemorrhoids, incontinence, kidney stones, lacrimation, ligament tears, menorrhagia, nail weakness, nephritis, osteoporosis, rectal prolapse, prostatitis, spermatorrhea, tendonitis, tooth weakness, tuberculosis, ulcers, urethritis, urinary tract infection, and venereal disease. It is also used to facilitate convalescence.

Topically, horsetail can be prepared as a poultice to stop bleeding and promote healing; a douche to treat leukorrhea; an eyewash or compress to treat conjunctivitis and eye inflammation; a hair rinse to strengthen weak hair and decrease dandruff and oily conditions; a mouthwash to treat gingivitis and canker sores; a foot soak to freshen malodorous and sweaty feet; or a bath herb to treat poor circulation and weak skin tone. Ashes of horsetail can be applied to burns and wounds to speed the healing of tissues.

As a flower essence, horsetail improves communication on various levels and helps one to make genuine contact with others.

Edible Uses

When the plant is young its outer stem can be peeled and the inner pulp eaten. The young heads can also be eaten: boil for 20 minutes, change the water, and boil another 20 minutes to eliminate bitter principles, and then eat them like asparagus. The roots are tuberous and can be eaten raw in the early spring or boiled later in the year; they contain a nourishing starch. The fresh plant can also be juiced.

Other Uses

Horsetail is fibrous and has been used to polish wood, arrowheads, cookware, and metals. The powdered stems were once placed in moccasins or shoes to prevent foot cramps from traveling long distances. The Missouri Indians wove the plant into mats. Horsetail tea is used to water plants as a nourishing tonic and to strengthen those susceptible to mildew and blight such as roses and tomatoes.

Constituents

Beta-carotene, ascorbic acid, calcium, manganese, magnesium, potassium, selenium, silica, sulfur, alkaloids (nicotine, palustrine, palustrinine, relustrine), glycosides (isoquercitrin, luteolin, rutin, kaempferol), saponin (equisetonin), phytosterols, tannin, acontic acid, thiaminase

Energetic Correspondences

- Flavor: sweet, bitter
- Temperature: cool
- Moisture: dry
- Polarity: yin
- Planet: Saturn/Moon
- Element: earth

Contraindications

Large amounts of the fresh herb can be toxic due to the presence of the enzyme thiaminase, which, if ingested over a long period of time, can cause a deficiency in B vitamins. However, drying, cooking, or tincturing horsetail destroys that enzyme, making horsetail safe, and the fresh herb is safe in small amounts. Avoid long-term use during pregnancy.

If you are wildcrafting, collect horsetail only in the spring to avoid plants with an excessive selenium and nitrate content. Never collect horsetail plants with brown spots, which are fungi.

Range and Appearance

Most horsetail varieties are perennials, though some are annuals. The plant grows in damp acidic soil areas near streams, ditches, and roadsides; it is native to Eurasia, Africa, and North America. In early spring the hollow stems rise to a height of 2 to 3 feet; they are unbranched and look like multijointed bamboo. At the top of some plants is a conelike strobile, where the reproductive spores are produced. Horsetails bearing a cone are considered fertile; those without are infertile. Later in the season, the unbranched stems wither away, and new, profusely branching ones appear, with green whorls of branches radiating from the nodes (joints), resembling miniature trees.

HO SHOU WU

Botanical Name

Polygonum multiflorum

Family

Polygonaceae (Rhubarb Family)

Etymology

The genus name, *Polygonum,* is Latin for "many knees," in reference to the many joints on the stems. The species name, *multiflorum,* is Latin for "multi-flowered."

The Mandarin common name *he shou wu,* from which the English common name *ho shou wu* is derived, means "black-haired Mr. He," a reference to a story about the fifty-six-year-old, gray-haired Mr. He who ate ho shou wu root for a year, then fathered a son and grew a full head of black hair.

Also Known As

Cantonese: ho sau wu, sao wu
English: Chinese cornbind, climbing knotweed, flowery knotweed, fo-ti, he shou wu, tangled vine
Japanese: kashuu, yakoto
Korean: hasua, yagyodûng
Mandarin: he shou wu, shou wu, ye jiao téng

Part Used

Root (raw or cooked)

Physiological Effects

Alterative, antibacterial, antidepressant, anti-inflammatory, antioxidant (when raw), antispasmodic, antitumor, antiviral, aphrodisiac, astringent, blood tonic, cardiotonic, chi tonic, demulcent, deobstruent, diuretic, febrifuge, hepatic, hypoglycemic, immune tonic, interferon stimulant (when cooked), laxative (when raw), liver tonic (when raw), kidney tonic, rejuvenative (when cooked), restorative, sedative, yin tonic

Medicinal Uses

Ho shou wu root is available either raw and dried or cooked in a black soybean broth. It is one of China's most common blood tonics. It strengthens the bones and muscles, moistens the intestines, builds bone marrow, and calms the spirit.

Cooked ho shou wu root is used to treat anemia, atherosclerosis, blurred vision, constipation (due to dry intestines), diabetes, dizziness, exhaustion, goiter, hair loss, high cholesterol, infertility, high cholesterol, hot flashes, hypertension, hypoglycemia, infertility, knee weakness, low sperm count, lumbago, scrofula, insomnia, malaria, menopausal complaints, numbness, premature aging, premature gray hair, premature menopause, rickets, schizophrenia, spermatorrhea, spleen weakness, tinnitus, tuberculosis, vaginal discharge, and vertigo.

Raw ho shou wu root is used to treat carbuncles and swollen lymph glands or nodes.

Edible Uses

Ho shou wu roots are edible and are nourishing to the liver, blood, and kidneys; they are often added to soups. The young shoots can also be eaten; like their cousin rhubarb, though, they contain oxalic acid, and if they are a bit mature, they should be either cooked or soaked in water for a couple of hours and then rinsed before consumption.

Other Uses

None known

Constituents

Magnesium, phosphorous, potassium, unsaturated fatty acids, lecithin, anthraquinones (chysophanol, emodin, rhapontin), phenolic glucosides, allantoin, tannins

Energetic Correspondences

- Flavor: sour, bitter, sweet
- Temperature: warm
- Moisture: dry
- Polarity: yin
- Planet: Mars/Saturn
- Element: water

Contraindications

Avoid ho shou wu during bouts of diarrhea and excessive phlegm. The raw root is more laxative than the cooked variety. If using the cooked root and suffering from weak digestion, combine it with a digestive tonic herb such as ginger or dried orange peel. There have been rare reports of dermatitis or numbness in the extremities after ingestion of large doses.

Range and Appearance

Ho shou wu is a perennial deciduous vine native to China, Japan, Vietnam, and Taiwan. It grows along streambanks and in valley thickets and thrives in poor soil. The leaves are heart shaped, singular, and alternate. White flowers bloom in inflorescences.

When purchasing ho shou wu, look for dark roots, not those streaked with white, which are of inferior quality.

HYDRANGEA

Botanical Name

Hydrangea arborescens

Family

Saxifragaceae (Rockfoil Family)

Etymology

The genus name, *Hydrangea,* derives from the Greek *hydro,* "water," and *angeion,* "vessel." The common name *seven barks* refers to the fact that when the bark peels off, it does so in several layers of various colors.

Also Known As

English: seven bark, smooth hydrangea, tree
  hydrangea
Finnish: pallohortensia
French: hortensie, hydrangelle de Virginie
German: baumartige hydrangie, grosser
  wasserstrauch, hortensie, kehlopf
Swedish: vidjehortensia

Parts Used

Root (dried), rhizome (dried)

Physiological Effects

Cathartic, demulcent, diuretic, laxative, lithotriptic, sialagogue, stomachic, tonic

Medicinal Uses

Hydrangea was used widely by the Cherokee Indians and, later, European settlers to treat stones in the urinary tract. It is known to help remove uric acid accumulations from the body, cleanse the kidneys, and soften deposits. It aids in the passage of stones and helps prevent their reoccurrence. It also deters infection, soothes inflammation, and strengthens the capillaries. Hydrangea is used in the treatment of arteriosclerosis, arthritis, bladder stones, backache due to kidney problems, capillary fragility, cystitis, dropsy, dysuria, gout, kidney stones, nephritis, prostatitis, urethritis, and urinary tract infection.

Topically, hydrangea can be used as a compress or poultice to treat burns, sprains, tumors, and wounds.

Edible Uses

The roots and rhizomes are not generally considered edible. The young shoots and leaves, however, are edible after being cooked.

Other Uses

In magical traditions, hydrangea is said to offer protection against negative energies when burned as incense, scattered around the home, or carried.

Constituents

Rutin, quercetin, kaempferol, glycosides (hydrangin), saponins, resins, albumen, essential oils

Energetic Correspondences

- Flavor: pungent, sweet
- Temperature: cool
- Moisture: moist
- Polarity: yin
- Planet: Venus/Moon
- Element: earth

Contraindications

Excessive amounts can cause gastrointestinal distress, dizziness, and chest congestion. Hydrangea is not recommended for long-term use or during pregnancy. Use just the root or rhizome; there have been some reports of the flowers and leaves causing toxicity in humans.

Range and Appearance

Hydrangea is a Native American decidious shrub that can grow 5 to 10 feet tall. It grows in the wild along streams, hills, and woodlands and is a popular ornamental. The leaves are opposite, mostly ovate, pointed, and toothed. The numerous, small, beautiful flowers are borne on cymes and are usually white but sometimes pink or purple, depending on soil alkalinity. Most hydrangeas do best in rich, moist soil and prefer full sun, though they will tolerate partial shade.

HYSSOP

Botanical Name

Hyssopus officinalis

Family

Lamiaceae (Mint Family)

Etymology

The genus name, *Hyssopus*, derives from the Greek name for the plant, *hyssopus*, a term that is itself of Semitic origin and perhaps deriving from the Hebrew *ezobh*, meaning "holy herb," in reference to the plant's use in purifying places of worship.

Also Known As

Bulgarian: isop
Cantonese: niu xi cao
Croatian: ljekoviti
Czech: yzop
Danish: isop
Dutch: hyssop
Esperanto: hisopo
Estonian: harilik iisop
Finish: iisoppi
French: hysope
German: eisop
Greek: issopos
Hebrew: esov
Hungarian: izsóp
Icelandic: ísópur
Italian: issopo
Japanese: hissopu
Korean: hasop
Lithuanian: vaistinis isopas

Norwegian: isop
Polish: hyzop lekarski
Portuguese: hissopo
Romanian: isop
Russian: issop
Sanskrit: jufa
Serbian: izop
Slovak: yzop lekársky
Slovenian: izop
Spanish: hisopo
Swedish: isop
Turkish: çördük out
Ukrainian: isop zvichajnyj
Yiddish: ezev

Part Used

Aboveground plant

Physiological Effects

Anthelmintic, antiseptic, antispasmodic, antiviral, aperient, aromatic, astringent, carminative, chi tonic, cholagogue, circulatory stimulant, diaphoretic, diuretic, emmenagogue, expectorant, febrifuge, lithotriptic, lung tonic, mucolytic, pectoral, sedative, spleen tonic, stimulant, stomachic, sudorific, vasodilator, vermifuge, vulnerary

Medicinal Uses

Hyssop warms and stimulates the lungs, helps the body expel phlegm, increases respiratory capacity, balances circulation, and cleanses the kidneys. It is being researched for its beneficial effects in cases of HIV. It is used in the treatment of amenorrhea, anxiety, asthma, bronchitis, catarrh, chicken pox, colds, congestion, cough, debility, depression, dropsy, dyspepsia, fever, flatulence, flu, grief, hay fever, headache, herpes, hoarseness, hysteria, indigestion, jaundice, parasites, phlegm, rheumatism, scarlet fever, scrofula, shortness of breath, smallpox, sore throat, tuberculosis, and whooping cough.

Topically, hyssop tea can be used as a gargle to soothe sore throat; as a compress to treat black eyes, bruises, insect bites, sprains, and wounds; and as deodorant wash. Hyssop as a bath herb or compress can be used to relieve rheumatism and muscle soreness.

As a flower essence hyssop encourages the release of guilt and aids forgiveness.

Edible Uses

The young leaves and tips of the shoots are edible. Some use the fresh herb as a seasoning substitute for sage. The flowers are both edible and decorative. As a tea, hyssop is light and aromatic.

Other Uses

Hyssop was once used as a strewing herb and to deter bugs and the spread of infection. The essential oil is used in perfumery.

Constituents

Potassium, silicon, malic acid, flavonoids (hesperidin, hyssopin), essential oils (borneol, cineol, limonene, geraniol, thujone, pinene, camphene, pinocarvone, terpenens), tannin, glycoside (diosmin), bitter lactones (marrubiin, ursolic acid)

Energetic Correspondences

- Flavor: bitter, pungent
- Temperature: warm
- Moisture: dry
- Polarity: yang
- Planet: Jupiter
- Element: fire

Contraindications

Avoid during pregnancy and in cases of epilepsy or high blood pressure.

Range and Appearance

Hyssop is a highly aromatic, mostly evergreen perennial native to Eurasia. It is woody at the base, has square stems and rodlike branches, and can grow to 2 feet in height. The leaves are opposite, lanceolate to linear, and thick, with one rib underneath. The flowers are usually purplish blue but sometimes are white or pink, and they grow in whorls of six to fifteen flowers.

The plant prefers full sun to partial shade, has low water requirements, and does well in sandy, well-drained soil. The flowers are much relished by bees and butterflies.

IRISH MOSS

Botanical Name

Chondrus crispus

Family

Gigartinaceae (Gigartina Family)

Etymology

The genus name, *Chondrus,* derives from the Greek *chondros,* "cartilage" or "grain." The species name, *crispus,* is Latin for "curly." The common name *Irish moss* references the plant's use in Ireland.

Also Known As

English: carrageenan, carragheen, chrondus, jelly moss, pearl moss
Finnish: karrageenilevä
French: mousse de Chine
German: irländisches moos, knorpeltang
Swedish: karragentång

Part Used

Entire plant (frond)

Physiological Effects

Alterative, anti-inflammatory, antiviral, demulcent, emollient, expectorant, laxative, nutritive, yin tonic

Medicinal Uses

This gentle herb cools and soothes the gastrointestinal tract. It can help alleviate both duodenal and peptic ulcers without any negative effects upon the colon. It also helps reduce gastric secretions. It is used in the treatment of acid indigestion, bronchitis, colds, coughs, cystitis, debility, diarrhea, dysentery, flu, gastritis, goiter, lung dryness, sore throat, and ulcers.

Topically, Irish moss is sometimes included in lotions to soften the skin and prevent premature wrinkling. As a compress or poultice it can soothe inflamed tissues.

Edible Uses

Irish moss is edible has been regarded mainly as a survival food; it was an important food source for the Irish during the famine of the nineteenth century. It must be soaked or cooked first. It is used by the food industry to add texture and stability to ice cream, whipped cream, jellies, puddings, soups, and salad dressings. It is now popular in raw cuisine as a thickening agent.

Other Uses

Irish moss was once used to stuff mattresses, as cattle feed, and to thicken colored inks to be used in printing. It is sometimes used today to thicken cosmetics and as a binding agent in products such as toothpaste.

In magical traditions, Irish moss is placed under rugs or in one's pocket to attract prosperity and is carried on voyages to ensure safe journeying.

Constituents

Protein, polysaccharides, iodine, sulfur, bromine, mucilage, carrageenans, beta-carotene, vitamin B_1

Energetic Correspondences

- Flavor: sweet, salty
- Temperature: cool
- Moisture: moist
- Polarity: yin
- Planet: Moon
- Element: water

Contraindications

Because Irish moss has some blood-thinning properties, people who are on anticoagulating medications should avoid its use.

Range and Appearance

Irish moss is a seaweed that prevails on the rocky coasts of the North Atlantic. It can appear in a wide range of colors, from white to yellow, red, or purple. It has long, thin, tufted fronds 2–10 inches in length.

ISATIS

Botanical Name

Isatis tinctoria (syn. *I. indigotica*)

Family

Brassicaceae (Cabbage Family)

Etymology

Isatis, the genus and common name, is a Greek term denoting a plant producing a dark dye. *Tinctoria,* the species name, derives from the Latin *tingere,* "to tinge," in reference to this plant being a source of a blue dye.

Also Known As

Cantonese: baan laam gan (root), daii ching yip (leaf)
English: asp of Jerusalem, dyer's woad, istan, woad
German: waid
Japanese: banrankon (root), taiseiyo (leaf)
Korean: p'allamgûn
Mandarin: ban lán gen (root), da qing ye (leaf)
Sanskrit: nila

Parts Used

Root (primarily), leaf

Physiological Effects

Alterative, antibiotic, anti-inflammatory, antimicrobial, antiseptic, antiviral, astringent, febrifuge

Medicinal Uses

Isatis was once used in war paint during the Roman Empire, where it served the double purpose of stopping bleeding and healing wounds.

The root is most commonly used, though the leaves are used as well. The leaves are said to be best for the upper portions of the body, such as the throat and lungs. Isatis diminishes the activity of bacteria, fungi, and viruses; it exhibits in vitro activity against *E. coli,* salmonella, shigella, neissera, staph, and strep bacteria. It clears heat, reduces inflammation, and increases the number and activity of phagocytes. It is used to treat AIDS, blood poisoning, boils, bronchitis, cancer, chicken pox, conjunctivitis, cough, encephalitis, fever, hepatitis, herpes, HIV, infection, jaundice, laryngitis, leukopenia (low white-blood-cell count), measles, meningitis (viral), mononucleosis, mumps, pneumonia, scarlet fever, shingles, sore throat, tonsillitis, and typhoid.

Topically, isatis can be used as a poultice to prevent infection in wounds.

Edible Uses

The root is not generally considered edible. The leaves can be consumed but are very bitter; they are best if soaked first and rinsed.

Other Uses

After a double-fermentation process, the above-ground portions of the plant produce a blue dye, which was used in ancient times, among other purposes, by peoples of Britain to dye their bodies blue in order to present a terrifying appearance to their enemies in battle. The dye is still in use today, though for tamer purposes, such as to enhance indigo dyes and to dye cotton a dark blue.

Constituents

Arginine, glutamine, proline, tyrosine, polysaccharides, sitosterol, isatin, pigments (indirubin), resin

Energetic Correspondences

- Flavor: bitter
- Temperature: cold
- Moisture: dry
- Polarity: yin
- Planet: Saturn
- Element: earth

Contraindications

Do not use isatis for more than three weeks at a time. Long-term use can deplete the body of friendly intestinal flora, weaken digestion, and cause internal coldness. There are some reports of isatis causing nausea. Do not use in cases of general weakness.

Range and Appearance

Isatis is a biennial or perennial native to Eurasia that

grows in moist, alkaline soil in full sun to partial shade. The first year it bears a rosette of leaves; in its second year it produces a stem of about 2 feet in height bearing small, four-petaled, hermaphroditic yellow flowers. The leaves are pointed and oblong. The seed capsules turn black when ripe. Isatis is widely naturalized in North America and is considered a noxious weed in many regions.

JASMINE

Botanical Name

Jasminum grandiflorum, J. officinale, J. sambac

Family

Oleaceae (Olive Family)

Etymology

Jasminum, the genus name and source of the common name *jasmine,* derives from the Persian *yasmin,* "white flower."

Also Known As

Cantonese: yeh-hsi-ming
English: pikake, queen of the night, sambac
Filipino: sampaguita
French: jasmin
German: jasmin
Hindi: johi, mogra
Indonesian: melati
Italian: gelsomino
Malaysian: melor, pekkan
Sanskrit: jati
Turkish: yasemin

Part Used

Flower

Physiological Effects

Alterative, anodyne, antibacterial, aphrodisiac, sedative

Medicinal Uses

Jasmine flowers relax and warm the genitals and intestines, harmonize the menstrual cycle, promote tissue repair, moisten the skin, and relieve pain. They are used to treat breast cancer, cough, depression, erectile dysfunction, headache, and low libido.

Topically, jasmine is used in lotions to soothe dry and sensitive skin. The dried or fresh flower makes a relaxing bath herb. The flowers can be prepared as poultice that is applied to the breasts to decrease milk production or as a cool compress to calm inflammation in the eyes. The leaves can be made into a mouthwash to treat mouth sores; the juice pressed from the leaves can be used to help remove corns.

Many consider the aroma of the flowers itself to be an aphrodisiac as well as to foster feelings of love, confidence, compassion, receptivity, and physical and emotional well-being. The essential oil of jasmine has a chemical structure similar to that of human sweat, and it has been shown to stimulate dopamine production. Smelling the essential oil of jasmine has been shown to abate seizures and lift depression. Also, the essential oil is believed to increase the attractiveness of whoever wears it.

As a flower essence, jasmine helps those who have lost their sense of purpose and lack of ambition toward true soul destiny, as well as loners who have issues with authority figures and cannot get along with others and those who are prone to accidents. It helps them replace feelings of alienation with a sense of peace in their environment.

> Pure jasmine essential oil is very expensive. If you pay a cheap price for it, expect it to be adulterated.

Edible Uses

Jasmine flowers are not only edible but wonderfully decorative. They have a delightful aroma and flavor.

Other Uses

Jasmine is used to scent soaps, perfumes, and incenses. In some cultures a garland of jasmine flowers is given to honored guests; it is also used in religious offerings, especially in the Hindu and Buddhist traditions.

In magical traditions, burning jasmine as an incense is said to induce prophetic dreams.

Constituents

Essential oils (benzyl alcohol, benzyl acetate, linalol, linalyl acetate), salicylic acid, alkaloids (jasminine)

Energetic Correspondences

- Flavor: pungent, bitter, sweet
- Temperature: neutral
- Moisture: moist
- Polarity: yin
- Planet: Venus/Jupiter/Pluto/Moon
- Element: water

Contraindications

Avoid jasmine during pregnancy. Do not confuse jasmine with yellow jasmine (*Gelsemium semipervirens*), which is toxic.

Range and Appearance

Jasmine, long considered to have one of the most beautiful and fragrant flowers on earth, is native to Asia and Africa. The genus comprises more than three hundred species of climbing vines and shrubs, both deciduous and evergreen. The leaves are opposite and usually pinnate. The flowers are long and tubular, with five to eight clefts and four corolla lobes, and they are usually white or yellow in color. The flowers are especially fragrant at night, becoming more so as the moon becomes full.

JUJUBE

Botanical Name

Ziziphus jujuba (syn. *Z. zizyphus, Z. vulgaris, Z. sativa*)

Family

Rhamnaceae (Buckthorn Family)

Etymology

Both the genus name, *Ziziphus,* and the species name, *jujube,* derive from the Greek *zizyphon,* the name of an ancient North African tree.

Also Known As

Cantonese: daai jou
English: Chinese date, jujube date, red date, sweet jujube
French: jujube de chine, jujubier de berbérie
German: brustbeere, judendom
Hindi: badara
Italian: giuggiole
Japanese: sanebuto natsume, taiso
Mandarin: da zao, mei zao
Spanish: azufaifo chino
Thai: phutsaa cheen

Parts Used

Fruit

Physiological Effects

Analgesic, anodyne, cardiotonic, chi tonic, demulcent, diuretic, emollient, expectorant, hepatoprotective, hypnotic, hypotensive, immune tonic, laxative, liver tonic, nervous system tonic, nutritive, pectoral, refrigerant, rejuvenative, sedative (mild), spleen tonic, stomach tonic, yang tonic, yin tonic

Medicinal Uses

There are both red and black varieties of jujube dates; the black variety is considered more of a chi tonic and the red one more of a blood tonic.

Jujube dates offer excellent support for the adrenal glands. They help tonify the heart, calm the spirit, strengthen the stomach and spleen, normalize bodily functions, invigorate chi, enhance the secretion of body fluids, nourish blood and chi, and improve the complexion. They can be used to help a person gain weight and have more energy, and they are added to many strong yang tonic formulas to buffer their effects.

Jujube dates are used in the treatment of allergies, anemia, anxiety, appetite loss, cancer, depression, diarrhea, dry skin, emotional instability, fatigue, heart palpitations, hypertension, hysteria, insomnia, malnutrition, moodiness, night sweats, pain, shortness of breath, stress, and underweight conditions.

Topically, jujube dates can be made into a wash,

powder, paste, or salve to soothe wounds or irritated tissues.

As a flower essence, jujube helps calm those prone to nervous stomachs and relieves nausea and anxiety.

Edible Uses

Jujube dates are as important a staple in China as apples are in North America. They can be eaten plain or prepared as ingredients in other dishes, such as oatmeal or soups. The dates can also be made into wine. The flowers of the plant are sometimes infused in honey. The leaves of the plant are also edible when cooked but are generally considered only a survival food, for emergency situations.

Other Uses

Jujube wood is used to make agricultural tools and also charcoal.

Constituents

Beta-carotene, vitamin B complex, vitamin C, calcium, iron, phosphorous, saponins, flavonoids (rutin), mucilage, triterpenes (ursolic acid, oleanolic acid), sterols, sugars, fat, zizyphic acid, pectin

Energetic Correspondences

- Flavor: sweet
- Temperature: warm
- Moisture: moist
- Polarity: yang
- Planet: Mars/Jupiter/Pluto
- Element: fire

Contraindications

Avoid jujube in cases of dampness, bloating, or intestinal parasites.

Range and Appearance

Jujube is a deciduous large shrub or tree that can grow to 30 feet tall. It is cultivated and naturalized in Eurasia, where it thrives in hot, dry climates. The leaves are smooth and firm. Many varieties have spines. The fragrant, hermaphroditic, greenish yellow flowers are borne on cymes. The oblong or oval fruits become dark red to purplish black when ripe.

JUNIPER

Botanical Name

Juniperus communis

Family

Cupressaceae (Cypress Family)

Etymology

The origin of the name is uncertain. The Latin name for the plant, *juniperus,* may derive from an earlier Celtic term; it may also derive from the Latin *iuveniparus,* "early bearing." The species name *communis* is Latin for "common."

Also Known As

Arabic: arar
Czech: jalovec
Danish: junipero
Dutch: jenever, jeneverbes
English: common juniper, gin plant
Finnish: kataja
French: genévrier
German: wacholder
Greek: arkevthos
Hebrew: ar-ar, guniper
Italian: ginepro
Japanese: junipa, seiyo-suzo
Korean: junipeo, kophyang-namu
Mandarin: du song
Norwegian: einer
Portuguese: junípero
Russian: mozhzhevelnik
Sanskrit: hapusha
Spanish: enebro, junípero
Swahili: mreteni
Swedish: en, enbär
Turkish: ardiç
Ukrainian: yalivets zvychajnyj
Vietnamese: cây bách xù
Yiddish: kadik, yalovets

Part Used

Ripe berry (ripe when blue)

Physiological Effects

Antifungal, anti-inflammatory, antirheumatic, antiscorbutic, antiseptic, carminative, diaphoretic, digestive, diuretic, emmenagogue, hypoglycemic, stomachic, urinary antiseptic

Medicinal Uses

Juniper berry stimulates the flow of urine by increasing the glomerular filtration rate, the process by which blood and wastes are purified. A small amount of the berries (five to seven) eaten before a meal helps stimulate hydrochloric acid production; eaten every day, they help clean out residues of tar and nicotine in the lungs for smokers who are quitting that habit. Juniper berry is used in the treatment of appetite loss, arthritis, catarrh, cholera, cystitis, diabetes, dysentery, flatulence, flu, gonorrhea, gout, kidney stones, tapeworm typhoid, and urinary tract infection.

Topically, juniper can be added to massage oil or used as bath herb in the treatment of joint and muscle soreness, rheumatism, and cellulite; it also can be added to salves to treat acne, eczema, or psoriasis or, as a chest rub, congestion. Juniper berry tea can be used as a gargle to relieve sore throat, as a hair rinse to treat dandruff or alopecia, as a douche to treat yeast infection, or as a room spray or steam inhalation to treat lung infection.

Edible Uses

The berries are edible; they are ripe when blue. They are sometimes roasted and used as a coffee substitute; they also can be dried and ground and used as a spice, much like pepper. Along with the branches, the berries are also used to flavor gin, chartreuse, and other alcoholic beverages.

Other Uses

Juniper tea was once used to disinfect surgeons' tools. As an incense, juniper has been burned for its purifying properties, at times during epidemics. The essential oil repels insects and is included in some perfumes. In European and Native American folkloric traditions, juniper is said to offer protection against theft, accidents, wild animal attacks, sickness, and evil. It is also sometimes used as an ingredient in love incenses.

Constituents

Vitamin C, essential oils (camphene, cineole, myrcene, pinene), sesquiterpenes (cadinene, elemene), flavonoids, glycosides, tannins, podophyllotoxin, resin

Energetic Correspondences

- Flavor: pungent, bitter
- Temperature: hot
- Moisture: dry
- Polarity: yang
- Planet: sun
- Element: fire

Contraindications

Avoid during pregnancy or in cases of heavy menstrual bleeding. Long-term use may irritate the kidneys.

Range and Appearance

Native to Europe, North America, and northern Asia, juniper is an evergreen shrub growing 1 to 12 feet tall. It is densely branched with needlelike foliage jointed at the base. Scales of the female fruiting cones become fleshy and form a berry. The berries are green when young and become blue-black in eight to ten months. This shrub smells much like pine, with citrusy overtones. It prefers full sun and well-drained soil and can tolerate extremely cold weather.

KAVA KAVA

Botanical Name

Piper methysticum

Family

Piperaceae (Pepper Family)

Etymology

The genus name, *Piper,* derives from the Greek name for pepper, *peperi.* The species name, *methysticum,* is thought to be Latin for "intoxicating." The common name *kava* is Tongan for "bitter."

Also Known As

English: asava pepper, inebriating pepper, intoxicating long pepper, kava, kawa, kawa kawa, lawena, wati, yoqona
Fijian: waka, yanggona
French: kawa, poivrier
German: kawa pfeffer, rauschpfeffer
Hawaiian: awa
Italian: pepe kava
Spanish: kavaka
Turkish: kava biberi

Parts Used

Root, upper rhizome

Physiological Effects

Analgesic, anaphrodisiac (if used excessively), anesthetic, antifungal, antibacterial, anti-inflammatory, antiseptic, antispasmodic, aphrodisiac, diaphoretic, diuretic, euphoric, hypnotic, muscle relaxant, nervine, psychoactive, sedative, siliagogue, soporific, stimulant, tonic

Medicinal Uses

Kava calms the heart and respiration, reduces blood clotting, relaxes the muscles without blocking nerve signals, and calms physical tension without numbing mental processes. It is a spinal rather than cerebral depressant. Users claim it promotes increased sound sensitivity, more fluent speech, and feelings of euphoria. Part of its mood-elevating ability might be due to its activation of mesolimbic dopaminergic neurons. Kava kava is also said to increase tolerance of pain; Aborigines often took kava kava before being tattooed, and women in labor sometimes drink kava kava juice as a calmative and to facilitate birth.

Kava kava is used in the treatment of anger, anxiety, asthma, attention deficit disorder, bronchitis, convulsions, cramps, cystitis, depression, dysuria, epilepsy, facial neuralgia, fear, fibromyalgia, gleet, gonorrhea, gout, headache (tension), hot flashes, hyperactivity, incontinence (nocturnal), insomnia, irri-

table bladder, menstrual cramps, nervousness, pain, restlessness, rheumatism, sciatica, stress, urinary tract infection, uterine inflammation, withdrawal symptoms (from alcohol, nicotine, or tranquilizers), and vaginitis.

Topically, kava kava can be used as an antiseptic, anesthetic, and healing compress or poultice for painful wounds, headaches, and fungal infections. It also can be prepared as a mouthwash to ease gum and tooth pain. It has even been used topically as a salve or poultice to treat leprosy.

Edible Uses

Generally not considered edible, aside from as tea.

Other Uses

In the South Pacific, kava kava is used ceremoniously to celebrate marriages, births, deaths, and other types of beginnings and endings. It is often used to honor a guest or to enhance communication, such as in settling a dispute, counseling a couple, or sealing a business agreement. When Captain James Cook landed on Tahiti in 1768 on *The Endeavor*, the Tahitian natives offered him kava kava.

Kava kava is thought to have been cultivated for at least three thousand years in the South Pacific. It is said that the noble classes used kava for pleasure, the priests for ceremony, and the working classes for relaxation. When European missionaries began to have strong influence in the area, many thousands of kava plants were ripped out of the ground. Where this occurred, rates of alcoholism increased.

Traditionally the root was chopped and chewed by young women and men, who then spit the juice into a bowl for others' consumption. Nowadays the root is pounded and grated and not chewed by anyone. When served a cup of kava kava tea, good manners dictate that one must chug the entire cup while the audience claps three times and shouts "Maca!," which means "empty."

Kava kava helps warm the emotions, and small amounts can produce a pleasant euphoric sensation. It is also used for divination and to produce inspiration. Taking kava kava before bed can help induce pleasant sleep and vivid dreams.

Kava kava is fat soluble, so when preparing it as a tea, add coconut milk to the steeping solution to help the infusion assimilate kava's compounds.

Constituents

Flavonoids, sesquiterpene lactones (methysticin, yangonin, kavahin, dihydrokavain)

Energetic Correspondences

- Flavor: pungent, bitter
- Temperature: hot
- Moisture: dry
- Polarity: yin
- Planet: Saturn/Uranus/Venus/Pluto
- Element: water

Contraindications

Avoid during pregnancy and while nursing, and do not give to young children. Avoid in cases of Parkinson's disease and severe depression. Do not take in conjunction with alcohol, sedatives, tranquilizers, or antidepressants, as it can potentiate their effects. Remain aware of kava kava's soporific effects; try to avoid driving, operating heavy machinery, or other activities that require fast reaction times after taking kava kava. On the plus side, kava kava, unlike many sedatives, is not habit forming. Daily use of kava shouldn't exceed three months, though occasional use on an ongoing basis is fine for those in good health.

Kava kava may cause the tongue, mouth, and other body parts to feel somewhat numb and rubbery temporarily; this is normal. However, excess amounts can cause disturbed vision, dilated pupils, and difficulty walking. Large doses taken for extended periods can have a cumulative effect on the liver, causing kawaism, a condition marked by a yellowish tinge to the skin, a scaly rash, apathy, anorexia, and bloodshot eyes.

In Europe there have been some reports of severe liver damage resulting from use of kava kava, prompting a number of nations to ban sales of it. The problem appears to be caused by a compound, called pipermethystine, that is found in the stem peelings and leaves of the kava plant but not in the roots. Traditional kava preparations are extracted from the roots, and the peelings and leaves are discarded. However, some European pharmaceutical companies bought up the kava waste products when demand for kava extract soared in the early 2000s. The cases of liver damage appear to have involved people who took standardized extract capsules, which may have contained kava stem peelings and roots as well as chemical solvents. For this reason, avoid kava products made from the leaves or stems of the plant. The traditional tea prepared from the root appears to be quite safe.

Range and Appearance

Kava kava is native to the islands of the southern and western Pacific Ocean. It is a shrub that thrives at 500 to 1,000 feet above sea level in well-drained, sandy soil. The stems vary in color from green to black and have swollen nodules. The cordate leaves can grow to 8 inches in diameter. Flowering is rare. When flowers do appear, the male flowers are singular and axillary, while the female flowers form numerous spikes.

There are more than twenty varieties of kava kava, with white and black grades having the greatest social and commercial significance. Growers prefer the black grades, as they provide a quicker return on their investment, being ready to harvest in about two and a half years. Users prefer white grades, which take about four years to mature but have stronger effects.

LADY'S MANTLE

Botanical Name

Alchemilla vulgaris, A. xanthochlora

Family

Rosaceae (Rose Family)

Etymology

The genus name, *Alchemilla*, derives from the Arabic

alkemelych, "alchemy," as alchemists believed that the morning dewdrops on this plant, which they called "heaven's water," held magical powers to help them in their work. The "lady" in the common name *lady's mantle* is the Virgin Mary, with whom the plant was associated in the Middle Ages; the leaf of the plant was thought to resemble a cloak. In earlier times, however, this plant was linked to Freya, the Norse goddess of love and beauty.

Also Known As

Dutch: leeuwenvoet

English: bear's foot, dewcup, great sanicle, lion's foot, nine hooks, Our Lady's mantle

Finnish: poimulehti

French: alchémille, manteau de Notre Dame, patte de lapin, pied de lion, pinou, porte-rosé

German: frauenmantel, grosser sanikel, mutterkraut, ohmkraut, sinnau, taumantel

Italian: alchemilla comune, pie di lione

Spanish: alquimila

Swedish: daggkåpa

Parts Used

Leaf, flowering shoot

Physiological Effects

Anti-inflammatory, astringent, depurative, diuretic, emmenagogue, febrifuge, hemostatic, liver decongestant, nervine, styptic, tonic, vulnerary

Medicinal Uses

Lady's mantle breaks up congestion, removes excess dampness, clears heat and toxins, stops bleeding, promotes tissue healing, reduces pain, and calms the spirit. It also strengthens muscles and tissues and helps restore vitality after childbirth. It was used to staunch bleeding on the battlefields of the fifteenth and sixteenth centuries. Today, it is used in the treatment of appetite loss, cystitis, diarrhea, hemorrhage, irregular menses, leukorrhea, menorrhagia, menopausal flooding (heavy menstrual bleeding), postpartum hemorrhage, rheumatism, and uterine prolapse. It can be taken by a pregnant woman ten days before she expects to deliver to prevent excessive bleeding during childbirth; it also can be used to stimulate labor that has been delayed or to prevent miscarriage. However, such use should be supervised by a qualified health-care professional.

Topically, lady's mantle can be made into a healing poultice for wounds. It also can be prepared as a bolus, douche, or sitz bath to treat vaginal infection or leukorrhea. It can be used as an eyewash to treat conjunctivitis, as a mouthwash to heal sores and after dental extraction, and as a gargle to treat laryngitis. The juice or tea can be applied topically to dry up acne; the plant can be prepared as a facial steam for the same purpose.

Edible Uses

The flowers and leaves are edible when young and can be added to salads. The root is also edible.

Other Uses

Lady's mantle is often included in lotions to soften rough skin, lighten freckles, and minimize enlarged pores or birthmarks. In magical traditions it is used to attract love.

Constituents

Lecithin, tannin (ellagic acid), salicylic acid, saponins, phytosterols, essential oil

Energetic Correspondences

- Flavor: bitter
- Temperature: warm
- Moisture: dry
- Polarity: yin
- Planet: Venus/Uranus/Mars
- Element: water

Contraindications

Avoid during pregnancy, except under the guidance of a qualified health-care professional. Do not use in conjunction with oxytocin.

Range and Appearance

Lady's mantle is a perennial, native to Eurasia but widely naturalized, can grow 4 to 18 inches in height. The stems are bluish green when young and become reddish brown as they mature. The toothed, palmate, almost circular leaves have seven to eleven lobes each. The greenish yellow flowers are small and grow in umbellate panicles. The plant prefers moist, shady conditions.

LARCH

Botanical Name

Larix spp., including *L. americana* (American larch), *L. decidua* (European larch), *L. gmelinii* (Dahurian larch), *L. laricina* (syn. *Pinus laricina*, *L. alaskensis*), *L. lyallii* (subalpine larch), *L. occidentalis* (western larch), *L. sibirica* (Russian larch)

Family

Pinaceae (Pine Family)

Etymology

The genus name, *Larix*, and the common name *larch* derive from the Latin name for larch, *laricina*.

Also Known As

Cantonese: luò yè song
English: black larch, hackmatack, tamarack, violon
Finnish: lehyikuusi
French: mélèze laricin
German: lärche
Italian: larice
Japanese: karamatsu
Russian: listvennitza sibirsky
Swedish: lärk, lärkträd

Part Used

Inner bark

Physiological Effects

Alterative, anti-inflammatory, astringent, diuretic, immune stimulant, laxative, tonic, vulnerary

Medicinal Uses

Larch's active component, arabinogalactan, is a naturally occurring carbohydrate that activates macro-phage production and exhibits antiviral properties. It also prevents "unfriendly" bacteria from adhering to cells and encourages the increase in populations of "friendly" bacteria that support the immune system. Larch is used in the treatment of asthma, bleeding, bronchitis, colds, cystitis, depression, diarrhea, dysentery, ear infection, flu, jaundice, poisonous insect bites, and rheumatism.

Topically, larch can be used as a poultice to reduce inflammation; to treat boils, frostbite, hemorrhoids, and wounds, it can be prepared as a salve, sitz bath, or poultice. The oil distilled from larch has anthelmintic, emmenagogue, and vulnerary properties, and it can be applied topically to treat gout, neuralgia, and rheumatism. However, large amounts of the distilled oil, even applied topically, can irritate the kidneys.

Edible Uses

The inner bark is not generally considered edible, aside from as tea. The young shoots are edible raw or cooked. The gummy sap that exudes from the tree can be chewed as a gum.

Other Uses

Larch was once a common material for making snowshoes. It is valued for its ability to resist decay, and it is popular for building boats. The yellowed autumn leaves can be processed to produce a brown dye for wool.

Constituents

Polysaccharide (arabinogalactan), lignan, lariciresinol, liovil, secoisolariciresinol, resins (larinolic acid, laricinolic acid), volatile oils (pinene, limonene, phellandrene, borneol)

Energetic Correspondences

- Flavor: bitter
- Temperature: warm
- Moisture: dry
- Polarity: yang
- Planet: Mars/Saturn/Sun/Jupiter
- Element: air

Contraindications

The use of larch by pregnant and nursing women has not been studied comprehensively, so until such time as studies have shown larch to be safe, it would be best to avoid it at these times. Those on a low-galactose diet should avoid using preparations of concentrated arabinogalactans, such as those in some commercial products.

Range and Appearance

Larch trees are native to Eurasia and northern North America and prefer cold, moist areas; they are often found near bogs and swamps. They can reach a height of 80 to 100 feet. The trees have a silver-gray to gray-brown bark when young, that changes to reddish brown to brown on mature trees. The trees are deciduous, with soft, 1- to 2-inch-long leaves that grow in clusters.

LAVENDER

Botanical Name

Lavandula spp., including *L. angustifolia* (syn. *L. officinalis, L. vera, L. spica*), *L. stoechas* (French lavender), *L. viridis*

Family

Lamiaceae (Mint Family)

Etymology

The genus name, *Lavandula,* and common name *lavender* derive from the Latin *lavare,* "to wash," as this herb was added to baths for its therapeutic properties and delightful fragrance.

Also Known As

Arabic: khuzaama, lafand
Armenian: hoosam
Bulgarian: lavandula
Cantonese: fàn yì chóu
Croatian: ljekovita lavanda
Czech: levandule
Danish: lavendel
Dutch: lavendel

English: elf lead, lavers, nard, spike
Estonian: tähklavendel
Finnish: tupsupäälaventeli
French: lavende
German: kopfwehblume, lavendel, tabakblumen
Greek: levanta
Hebrew: lavender
Hungarian: levendula
Icelandic: lofnarblóm
Italian: lavanda, nardo, spigo
Japanese: rabenda
Korean: rabandin
Lithuanian: tikroju levanda
Mandarin: xun yi cao
Norwegian: lavendel
Polish: lawenda waskolistna
Portuguese: alfazema
Russian: lavanda
Sanskrit: dharu
Serbian: lavanda
Spanish: espliego, lavanda alhuccema, lhucema
Swedish: lavendel
Thai: lawendeort
Turkish: lavânta çiçegi
Ukrainian: lavanda
Vietnamese: hoa oai huong
Yiddish: lavendl

Part Used

Flower

Physiological Effects

Analgesic, anaphrodisiac, antibacterial, antidepressant, antifungal, anti-inflammatory, antiseptic, antispasmodic, aromatic, bitter, carminative, cholagogue, digestive, diuretic (mild), expectorant, nervine, rubefacient, sedative, stimulant, tonic

Medicinal Uses

Before World War II lavender was commonly used as an antiseptic dressing for wounds and to get rid of parasites. In addition to its wound-healing properties, lavender has been shown to exhibit activity against diphtheria, typhoid, pneumonia, staph, strep, and many flu viruses. The herb clears heat, calms the nerves, and settles digestion. It also appears to stabilize or inhibit mast cell activity. It is used to treat amenorrhea, anxiety, asthma (related to nerves), colic, convulsions, cough, depression, dizziness, fainting, fear, fever, flatulence, halitosis, headache (tension or migraine), hypertension, hysteria, insomnia, irritability, muscle spasms, nausea, nervous exhaustion, nervousness, pain, and stress.

Topically, lavender tea can be used as a mouthwash to get rid of bad breath, a footbath to relieve fatigue, or a douche, sitz bath, or enema to treat yeast infections, trichomonas, gardnerella, or other types of infection. Lavender can also be used as a bath herb to soothe cranky children. It can be prepared as a fragrant shampoo or rinse to help prevent hair loss, as a salve to relieve inflammation (including that related to eczema and psoriasis), or as a massage oil to treat cellulite, earache, edema, rheumatism, and sore muscles.

Lavender essential oil is an excellent remedy for relieving pain, promoting healing, and preventing infection and scarring. It can be applied topically, undiluted, to treat acne, athlete's foot, bee stings, boils, burns, cold sores, headache, infected wounds, insect and spider bites, joint soreness, scabies, and toothache. Placing a drop of lavender essential oil on the edge of the mattress of a teething baby can help calm him or her. Simply inhaling the scent of lavender essential oil from the bottle helps prevent fainting and relieves stress and depression.

Edible Uses

Lavender flowers are edible and, in fact, are an essential ingredient in Herbes de Provence. They are often added in small amounts to various dishes and can be candied or crystallized. Lavender-infused honey is a superb delicacy. Lavender leaves have a strong flavor but can be eaten in small amounts.

Other Uses

In the Middle Ages lavender was a popular strewing herb and was a common ingredient in sachets to repel moths and bugs from stored clothing. In the days when corsets were the fashion, ladies would tuck some lavender oil in a bottle around their necks to revive them when they were feeling faint. And when the world was in the throes of the bubonic plague, lavender was burned in sick rooms to help prevent the spread of the disease.

Today, lavender is popular as a spirit lifting, nerve-relaxing, calming fragrance. It is popular in baths, sachets, potpourris, sleep pillows, soaps, perfumes, and other aromatic products. It is a helpful fragrance in a birthing room, as it can help calm the laboring woman, and also in a death room, where it helps calm all present.

The dried leaves of the plant are sometimes included in smoking mixtures.

Constituents

Flavonoids (luteolin), essential oils (linalool, camphor, eucalyptol, geraniol, limonene, cineole), tannins, coumarins, triterpenoids

Energetic Correspondences

- Flavor: bitter, pungent, sweet
- Temperature: cool
- Moisture: dry
- Polarity: yang
- Planet: Sun/Mercury/Jupiter
- Element: air

Contraindications

Avoid large doses of lavender during pregnancy, as its effect on the developing fetus has not yet been determined.

Range and Appearance

Lavender is a small, tender, perennial shrub, native to the Mediterranean region, that prefers dry soil and full sun; it is common in scrubland and on grassy hillsides. It grows to a height of 1 to 4 feet, though on occasion it reaches up to 6 feet. The plant appears to be covered with a grayish down. The leaves are opposite and narrow. The aromatic purple flowers grow in terminal spikes and attract bees and butterflies.

LEMON BALM

Botanical Name
Melissa officinalis

Family
Lamiaceae (Mint Family)

Etymology
Melissa, the genus name, derives from the Greek *melisso-phyllum,* "bee leaf," in reference to the flower being a favorite of bees. The species name, *officinalis,* is Latin and means that the plant has long been an official herb of the apothecaries.

Also Known As
Arabic: hashisha-al-namal, turijan
Bulgarian: matochina
Cantonese: heung fung chou
Czech: medunka
Danish: citronmrlisse
English: balm, bee balm, dropsy plant, heart's delight, melissa
Esperanto: meliso
Estonian: meliss
Finnish: sitruunamelissa
French: mélisse
German: melisse, zitronenmelisse
Greek: melissophyllon
Hebrew: melissa
Hungarian: melissza
Icelandic: sítrónumelissa
Italian: melissa
Japanese: remonbamu, seiyo-yamahakka
Korean: mellisa
Mandarin: xiang feng cao
Norwegian: sitronmelisse
Polish: melisa lekarska
Portuguese: erva-cidreira, melissa
Romanian: roinita
Russian: melissa limonnaya, limonnik
Serbian: melisa
Spanish: balsamita maior, toronjil
Swedish: citronmeliss, hjärtansfröjd
Turkish: limon nanesi, melisa otu
Ukrainian: melisa likarska
Yiddish: melise

Part Used
Aboveground plant

Physiological Effects
Antibacterial, antidepressant, antihistamine, anti-inflammatory, antioxidant, antispasmodic, antiviral, aromatic, carminative, cephalic, cholagogue, diaphoretic, digestive, emmenagogoue, febrifuge, hypotensive (mild), nervine, parturient, rejuvenative, sedative, stomachic, tonic, vasodilator

Medicinal Uses
Lemon balm was widely used in ancient Greece and Rome. Avicenna, the great Arabic physician (980–1037), said that lemon balm caused "the mind and heart to be merry."

Lemon balm clears heat, calms the heart, improves concentration, cleanses the liver, improves chi circulation, and lifts the spirits. German studies indicate that lemon balm's volatile oils help protect the cerebrum from excess external stimuli. It is a good herb for children; a cup of tea before bed can help prevent nightmares and allow for a good night's sleep, and it is excellent to calm the nerves and boost the mood of schoolchildren who are anxious about upcoming tests.

Lemon balm is used in the treatment of allergies, amenorrhea, anxiety, asthma, attention deficit disorder, bronchitis, chicken pox, chronic fatigue, colic, colds, depression, fever, flatulence, flu, Grave's disease, headache, heart palpitations, herpes, homesickness, hyperactivity, hypertension, hysteria, indigestion, insomnia, menstrual cramps, migraine, mumps, muscle spasms, nausea, nervousness, Newcastle disease, nightmares, pain, restlessness, senility, shingles, smallpox, stomachache, and teething.

Topically, lemon balm can be used as a compress to treat boils, burns, eczema, gout, headache, insect bites, sunburn, tumors, and wounds. It makes an uplifting bath herb. The essential oil can be added to salves to treat herpes.

Edible Uses

Lemon balm is certainly edible. The chopped leaves are used to season many dishes and as a garnish. The dried leaves are not as flavorful as the fresh, so use the fresh plant whenever possible.

The tea made from the fresh leaves is flavorful and refreshing, with a lemon scent. The herb can be steeped for ten minutes or longer, as it does not become bitter with longer steeping. Lemon balm tea is lovely hot or iced and is suitable for daily use. It goes well with the addition of mint or a squeeze of lime.

Other Uses

Lemon balm is used to make Eau des Carmes, a reviving wine made by the Carmelites and dating from the seventeenth century. It was once used as a strewing herb. The leaves are rubbed on wood to produce a lovely shine. Beekeepers rub lemon balm inside hives to attract new bees and keep established ones home. In magical traditions, lemon balm is burned as incense or placed in sachets to attract love and protection from negative energies.

Constituents

Vitamin C, calcium, magnesium, essential oils (citral, linalool, eugenol, citronellal, geraniol), tannins (catechin), bitter principle, resin, flavonoids (polyphenols), succinic acid, rosmarinic acid

Energetic Correspondences

- Flavor: sour
- Temperature: cool
- Moisture: dry
- Polarity: yin
- Planet: Moon/Venus/Jupiter
- Element: water

Contraindications

Lemon balm is generally considered very safe and is a favorite herb for children. It can lower thyroid function, however, which is beneficial in some cases but not for those with a hypothyroid condition.

Range and Appearance

Lemon balm, a perennial native to Europe but widely cultivated in North America, prefers to grow in disturbed areas and open woods. The plant grows to about 2 feet in height and has a four-sided stem. Its lemon-scented leaves are opposite, oval, pointed, and round-toothed. The light yellow, white, or lavender flowers are borne on auxiliary stems.

The herb thrives in full sun to partial shade, needs only moderate watering, and prefers well-drained soil. Bees love it; growing lemon balm in the garden will help attract them to the garden. Lemon balm will also repel many pests from the garden.

LEMON VERBENA

Botanical Name

Aloysia citriodora (syn. *A. triphylla, Verbena triphylla, V. citriodora*)

Family

Verbenaceae (Teak Family)

Etymology

The genus name, *Aloysia*, was given in honor of Maria Louisa Teresa de Parma (1751–1819), the wife of Spain's King Charles IV. The species name, *citriodora*, derives from the Latin *citrus*, a name for citrus fruits, in reference to the plant's lemony scent.

Also Known As

Cantonese: nìhng mung mah bin chóu
Croatian: zeleni limun-sporis
Czech: sporys
Danish: jernurt
Dutch: citroenverbena
Estonian: sidrunaloisia
Finnish: lippia
French: verveine citronelle
German: zitronenverbene
Greek: louïza
Hebrew: lipia limonit, luizah
Hungarian: citrom verbéna
Japanese: boshu-boku

Korean: remon beobena
Lithuanian: citrininè aloyzija
Mandarin: ning meng ma bian cao
Polish: lippia trójlistna
Portuguese: limonete
Romanian: verbină
Russian: verbena limonnaya
Serbian: limun verbena
Spanish: hierbaluisa
Swedish: lippia
Yiddish: tsitrin-lippie

Part Used

Aboveground plant

Physiological Effects

Antibacterial, antispasmodic, aromatic, febrifuge, sedative, stomachic

Medicinal Uses

Lemon verbena clears heat, relaxes the nerves, and fights infection. It is used in the treatment of asthma, colds, diarrhea, dyspepsia, fever, flatulence, flu, heart palpitations, indigestion, menstrual cramps, migraines, neuralgia, nausea, restlessness, sinus congestion, stomachache, and vertigo.

Topically, it makes a refreshing lemon-scented bath herb, and it can be used as a compress to treat puffy eyes or as a gargle for sore throats and tonsillitis.

Edible Uses

Lemon verbena is used as a culinary herb. It has a lemony aroma and flavor, stronger and sweeter than that of lemon balm, with a hint of vanilla in the taste. Lemon verbena tea sweetened and served iced is popular in Spain. It is also lovely with the addition of mint.

Other Uses

Lemon verbena is popular in potpourris, as its leaves have a long-lasting scent. The essential oil is used to scent soaps, bath oils, cosmetics, and perfumes and to repel aphids, mosquitoes, and mites. In magical traditions, lemon verbena is used to make one attractive to the opposite sex.

Constituents

Flavonoids, essential oils (borneol, cineole, citral, geraniol, limonene, linalool), mucilage, tannin

Energetic Correspondences

- Flavor: sour
- Temperature: cool
- Moisture: dry
- Polarity: yang
- Planet: Mercury/Venus
- Element: air

Contraindications

Large or prolonged dosages can irritate the digestive tract.

Range and Appearance

A perennial native to the South, lemon verbena has pale green, fragrant, lanceolate, 3- to 4-inch-long leaves arranged in threes. The leaves have parallel veins at right angles to the midrib. The flowers are pale purple and grow in terminal panicles.

The plant prefers full sun, moderate to large amounts of water, and light, well-drained, alkaline soil.

LEMONGRASS

Botanical Name

Cymbopogon citratus (formerly *Andropogon nardus*)

Family

Poaceae (Grass) Family

Etymology

The genus name, *Cymbopogon*, derives from the Greek *kumbo*, "cup," and *pogon*, "beard." *Citratus*, the species name, refers to its fresh lemony scent.

Also Known As

Arabic: hashisha al-limun
Bulgarian: limonova treva
Cantonese: chóu gèung, fùng màauh

Croatian: vlaska

Czech: citrónová tráva

Danish: citrongræs

Dutch: citroengras

English: citronella, fever grass, squinant

Esperanto: citronelo

Estonian: harilik sidrunhein

Finnish: sitruunaruoho

French: verveine des Indes

German: zitronengras

Greek: lemonochorto

Hebrew: essef limon, limonit rehanit

Hindi: khawi, sera, verveine

Hungarian: citronella

Icelandic: sítrónugras

Indonesian: sereh

Italian: cimbopogone

Japanese: remonso

Khmer: bai mak nao

Korean: remon-gurasu

Mandarin: chao jiang, feng mao

Nepali: pirhe ghaans

Polish: palczatka cytrynowa

Portuguese: capim-santo, erva-cidreira

Romanian: citronella

Russian: limmononaya trava

Serbian: limun trava

Spanish: hierba de limón, té limón, zacxate-limón

Swedish: citrongräs

Thai: cha khrai, ta krai

Turkish: limon out

Vietnamese: sà, sa chanh

Part Used

Leaf

Physiological Effects

Antibacterial, antifungal, antioxidant, antiseptic, antispasmodic, antiviral, aromatic, astringent, diaphoretic, digestive, diuretic, febrifuge, refrigerant, rubefacient, sedative, stimulant, sudorific

Medicinal Uses

Lemongrass essential oil has exhibited activity against *E. coli* and *Staphylococcus aureus*. The herb contains five components that help prevent blood platelet aggregation. It is used in the treatment of cholera, colds, colic, diarrhea, fever, flatulence, flu, headache, herpes, insomnia, parasites (especially nematodes), and stomachache. It is also considered a cancer preventive.

Topically, lemongrass can be used as a compress to relieve arthritis pain and as a bath herb to soothe sore muscles.

Edible Uses

Lemongrass is commonly used in South Asian cuisine. It has a delightful lemonade-like flavor.

Other Uses

Lemongrass is sometimes planted around homes to deter snakes. In magical traditions, it is used to encourage passion and psychic development.

Constituents

Vitamin C, silica, essential oils (borneol, citral, citronellal, geraniol), monoterpene (myrcene), alkaloids, saponins

Energetic Correspondences

- Flavor: sour, pungent, bitter
- Temperature: cool
- Moisture: dry
- Polarity: yang
- Planet: Mercury
- Element: air

Contraindications

Avoid large doses during pregnancy, as it can stimulate the uterus.

Range and Appearance

Native to the tropics of Southeast Asia, lemongrass, a tender perennial, can grow up to 6 feet in height. It has long, narrow, pointed leaves that are rough and sawlike to the touch. The leaves grow in groups and sheath the stem at the plant's base, which is bulbous and fibrous. When the leaves are crushed they give off a distinct aroma of lemon. The flowers grow in a bunched panicle.

Lemongrass thrives in a hot, sunny environment with sandy soil, but it will tolerate full sun to full shade. It requires moderate to high amounts of water and rich loam or sandy soil.

LICORICE

Botanical Name

Glycyrrhiza glabra (European licorice), *G. inflata, G. lepidota* (American licorice), *G. uralensis* (Chinese licorice)

Family

Fabaceae (Pea Family)

Etymology

The genus name, *Glycyrrhiza,* derives from the Greek *glyky ryhiza,* "sweet root," as does the common name *licorice. Glabra,* the species name, is Latin for "smooth," in reference to the smooth seed-pods.

Also Known As

Afrikaans: soethoutwortel
Arabic: irg as-sus, sous
Armenian: madoodag
Bengali: jashtimodhu
Bulgarian: sladnik
Cantonese: gam chou
Croatian: sladki korijen
Czech: lé korice
Danish: lakrids
Dutch: zoethout
English: black sugar, great harmonizer, grandfather herb, honeygrass, lacris, liquorice, Spanish juice, sweet root
Esperanto: glicirizo
Estonian: lagrits, magusjuur
Farsi: shirin bayan
Finnish: lakritsikasvi
French: réglisse
German: lakritze
Greek: glykoriza
Hebrew: shush, shush kireah

Hindi: mulhathi
Hungarian: édesfa
Icelandic: lakkrís
Italian: liguiririzia, regolizia
Japanese: rikorisu, uraru-kanzo
Korean: kamcho, rikorisu
Latvian: lakrica
Mandarin: gan cao, kan tsau
Norwegian: lakrisrot
Polish: korzen lukrecji
Portuguese: alcaçuz
Romanian: lemn dulce, reglisa
Russian: lakrichnik, lakrista
Sanskrit: madhuuka, yashtimadhu
Serbian: konjeda
Spanish: orozuz, ragaliz
Swahili: susu
Swedish: lakrits
Thai: chaometes
Turkish: meyan kökü
Ukrainian: lokrytsya
Urdu: mulhati
Vietnamese: cam thao
Yiddish: lakrets
Zulu: mlomo-mnandi

Part Used

Root (stolon)

Physiological Effects

Adrenal tonic, alterative, antacid, antiarthritic, antibacterial, antifungal, anti-inflammatory, antimutagenic, antioxidant, antiseptic, antispasmodic, antitumor, antitussive, antivenomous, antiviral, aperient, aphrodisiac, chi tonic, demulcent, emollient, expectorant, febrifuge, galactagogue, hepatoprotective, immune tonic, laxative (mild), lung tonic, nutritive, pectoral, phytoestrogenic, rejuvenative, sedative, sialogogue, tonic

Medicinal Uses

Licorice is one of the most commonly used herbs in traditional Chinese medicine. It enters all twelve meridians and harmonizes the effects of other herbs, helping to prolong their effects. Licorice clears heat and encourages the movement of leukocytes toward areas of inflammation. Its constituent glycyrrhizin (which is similar to the human hormone cortisol) inhibits the production of the inflammatory prostaglandin E2. Licorice stimulates interferon production, soothes irritated mucous membranes, restores pituitary activity, and helps normalize the function of glands and organs. It also helps induce feelings of calmness, peace, and harmony.

Licorice is used in the treatment of acid indigestion, Addison's disease, adrenal weakness, age spots, AIDS, alcoholism, allergies, arthritis, asthma, bladder infection, bronchitis, bursitis, cancer, candida, carbuncles, catarrh, chronic fatigue, cirrhosis, colds, constipation, cough (dry), debility, depression, diarrhea, dry cough, dropsy, dyspnea, dysuria, eczema, Epstein-Barr virus, emotional instability, emphysema, fatigue, fever, gallbladder inflammation, gastritis, gout, Grave's disease, hair loss, hay fever, heartburn, hemorrhoids, hepatitis, herpes, HIV, hives, hoarseness, hypoglycemia, hysteria, immune system weakness, infertility (male and female), irregular ovulation, irritability, irritable bowel, laryngitis, Lyme disease, menstrual cramps, Parkinson's disease, pharyngitis, poisoning (from food or chemicals), prostatitis, psoriasis, shortness of breath, sore throat, stomachache, stress, tendonitis, thirst, tuberculosis, tumors, ulcers, underweight conditions, and wheezing.

In hair rinses, it can help prevent hair loss and dandruff. It also can be used as a lubricating enema or douche. Licorice is used in lotions and salves for inflamed eyelids and dry eyes, eczema, psoriasis, shingles, and wounds. It is included in mouthwashes for tooth decay prevention, gingivitis, and mouth sores. It can be used as a wash for itchy skin, and rashes. It is found in hair rinses for hair loss and dandruff. Also used as a lubricating enema or douche.

Edible Uses

Licorice root contains glycyrrhizin, which is fifty times sweeter than sugar, and as a result licorice is a common sweetener, one that can be safely consumed even by most diabetics. However, most licorice candies contain essential oil of anise or synthetic flavorings and not licorice, so don't depend on "licorice" bonbons for therapeutic value.

Licorice has a sweet, woody flavor and is an excellent thirst quencher. It is often added to other herbs and medicines to improve their flavor.

Other Uses

Ninety percent of the licorice imported into the United States is used to flavor tobacco. Licorice can also be used to make a fabric dye. In magical traditions, licorice is used in love charms and to promote fidelity.

Constituents

B-complex vitamins, choline, phosphorous, potassium, glycosides (glycyrrhizin, also known as glycyrrhic acid), saponins, phytoestrogens, coumarins, flavonoids (isoflavones, liquiritin, isoliquiritin), amines (asparagine, betaine), essential oil, protein, fat

Energetic Correspondences

- Flavor: sweet, slightly bitter
- Temperature: neutral
- Moisture: moist
- Polarity: yin
- Planet: Venus
- Element: water

Contraindications

Avoid licorice in cases of edema, nausea, vomiting, and rapid heartbeat. Licorice is not recommended during pregnancy or in combination with steroid or digoxin medications. Large doses may cause sodium retention and potassium depletion and may be emetic. Prolonged or excessive use may elevate blood pressure and cause headache and vertigo. Continuous use is not recommended in excess of six weeks, except under the guidance of a qualified health-care practitioner. Chinese licorice (*G. uralensis*) is said to be less likely to cause side effects than the European variety (*G. glabra*).

All these precautions notwithstanding, licorice is often added in very small amounts to other herbal formulas to harmonize them and prevent undesirable side effects.

Range and Appearance

There are about twenty species of licorice native to Eurasia, Australia, and North and South America. These perennial herbs or small shrubs have alternate, oddly pinnate leaves. Many of the species have sticky hairs. The small whitish, yellow, or purplish pealike flowers grow in spikes or racemes from the leaf axils. Licorice is often found in the wild in grassy areas with salty, alkaline soil. It prefers full sun to partial shade, moderate amounts of water, and well-drained or sandy soil. It fixes nitrogen and can be cultivated and turned into the soil to enrich it.

LINDEN

Botanical Name

Tilia spp., including *T. americana, T. cordata, T.* x *europea, T. platyphyllos*

Family

Tiliaceae (Tilia Family)

Etymology

Tilia, the genus name, is the classical Latin name for this tree. The common name *linden* derives from the Old English name for the tree, *lind.*

Also Known As

English: lime tree
Finnish: svartlind
French: tilleul
German: kleinblättrige
Italian: tiglio
Italian: tilia
Spanish: flor de tila
Swedish: lind, skogslind

Part Used

Flower

Physiological Effects

Antidepressant, antispasmodic, cephalic, cholagogue, choleretic, diaphoretic, diuretic, emollient, expectorant, hypotensive, nervine, sedative, stomachic, sudorific, tonic, vasodilator, vulnerary

Medicinal Uses

Linden moves stagnant chi, calms the nerves, and promotes rest. It also helps heal blood vessel walls, and its high mucilage content helps soothe irritated respiratory passages. It is used in the treatment of anxiety, arteriosclerosis, asthma, bronchitis, catarrh, colds, cough, diarrhea, fever, flu, headache, high cholesterol, hypertension, hysteria, indigestion, insomnia, migraine, pain, sore throat, and stress.

Topically, linden helps regenerate the skin. It can be used as a compress to treat boils, burns, and rashes and as a gargle for mouth sores. It is often included in facial washes to clear acne, freckles, and wrinkles. As a bath herb, it promotes relaxation and is often used to calm restless children.

Edible Uses

The flowers are edible and have a fragrant, jasmine-like aroma and pleasant flavor. The young leaves are also edible. The sap of the tree can be used as a sweetener or concentrated like maple syrup. Linden flower tea is one of the most popular herbal teas in Europe, where it is enjoyed to calm the nerves and aid digestion. It is a safe and suitable tea for children as well as adults.

Other Uses

The inner bark yields fibers that can be used to make paper, rope, baskets, mats, and cloth. The soft wood is favored by wood carvers. The flowers are sometimes added to sleep pillows.

Constituents

Vitamin C, iodine, manganese, essential oil (farnesol), flavonoids (herperidin, quercitin, kaempferol, astralagin), mucilage, phenolic acids (chlorogenic, caffeic), tannins

Energetic Correspondences

* Flavor: pungent, sweet
* Temperature: warm

- Moisture: dry
- Polarity: yang
- Planet: Jupiter/Saturn
- Element: air

Contraindications

Tilia americana should be consumed only in moderation, as large doses may cause nausea and excess use may damage the heart.

Range and Appearance

Linden trees, of which about thirty species exist, are native to Europe, western Asia, and North America. The trees prefer slightly acidic soil and moderate shade and water. They can grow to 130 feet in height. The leaves are alternate, heart shaped, uneven, and darker green on top and paler green underneath. The yellowish white, five-petaled flowers hang in clusters from peduncles and are beloved by bees.

LOBELIA

Botanical Name

Lobelia cardinalis (red lobelia, cardinal flower),
  L. inflata, L. siphilitica (blue lobelia)

Family

Campanulaceae (Bellflower Family)

Etymology

The genus name, *Lobelia*, honors the Flemish botanist Mathias l'Obel.

Also Known As

English: asthma weed, bladderpod, cardinal flower,
  emetic weed, eyebright, gag weed, Indian
  tobacco, pukeweed, vomit weed, vomitwort
Finnish: rohtolobelia
French: lobélie enflée, tabac Indien
German: aufgeblasene lobelie
Japanese: hanpenren
Sanskrit: dhavala
Swedish: läkelobelia

Parts Used

Leaf, flower, seed , root (rarely)

Physiological Effects

Alterative, antispasmodic, antivenomous, astringent, bronchial dilator, cathartic, diaphoretic, diuretic, emetic, emmenagogue, expectorant, muscle relaxant, narcotic, nervine, respiratory stimulant, sialagogue, sedative (in larger doses), stimulant (in smaller doses)

Medicinal Uses

The root of Lobelia was used by the Iroquois to treat syphilis, hence the species name *siphilitica*. Lobelia was included in the United States Pharmacopoeia from 1820 until 1936 and in the National Formulary from 1936 until 1960. Lobelia moves stagnant chi, relaxes and strengthens the nerves, calms spasms, opens and relaxes the respiratory system, allowing oxygen to flow more freely, and stimulates the vagus nerve, thereby having an emetic action when used in large amounts. Midwives once used lobelia to relax the pelvic muscles of the woman in labor. Lobelia also enhances the activity of other herbs.

Lobelia is used to treat allergies, asthma, bronchial spasms, bronchitis, catarrh, convulsions, diphtheria, dyspnea, edema, epilepsy, hysteria, laryngitis, muscle spasms, rheumatoid pain, pleurisy, sciatica, syphilis (root), tetanus, tonsillitis, wheezing, and whooping cough. It is sometimes smoked in a water pipe to treat asthma or bronchitis.

Topically, lobelia can be used as a gargle to soothe sore throat or a wash, compress, liniment, or poultice to treat boils, eczema, herpes, poison ivy or oak, and sore muscles. The freshly pressed juice of the plant can be applied topically to ease the pain of toothache.

Edible Uses

Not generally considered edible.

Other Uses

Some Native American tribes believed that placing a leaf in the bed of a quarreling couple would help them regain their love. Lobelia was both chewed and smoked by Native Americans. The alkaloid lobeline mimics the effects of nicotine, and thus this herb can be helpful for people wanting to give up tobacco.

Constituents

Niacin, magnesium, potassium, sulfur, piperidine alkaloids (lobeline, isolobeline), lobelic acid, chelidonic acid, glycoside (lobelacrin), essential oil (lobelianin), fats, lignin, resin

Energetic Correspondences

- Flavor: bitter, pungent
- Temperature: neutral
- Moisture: dry
- Polarity: yin
- Planet: Mercury/Saturn/Neptune
- Element: water

Contraindications

Avoid overdosing, as overdose can cause sweating, nausea, vomiting, pain, paralysis, lowered body temperature, rapid pulse, coma, and even death. Lobelia is best used in combination with other herbs and in small amounts, one-fifth to one-third the amount of other herbs used in a formula.

Avoid during pregancy or in cases of hypotension, hypertension, fainting, paralysis, shock, pneumonia, or fluid surrounding the heart or lungs.

Lobelia inflata is much more emetic than other varieties; *Lobelia siphilitica* is milder and less likely to cause vomiting. However, an emetic, which causes vomiting, is sometimes a desirable therapy to help the body eliminate a poison or to stop an asthma attack.

The fresh leaf has caused contact dermatitis in rare cases.

Range and Appearance

Lobelia is native to eastern North America and Europe. It can be either an annual or biennial and ranges from 6 inches to 2 feet in height. The leaves are alternate, sessile, ovate-lanceolate, veiny, and covered with hairs. The numerous tubular, five-lobed, hermaphroditic flowers are pale blue and originate from the leaf axil. Lobelia grows along roadsides and in both pastures and woodlands. The plant flourishes in moist, partially shady conditions in most types of soil.

MACA

Botanical Name

Lepidium meyenii, L. peruvianum

Family

Brassicaceae (Mustard Family)

Etymology

The genus name, *Lepidium,* derives from the Greek *lepis,* "scale," perhaps in reference to the heavy root. The common name *maca* is a Quechua word for the plant.

Also Known As

English: ayak, ayuk willku, chichira, maca-maca, maka, pepperweed, Peruvian ginseng, quechua
Quechua: ayak chichira, ayak willku, maca maca
Spanish: maino

Part Used

Root

Physiological Effects

Adaptogen, antioxidant, aphrodisiac, immune tonic, nutritive, rejuvenative, tonic

Medicinal Uses

Alkaloids in maca are believed to affect the hypothalamus-pituitary axis, which has a positive effect on the adrenals, thyroid, and pancreas. Maca increases the production of estrogen, testosterone, and progesterone. It also increases the quantity of semen men produce and the motility of their sperm. In animal studies it has been shown to stimulate the maturation of multiple egg follicles. It is also used as a tonic for recovering alcoholics, helping to decrease cravings for alcohol.

Maca is used in the treatment of adrenal exhaustion, anemia, chronic fatigue, erectile dysfunction, fatigue, infertility, irregular menses, low sperm count, memory loss, menopause symptoms (hot flashes, night sweats, mood swings), osteoporosis, premature aging, rheumatism, stomach cancer, tuberculosis, and vaginal dryness. It is also used to support convalescence.

Edible Uses

Maca roots can be eaten much like sweet potatoes, raw or cooked. They have a flavor like that of butterscotch and are often baked, roasted or made into a porridge known as mazamorra. They are also used to make a sweet fermented drink called maca chicha. Maca powder is often added to smoothies and "superfood" confections.

The leaves are also edible and can be eaten raw or cooked.

Other Uses

The Inca cultivated maca over two thousand years ago. Legend has it that Incan warriors would consume it before battle as a strengthening tonic. During the Spanish colonialization of Peru, maca was used as a currency. There are chronicles of Spanish conquistadors finding that their horses and pigs became infertile at the high altitude (a common phenomenon). Incan farmers recommended that the Spaniards feed the animals maca, as they had found that it increased reproduction in their own llamas and alpacas.

Constituents

Vitamin B_1, vitamin B_2, vitamin B_{12}, vitamin C, vitamin E, calcium, iodine, iron, phosphorous, zinc, fatty acids (linolenic, palmitic, oleic), amino acids (histidine, glycine, tyrosine, lysine, phenylalanine, valine, methionine), carbohydrates, saponins, alkaloids, phytosterols (sitosterol, stigmasterol, campesterol, ergosterol), isothiocyanates (benzyl and p-methoxybenzyl glucosinolates), tannins

Energetic Correspondences

- Flavor: sweet
- Temperature: warm
- Moisture: moist
- Polarity: yin
- Planet: Venus/Jupiter
- Element: air

Contraindications

Generally regarded as safe. High doses may contribute to insomnia.

Range and Appearance

Maca is a hardy biennial or perennial that grows in the Peruvian Andes Mountains at altitudes ranging from 11,000 to 14,500 feet. It has a very high tolerance for frost, sun, and wind but requires moist soil. It grows in a low-lying mat, with scalloped leaves. The four-petaled hermaphroditic flowers are off-white. The radishlike tubers can be cream, yellow banded with purple, purple, or black.

> Maca roots have a long shelf life. Once dried, they will remain viable in storage for up to seven years.

MARIJUANA

Botanical Name

Cannabis sativa

Family

Cannabaceae (Cannabis Family)

Etymology

The genus name, *Cannabis,* is thought to derive from the Hebrew *kaneh-bosm,* meaning "aromatic reed," and/or the Greek name for this plant, *kannabis,* which means "two dog"; legends from ancient Egypt and the Dogon people of Africa hold that this plant came from the constellation Canis Minor, or "small dog," the companion to Canis Major. The species name, *sativa,* derives from the Latin *satus,* "planting," and denotes the plant's long history of cultivation.

Also Known As

Afrikaans: dagga
Arabuc: qinnib, tîl
Cantonese: fa ma yan
Danish: indisk hamp
Dutch: indische hennep

English: cannabis, charas (resin), dagga, grass, hemp, Indian dreamer, Mary Jane, pot
Finnish: hamppu
French: chanvre, herbe
German: hanf, marihuana
Hindi: bhang, ganja
Italian: canapa indica
Japanese: kamanin, mashinin, taima
Korean: arnain, hwamain
Mandarin: ma ren
Nepali: bhaang, cares, gaanjaa
Russian: kannabis sativa, penek
Sanskrit: ganja, vijaya
Spanish: cañamo, marihuana
Swedish: hampa
Thai: porkanchaa
Turkish: kinnab
Zulu: nsangu

Parts Used

Bud (flowering top of female plant), resin, leaf, seed

Physiological Effects

Bud, resin, leaf: analgesic, anesthetic, anticonvulsant, antidepressant, antiemetic, anti-inflammatory, antispasmodic, aphrodisiac (but can also be anaphrodisiac, depending on dosage and circumstance), appetite stimulant, bronchial dilator, cataleptic, cerebral sedative, euphoric, hallucinogen, hypnotic, hypotensive, vasodilator
Seed: demulcent, laxative, nutritive, yin tonic

Medicinal Uses

Marijuana bud's effects can vary in different people, but most noted are the dilation of blood vessels and alveoli sacs in the lungs, resulting in deeper respiration and an increase in heart rate. Low doses tend to promote a sense of relaxation. The bud increases levels of phenylethylamine, a neurotransmitter that makes us feel more in love. The bud is used in the treatment of AIDS, anorexia, asthma, cerebral palsy, chemotherapy nausea, coughs (spasmodic), depression, epilepsy, glaucoma, insomnia, menstrual cramps, migraines, multiple sclerosis, muscle spasms, nausea, nervousness in the elderly, nightmares, pain (from arthritis, childbirth, rheumatism, and so on), piritis (chronic itching), and spastic paralysis.

Marijuana seed lubricates and nourishes the colon. It is an essential component of Asian patent formulas for constipation due to dryness, and as a laxative it is considered gentle enough even for the elderly and postpartum women. It is also indicated for menstrual irregularities, postpartum recovery, recovery from fever, severe vomiting, wasting diseases, and "blood deficiency," such as anemia. The seed is also used to clear heat, promote wound healing, and nourish the yin fluids of the body. It can be used both orally and topically.

Between 1840 and 1900 over a hundred published medical papers recommended marijuana leaf to aid sleep, calm the nerves, relieve pain and nausea, and stimulate appetite. The leaves are not psychoactive unless processed with heat, such as by cooking them in oil, although vaporizing is a new technique that does not burn the herb and reduces smoke inhalation.

Though marijuana is most often smoked to achieve therapeutic effect, it can also be consumed as food, tinctured, encapsulated, or made into a sublingual spray.

In terms of topical applications, marijuana leaves can be used as a poultice or liniment to ease muscle spasms.

Edible Uses

The buds, young leaves, and seeds are all edible. In India marijuana is used to prepare *bhang*, an herbal milkshake that is traditionally served at wedding banquets to produce great joy. The seeds have no psychoactive properties and are rich in protein and omega-3 fatty acids.

Other Uses

Marijuana seeds were first brought to the Americas in 1632 by the Pilgrims. By 1762 Virginia farmers were being penalized for not growing this plant, as it was such an economically important crop. The stalks of the plant produce a very strong fiber that can be used to make cloth, rope, and paper. The oil from the seeds is used to make hair tonics (to prevent baldness), paint, varnish, lamp oil, and fuel for automobiles and airplanes. The resin is the source of the psychoactive hashish.

A myth from Nepal tells that Shiva, the world's creator and destroyer, lived with his goddess wife Parvati in the Himalayas. Yet Shiva wandered, amusing himself with nymphs and other goddesses. This displeased Parvati, so she sought a way to keep her husband close to home. She took the resin from a female hemp plant, and when Shiva returned home she offered him its smoke. He was filled with joy and arousal and they experienced divine bliss together. After this, he remained with his wife and proclaimed that the doors to paradise were now open to his devotees.

Constituents

Bud, resin, leaf: cannabinoids (tetrahydrocannbinol), flavonoids, essential oils, alkaloids (cannabisativine, muscarinem trigonelline), calcium
Seed: protein, lipids, choline, inositol, enzymes

Energetic Correspondences

- Flavor: bud, resin—sweet, pungent; leaf, seed—sweet
- Temperature: bud, resin—warm; leaf, seed—neutral
- Moisture: bud, resin, leaf—dry; seed—moist
- Polarity: yin
- Planet: Saturn/Mars/Neptune
- Element: fire/water

Contraindications

Smoking marijuana buds may affect some people adversely, possibly inducing paranoia, personality deviations, short-term memory loss, and perceptual distortions. Because of these possible effects, and marijuana's sedative properties, try to avoid driving, operating heavy machinery, or other activities that requires fast reaction times after taking marijuana.

Smoking in general can be hard on the lungs, and though cannabis buds have been used to treat asthma and bronchitis, smoking them can aggravate those conditions. Marijuana buds can also inhibit testosterone production, cause hypoglycemic states,

and lower HCL production. Dryness in the mouth and eyes is a common side effect.

The seeds are generally regarded as safe.

Range and Appearance

Native to the mountainous regions west of the Himalayas but widely cultivated, cannabis is an annual that can grow from 3 to 8 feet tall in a single season. It is generally dioecious, meaning that male and female flowers are borne on different plants, though in rare cases plants can be monoecious, producing both female and male flowers. The distinctive leaves are palmate and usually composed of an odd number of leaflets, from three to nine. Male plants are usually taller than females. Female plants tend to be stockier and to have fewer branches, while male plants are heavily branched and have fewer leaves.

Cannabis can be found growing wild along ditches, fields, and roadsides. It tolerates even poor soil and prefers moderate sun and water. The seeds are relished by birds and encourage singing and mating among them.

Though marijuana has been used medicinally for centuries, it is currently illegal to grow or possess it in many countries. Products made from seeds and fibers, however, are legal and available in the United States.

MARSHMALLOW

Botanical Name

Althaea officinalis

Family

Malvaceae (Mallow Family)

Etymology

The genus name, *Althaea*, derives from the Greek *althe*, "to heal." *Officinalis*, the species name, indicates that this was an official drug of the old European apothecaries. The common name *malva* derives from the Greek *malake*, "soft," in reference to this plant's soothing properties.

Also Known As

English: cheeses, hock herb, mallards, malva,
mortification plant, schloss tea, sweet weed,
white mallow, wymote
Finnish: rohtosalkoruusu
French: guimauve
German: althee, altheewurzel, eibisch, stockmalve
Greek: iviscus
Italian: altea, bismalva
Sanskrit: gulkairo
Spanish: altea, malvaisco
Swedish: altearot, läkemalva
Turkish: hatmi

Part Used

Root, leaf

Physiological Effects

Alterative, antacid, anti-inflammatory, antispasmodic, antitussive, aphrodisiac, demulcent, diuretic, emollient, expectorant, galactagogue, hemostatic, immune tonic, laxative, lung tonic, nutritive, rejuvenative, vulnerary, yin tonic

Medicinal Uses

Marshmallow root and leaf have a high mucilage content, which calms inflammation, nourishes bone marrow, soothes and moistens the skin, and promotes tissue healing. Marshmallow is especially effective in soothing irritation in the respiratory, urinary, and gastrointestinal tracts. As a tonifying herb it can aid children's growth and development. It also can help calm an overactive immune system and, because it helps stimulate white blood cell production, can function as an immune tonic. It decreases the nerve sensitivity that causes coughs.

Marshmallow is used in the treatment of acid indigestion, AIDS, asthma, blood in the urine, bladder stones, bronchitis, burns, catarrh, colitis, constipation, coughs, cystitis, diabetes, diarrhea, dysentery, dysuria, eczema, edema, emaciation, gastritis, hemorrhoids, herpes, HIV, hot flashes, insomnia, interstitial cystitis, irritable bowel syndrome, kidney stones, laryngitis, mastitis, nephritis, neuralgia, pharyngitis, pleurisy, pneumonia, polyruria, prosta-

titis, psoriasis, rheumatism, rickets, sexual debility, sore throat, tuberculosis, ulcers, urinary tract infection, vaginal dryness, and whooping cough.

Topically, the root and leaf can be used in compresses to treat burns, eye irritation, gangrene, hemorrhoids, insect bites, mastitis, psoriasis, sunburn, varicose veins, and wounds. They also can be prepared as a gargle to relieve sore throat or as a douche or enema to relieve vaginal or rectal irritation.

As a flower essence, marshmallow fosters warmth and emotional openness. For those feeling lonely and isolated and unable to give or receive from others, it eases communication.

Edible Uses

Marshmallow was originally an ingredient in the candy we now know as marshmallow. It is still used in the Middle East to make the sesame confection halva. The leaves and root can be eaten raw or cooked. The flowers are very beautiful and can be sprinkled raw as a garnish on other dishes. The seeds (known as cheeses for their old-fashioned cheesewheel shape) have a nutty taste and may be eaten raw, cooked, or pickled.

Marshmallow makes pleasant, soothing, mucilaginous tea. The concentrated tea can be used as an egg white substitute in many recipes.

Other Uses

Marshmallow is a hydrating herb that can be used in the bath to moisturize dry skin and in hair rinses to moisturize and add luster to dry hair. It is commonly substituted for slippery elm bark in herbal remedies, as elm becomes endangered due to Dutch elm disease. The root and stem yield a fiber that can be used in papermaking. Marshmallow root powder has been used as a binding agent in the manufacture of pills; the root also yields a glue. The oil from the seed can be used to make paints and varnishes.

The peeled root can be given to teething babies for them to chew on (under supervision, of course). The peeled root can also be used as a toothbrush.

Constituents

Beta-carotene, vitamin B_1, vitamin B_2, niacin, vitamin B$_5$, vitamin C, calcium, iron, magnesium, phosphorous, potassium, unsaturated fatty acids, mucilage, polysaccharides, flavonoids (quercitin, kaempferol), betaine, asparagine, tannins, coumarin, phenolic acids, lecithin, pectin, malic acid

Energetic Correspondences
- Flavor: sweet, bitter
- Temperature: cool
- Moisture: moist
- Polarity: yin
- Planet: Venus
- Element: water

Contraindications
The mucilage in marshmallow may cause a delay in the effects of pharmaceuticals taken at the same time.

Range and Appearance
Native to Africa, Asia, and Europe but naturalized in the eastern United States, this perennial herb can be found growing in cool, damp lowlands. It can grow to 4 to 5 feet in height and has downy, lobed leaves and large, hermaphroditic, pink to purple flowers. The fruits mature into buttonlike achenes. Marshmallow thrives in partial sun to full shade, prefers a rich loam soil, and requires only moderate amounts of water.

MEADOWSWEET

Botanical Name
Filipendula ulmaria (formerly *Spiraea betulifolia, S. lucida, S. ulmaria*)

Family
Rosaceae (Rose Family)

Etymology
The genus name, *Filipendula,* derives from the Latin *filum,* "thread," and *pendulum,* "hanging," in reference to the threads that connect the roots. The species name, *ulmaria,* refers to the resemblance of this species' leaves to those of the elm tree (*Ulmus*), which

are wrinkled on top. The common name *meadowsweet* refers to this herb's use in mead making.

Also Known As
English: bridewort, dolloff, goat's beard, lady of the meadow, meadwort, pride of the meadow, queen of the meadow, sweet hay
French: herbe aux abeilles, reine des près, spiraea, ulmaire, vignette
German: echtes mädesüss, geissleitern, moorspierstaude, wiesenkonigin
Italian: filipendula, olmaria, regina dei prati, pie di becco
Spanish: barbe de cabra, ulmaria

Part Used
Aboveground plant

Physiological Effects
Analgesic, anodyne, antacid, antibacterial, antiemetic, anti-inflammatory, antirheumatic, antispasmodic (mild), aromatic, astringent, cholagogue, diaphoretic, diuretic, febrifuge, sedative (mild), stomachic, urinary antiseptic

Medicinal Uses
Meadowsweet has a long history of use. It was held sacred among the Druids, being one of their three sacred herbs (along with vervain and mint). In his 1597 *Herbal,* John Gerard said of the herb, "The smell therof makes the heart merry and joyful and delighteth the senses." Meadowsweet has been shown to reduce inflammation, clear heat and toxins, and soothe irritation of the mucous membranes of the digestive tract. It also promotes the healing of tissue and reduces pain. In fact, like willow bark, meadowsweet was a forerunner of aspirin: salicylic acid was extracted from both in the 1830s. In fact, the name *aspirin* is derived from meadowsweet's former botanical genus name, *Spiraea.* However, meadowsweet is gentler on the stomach than aspirin, as it contains natural buffering agents.

Meadowsweet is used to treat arteriosclerosis, arthritis, cellulitis, cervicitis, colds, cystitis, diarrhea, dropsy, dyspepsia, edema, fever, flu, gastritis, gout, headache, heartburn, hyperacidity, insomnia, nausea, nephritis, pain, prostate enlargement, rheumatism, ulcers, urinary tract infection, and vaginitis.

Topically, meadowsweet can be used as an eyewash to treat conjunctivitis and eye inflammation and as a compress to relieve muscle aches and rheumatic joints and to heal wounds. It also can be used as a douche or enema to treat infection or as a relaxing bath herb.

As a flower essence, meadowsweet helps relax tension in the head and neck.

Edible Uses

Meadowsweet flowers can be eaten raw or cooked. They impart an almond fragrance to preparations they are used in, such as jam, stewed fruit, and wine. The leaves are often added to soups. The Shakers used this herb in beer brewing, as its natural sweetness enabled them to use less sugar.

Other Uses

The entire aboveground plant was used as a strewing herb during the time of Elizabeth I. The oil from the flower buds is used in perfume. The flowers themselves were once soaked in rainwater to create complexion water and are sometimes included in potpourri. They have also seen occasional use as paintbrushes for large surfaces. The root is used to dye wool black. In folkloric traditions, meadowsweet is said to promote happiness and to be a useful tool for divination.

Constituents

Vitamin C, calcium, iron, silica, sulfur, essential oils (salicyladehyde, methylsalicylate), salicylic acid, spireine, gaultherine, spiraeoside, flavonoids (quercetin, rutin, spiraeoside), vanillin, coumarin, glycoside, mucilage, tannin

Energetic Correspondences

- Flavor: bitter, sweet
- Temperature: cool
- Moisture: dry
- Polarity: yin
- Planet: Venus/Mercury/Jupiter/Saturn
- Element: air/water

Contraindications

Avoid meadowsweet in cases of sensitivity to salicylates, such as those found in aspirin.

Range and Appearance

Meadowsweet, a native of Europe and Asia, is a deciduous shrub that grows from 2 to 4 feet high and hybridizes easily. The ovate, pinnate leaves are dark green above and whitish and downy below. The tiny flowers are cream colored and clustered in irregular branched cymes. Meadowsweet prefers moist locations with loamy soils and partial shade to full sun.

MILK THISTLE

Botanical Name

Silybum marianum (formerly *Carduus marianus*)

Family

Asteraceae (Daisy Family)

Etymology

The genus name, *Silybum,* was given by the first-century Greek physician Dioscorides as a name to several edible thistles. The species name, *marianum,* honors the Virgin Mary. The common name *milk thistle* refers to the white veins on the leaves, which look as if milk was spilled upon them—according to legend, the milk of the Virgin Mary.

Also Known As

English: Marian thistle, Mary thistle, Mediterranean thistle, Our Lady's thistle, variegated thistle, Venus thistle, wild artichoke
Finnish: Maarianohdake
French: chardon béni, chardon Marie, lait de Notre Dame
German: benedikten distel, Mariendistel
Italian: cardo beneditto, cardo Mariano, cardo santo
Spanish: cardo lechoso, cardo Mariano
Swedish: Mariatistel
Turkish: mubarek dikeni

Part Used

Seed

Physiological Effects

Antidepressant, antioxidant, appetite stimulant, astringent, bitter tonic, cholagogue, demulcent, diaphoretic, digestive, diuretic, emetic, emmenagogue, galactagogue, hepatoprotective, stomachic, tonic

Medicinal Uses

Milk thistle seed has long been used medicinally; Dioscorides, who named the genus, wrote that milk thistle seed could be used to treat snakebite. Milk thistle seed helps protect the liver, prevents toxins from penetrating the interior of liver cells, promotes the growth of healthy liver cells, and improves the liver's function. It offers excellent support for the liver for those who need to take pharmaceutical drugs. After consumption of poisonous mushrooms such as death cap (*Amanita phalloides*) or exposure to carbon tetrachloride, which destroy liver cells and usually cause death, if intravenous applications of milk thistle seed compounds are given within 48 hours, the survival rate is almost 100 percent. Milk thistle seed has also been shown to stimulate and quicken liver regeneration in animals who have had partial hepatectomies. It also helps lower cholesterol levels and can help inhibit the growth of cancer cells in the breasts, cervix, and prostate.

Milk thistle seed is used in the treatment of alcohol abuse, bile duct inflammation, chemical exposure, chemotherapy side effects, cirrhosis, depression, drug abuse, environmental illness, hepatitis, high cholesterol, jaundice, liver damage, poisoning, and psoriasis.

Edible Uses

The seeds are edible; they are usually ground before being sprinkled onto culinary preparations. They can also be roasted and used as a coffee substitute, and an edible oil can be pressed from them.

Milk thistle leaves, with their spines removed, can be eaten as greens and are best when young and tender. The young stalks were once cultivated as a veg-etable; they can be eaten raw or cooked and are considered superior to cabbage. The flower buds, though small, yield a heart like an artichoke that can be eaten. The roots of the plant can be consumed raw, boiled, or steamed.

Other Uses

In magical traditions, milk thistle is worn as protection against negative energy and used in purifying baths.

Constituents

Flavonoids (silymarin), tyramine, histamine, gamma-linoleic acid, essential oil, mucilage, bitter principle

Energetic Correspondences

- Flavor: sweet, bitter
- Temperature: cool
- Moisture: moist
- Polarity: yang
- Planet: Moon
- Element: fire

Contraindications

There have been occasional reports of the seeds causing bloating or diarrhea or having a laxative effect.

Range and Appearance

Native to the Mediterranean region but naturalized throughout North America, milk thistle thrives on dry, rocky ground with full sun. The plant has shiny pale green leaves that are prickly at their outside edges and marked with "milky" white veins that run throughout the leaves. The flowers are red to purple.

MINT

Botanical Name

Mentha spp., including *M.* x *piperita* (peppermint), *M. spicata* (syn. *M. viridis;* spearmint)

Family

Lamiaceae (Mint Family)

Etymology

The genus name, *Mentha,* is taken from that of Minthe, in Greek mythology a nymph taken by Pluto as a lover. Pluto's jealous wife, Persephone, turned Minthe into a peppermint plant. The species name *piperita* is Latin for "like a pepper," in reference to the plant's peppery taste. The species name *spicata* is Latin for "like a spire," in reference to the terminal spikes of flowers.

Also Known As

Arabic: eqama (*M.* x *piperita*), nana (*M.* x *piperita*)

Armenian: ananookh (*M.* x *piperita*)

Bulgarian: giozum (*M. spicata*), menta (*M.* x *piperita*)

Cantonese: liu lan xiang (*M. spicata*), pak hom hoh (*M.* x *piperita*)

Croatian: paprena metvica (*M.* x *piperita*)

Czech: máta (*M.* x *piperita*), máta peprná (*M.* x *piperita*)

Danish: pebermynte (*M.* x *piperita*)

Dutch: pepermunt (*M.* x *piperita*)

English: brandy mint (*M.* x *piperita*), garden mint (*M. spicata*), lammint (*M.* x *piperita*), menthol mint (*M. spicata*), silver mint (*M. spicata*)

Esperanto: mento

Estonian: münt (*M.* x *piperita*)

Finnish: piparminttu (*M.* x *piperita*), viherminttu (*M. spicata*)

French: menthe poivrée (*M.* x *piperita*), menthe a epis (*M.* x *piperita*), menthe verte (*M.* x *piperita*), menthe vertebaume vert (*M. spicata*)

German: ackerminze (*M. spicata*), katzenkraut (*M. spicata*), grüne minze (*M. spicata*), pfefferminze gruene minze (*M.* x *piperita*), roemische minze (*M.* x *piperita*)

Greek: dyosmos (*M. spicata*), menta (*M.* x *piperita*)

Hebrew: menta (*M.* x *piperita*), na'na' (*M.* x *piperita*)

Hindi: podina (*M.* x *piperita*)

Hungarian: fodormenta (*M.* x *piperita*), menta (*M.* x *piperita*)

Icelandic: piparminta (*M.* x *piperita*)

Indonesian: bijanngut (*M.* x *piperita*), daun pudina (*M.* x *piperita*)

Italian: menta pepe (*M.* x *piperita*), menta peperina (*M.* x *piperita*)

Japanese: kakka (*M.* x *piperita*), minto (*M.* x *piperita*), pepaminto (*M.* x *piperita*), supeaminto (*M. spicata*)

Korean: hobu (*M.* x *piperita*), mintu (*M.* x *piperita*), pepeo-mintu (*M.* x *piperita*), spio-minto (*M. spicata*)

Mandarin: hu jiao bo he (*M.* x *piperita*)

Norwegian: peppermynte (*M.* x *piperita*)

Polish: mieta pieprzowa (*M.* x *piperita*)

Portuguese: hortelã-pimenta (*M.* x *piperita*)

Russian: myata perechnaya (*M.* x *piperita*)

Serbian: menta (*M.* x *piperita*), nana (*M.* x *piperita*)

Spanish: hierba buena (*M. spicata*), menta (*M. spicata*), menta romana (*M. spicata*), menta verde (*M. spicata*)

Spanish: piperita (*M.* x *piperita*)

Swahili: pereminde (*M.* x *piperita*)

Swedish: grönmynta (*M. spicata*), pepparmynta (*M.* x *piperita*)

Thai: bai saranai (*M.* x *piperita*), peppeort-mint (*M.* x *piperita*)

Turkish: nane (*M.* x *piperita*)

Ukrainian: myata pertseva (*M.* x *piperita*)

Vietnamese: rau tho'm (*M.* x *piperita*)

Yiddish: menta (*M.* x *piperita*)

Part Used

Aboveground plant

Physiological Effects

Analgesic (topically), anesthetic (topically), anodyne, antibacterial, antiemetic, anti-inflammatory, antioxidant, antiparasitic (especially peppermint), antiseptic, antispasmodic, antiviral (especially peppermint), aromatic, carminative, cholagogue, choleretic, diaphoretic, digestive, diuretic, emmenagogue, expectorant, refrigerant, stimulant, stomachic, tonic, vasodilator

Medicinal Uses

Mint relaxes the peripheral blood vessels, calms smooth muscle spasms, dries dampness, expels phlegm, and clears the head. It is regarded as an excellent remedy for stomach cramps due to its ability to reduce hypercontractability of the intestinal muscles. It is often added to formulas using laxative herbs, such as cascara sagrada, to prevent intestinal gripe.

Peppermint is considered the strongest mint medicinally, though the other mints have medicinal benefit as well. Peppermint has activity against a wide range of pathogens including streptococcus, staphylococcus, and candida. Spearmint is a better choice for culinary endeavors and is slightly less cooling than peppermint.

Mint is used the treatment of colds, colic, cough, diverticulitis, dizziness, dyspepsia, earache, emphysema, fainting, fatigue, fever, flatulence, flu, gallstones, halitosis, headache, heart palpitations, herpes, hiccups, hives, indigestion, irritable bowel, laryngitis, lung inflammation, measles, menstrual cramps, morning sickness, nausea, rash, sinusitis, sore throat, stomachache, and vomiting.

Topically, mint is analgesic and anesthetic. Warm compresses of mint can be used to treat back pain, joint inflammation, lung infection, neuralgia, rheumatism, and sinusitis, while cold compresses can be used to treat bruises, fever, headache, and hives. Mint can be used as a bath herb to cool and refresh the body and also to treat bug bites, chicken pox, itchy skin, and measles. The herb can also be prepared as a steam inhalation to treat asthma, bronchitis, laryngitis, nausea, shock, and sinus congestion. In a mouthwash, mint can freshen the breath and prevent gingivitis.

The essential oil of mint is sometimes added to massage oils for its ability to relieve chest congestion and pain. Its scent can be used to ease the symptoms of asthma, bronchitis, nausea, sinus congestion, and shock. The essential oil is often added to toothpastes and mouthwashes for its ability to combat bacteria, freshen breath, and prevent gingivitis.

As a flower essence, peppermint helps users to overcome lethargy and mental dullness by promoting clear and quick thinking. It helps users to see a future in which their desires are achieved. It can be helpful for those who have an excessive fear of losing their health, material goods, or loved ones.

Edible Uses

Although both are edible, spearmint is a better choice than peppermint for culinary arts, because it is slightly less cooling and less medicinal tasting. Mint leaves are edible raw or cooked and are popular especially in Asian and Middle Eastern cuisines.

Mint has a familiar, flavorful, fresh taste. It makes a refreshing, cooling iced tea and works well as a sun tea or cold-water infusion. It is often used to improve the flavor of other teas. Other beloved mints that make wonderful teas include apple mint (*Mentha suaveolens*), chocolate mint (a cultivar of *Mentha x piperita*), Corsican mint (*Mentha requienii*), field mint (*Mentha arvensis*), ginger mint (*Mentha x gracilis*), horsemint (*Mentha x villosa alopecuroides*), orange mint (*Mentha x piperita citrata*), pineapple mint (*Mentha suaveolens* 'Variegata'), and water mint (*Mentha aquatica*).

Other Uses

Essential oil of mint is used to scent soaps and shampoos and in insect repellents. The smell of mint repels rats and mice and has long been used to keep them out of grain storage buildings; in the home, mint was once used as a strewing herb and stuffed into matresses to discourage bed bugs and other vermin. Peppermint oil is sometimes used by sanitary engineers to test the soundness of pipes, as its odor will pinpoint any leaks. Adding peppermint oil to pastes prevents mold and increases the shelf life of the product. Mint essential oil is used to make menthol tobacco products.

In magical traditions, peppermint is used to clear negative energy by burning it as an incense, rubbing it on furniture, strewing it in a room, or using it as potpourri. In folkloric traditions, it is used for purification, attracting love, promoting healing, and enhancing psychic abilities.

Constituents

Beta-carotene, B-complex vitamins, vitamin C, potassium, flavonoids (luteolin, rutin), essential oils (menthol, menthene, methyl acetate, limonene, cineol, pulegone, carvone), ketone (menthone), tannins, resin; menthol is more predominant in peppermint, and carvone is more predominant in spearmint

Energetic Correspondences

- Flavor: pungent, sweet
- Temperature: cool (at first), warm (subsequently)
- Moisture: dry
- Polarity: varies by species; *M. x piperita*—yang; *M. spicata*—yin
- Planet: varies by species; *M. x piperita*—Mercury; *M. spicata*—Venus
- Element: varies by species; *M. x piperita*—fire; *M. spicata*—water

Contraindications

Avoid mint in cases of coldness, such as chills or yin deficiency, and during acute gallstone attack. Pregnant women should ingest no more than 1 to 2 cups daily of peppermint tea. Nursing mothers should avoid large amounts of mint, which can dry breast milk.

Range and Appearance

There are about twenty true mints, but they hybridize readily and there are now hundreds of species (with as many as 2,300 botanical name variations, about half of which are synonyms) grown all around the world.

Peppermint is the result of crossing *M. spicata* and *M. aquatica* and was first described in 1696 by the English botanist John Ray. It grows up to 3 feet in height and has an erect, four-sided, often purplish stem, with opposite, lanceolate, epilliptical, dark green leaves. The pink flowers form in dense terminal spikes. This species has a distinct peppermint aroma.

Spearmint has a narrower spike of flowers, and its leaves are more wrinkled. The leaves are opposite and have either no stalks or very short ones. The flowers are pink to purple and are borne on slender elongated spikes, and the stem is green. Spearmint's aroma is sweeter and less spicy than that of peppermint.

Mints thrive in partial shade to full sun. They like moderate to high amounts of water and are not particular about what kind of soil they will grow in.

They are perennials and tend to grow in colonies. They attract bees and butterflies to the garden and, when planted near cabbages and tomatoes, will help keep them pest free. Plant mint in your garden where you don't mind it spreading, as it has a tendency to take over. And if mint is threatening the rest of your garden, put handfuls of it to good use!

MISTLETOE

Botanical Name

Viscum album

Family

Loranthaceae (Mistletoe Family)

Etymology

The genus name *Viscum* is the Latin name for the species; it also refers to birdlime, a sticky substance smeared on twigs to trap birds, in reference to the viscous juice of mistletoe's berries. The species name *album* is Latin for "white," in reference to the white berries. The common name *misteltoe* derives from the Anglo-Saxon *mistel,* "dung," and *tan,* "twig," meaning "dung on a twig."

Also Known As

English: birdlime mistletoe, Druid's herb, European mistletoe, golden bough, holy wood, thunderbesam, witch's broom, wood of the cross
Finnish: misteli
French: herbe de la croix
German: laubholz-mistel, mistel
Italian: vischio
Spanish: muerdago
Swedish: mistel

Parts Used

Young branches, leaf (gathered in spring before the berries appear)

Physiological Effects

Antispasmodic, antitumor, cardiotonic, diuretic, hypotensive, immune tonic, narcotic, nervine, sedative, vasodilator

Medicinal Uses

Mistletoe reduces the heart rate and at the same time strengthens the capillary walls, improves circulation, and relaxes the muscles. It has been shown to destroy cancer cells and stimulate the immune system. European mistletoe is used to treat anxiety, arteriosclerosis, arthritis, cancer, chorea (rapid, jerky movements), convulsions, epilepsy, gout, headache (due to high blood pressure), hypertension, hysteria, insomnia, migraine, seizures, varicose veins, and vertigo. It is available in Europe in products sold under the trade names Abnobaviscum, Eurixor, Helixor, Iscador, and Vysorel.

Topically, mistletoe leaves can be made into a poultice to relieve rheumatism pain.

As a flower essence, mistletoe aids transformation of the body and mind. It can be helpful to those going through radical changes.

Edible Uses

The plant and its berries are toxic and should not be eaten.

Other Uses

The Druids considered mistletoe a sacred plant. They celebrated the beginning of winter by having a high-ranking priest collect some of the plant, cutting it free from its host plant with a golden knife, and they hung it in their homes as protection against all evils.

Folkloric tradition holds that carrying mistletoe will bring men good fortune in hunting and women fertiltity. When placed at the bedroom door, it is said to promote restful sleep and positive dreams.

Constituents

Glycoproteins, polypeptides (viscotoxin), flavonoids, triterpene saponins, caffeic acid, lignans, choline, vitamin C, histamine; constituents may vary according to the plant mistletoe grows on

Energetic Correspondences

- Flavor: bitter
- Temperature: cold
- Moisture: moist
- Polarity: yang
- Planet: Sun/Jupiter
- Element: air

Contraindications

Raw, unprocessed mistletoe is toxic, as are its berries. It should be used only under the guidance of a qualified health-care practitioner, and then should be used only in small doses. Rather than making your own products and risking toxicity, purchase those of reputable companies, and use them according to the manufacturer's recommendations.

Mistletoe may cause temporary numbness, vomiting, and reduced heart rate. Avoid during pregnancy.

Range and Appearance

Mistletoe is an evergreen, semiparasitic plant native to Europe, Asia, and north Africa. It grows on fruit, poplar, chestnut, pine, spruce, and other trees. The host trees are usually at least twenty years old before mistletoe encroaches, and they are not usually killed by the mistletoe. The plant forms pendant bushes where it grows. Its leaves are thick, oval to round, and 1 to 2 inches long. Its small, inconspicuous, sticky, white flowers are about $1/4$ inch long. It is dioecious, meaning that male and female flowers are borne on different plants.

MOTHERWORT

Botanical Name

Leonurus cardiaca

Family

Lamiaceae (Mint Family)

Etymology

The genus name, *Leonurus,* is derived from the Latin *leo,* "lion," and the Greek *oura,* "tail," in reference to shape of the leaf, which resembles a shaggy tail. The species name, *cardiaca,* is from the Greek *kardiaca,* "heart." The *wort* part of the common name is from the Old English *wyrt,* "plant"; the *mother* part of the common name refers to the use of the plant to ease women's problems from all stages of life, from menstruation to menopause.

Also Known As

Dutch: aartespan

English: benefit mother plant, lion's ear, lion's tail, throw-wort

Finnish: nukula

French: agripaume cardiaque, creneuse, herbe battudo

German: gerzgold, herzgespan, löwenschwanz, wolfstrapp

Italian: agripalma, cardiaca, melissa salvatica

Russian: pustirnik serdechny

Sanskrit: guma

Spanish: agripalma

Swedish: hjärtstilla

Part Used

Aboveground plant (including the seed)

Physiological Effects

Analgesic, antibacterial, antifungal, antioxidant, antirheumatic, antispasmodic, astringent, bitter, cardiotonic, circulatory stimulant, diaphoretic, diuretic, emmenagogue, hemostatic, hypotensive, immune stimulant, laxative, nervine, parturient, sedative, stomachic, tonic, uterine tonic, vasodilator

Medicinal Uses

Motherwort slows a rapid heartbeat, improves circulation, prevents blood platelet aggregation, regulates the menstrual cycle, and calms anxiety and stress that may contribute to heart problems. It is especially beneficial to women's health. It can help relieve pain during childbirth and, when used for several days after birthing, can help prevent uterine infection. It is said to make mothers more joyful and also helps women who tend to "over mother" to let go.

Motherwort is used in the treatment of amenorrhea, angina, anxiety, arrhythmia, asthma, arteriosclerosis, atherosclerosis, breast tenderness, convulsions, cramps, cystitis (interstitial), delirium tremens, depression (including postpartum and bipolar), diarrhea, dysmenorrhea, edema, epilepsy, goiter, headache, heartbreak, heart palpitations, herpes, high cholesterol, hot flashes, hypertension, hyperthy-roidism, hysteria, insomnia, labor difficulty, low libido, melancholy, menopause symptoms, myocardial ischemia, infertility (female), irregular menses, nervous exhaustion, neuralgia, placenta retention, poor vision, postpartum pain, premenstrual syndrome, rapid pulse, restlessness, rheumatism, sciatica, shingles, skin hypersensitivity, shortness of breath, stomachache, tachycardia, and vaginismus.

The seeds are used to improve virility and vision.

Topically, motherwort can be used as a douche to treat vaginitis.

Edible Uses

The fresh or dried flowers and seeds are edible; they are sometimes used to flavor beer. The seeds of the plant were once used as a substitute for sesame seeds.

Other Uses

An olive green dye is made from the leaves.

Constituents

Aboveground plant: beta-carotene, calcium, potassium, flavonoids (quercitin, rutin), citric and malic acids, alkaloids (stachydrine, leonurinine, betonicine), bitter glycosides (leonurine, leonuridin), caffeic acid, essential oil, phytosterols, tannins, resin

Energetic Correspondences

- Flavor: plant—pungent, bitter; seed—sweet
- Temperature: plant—cool; seed—cold
- Moisture: dry
- Polarity: yin
- Planet: Sun/Venus/Saturn
- Element: air

Contraindications

Avoid motherwort in cases of excessive menstrual bleeding. Avoid during pregnancy (but note that motherwort can be helpful during labor, under the guidance of a qualified health-care practitioner). The plant may cause contact dermatitis in some people.

Range and Appearance

Motherwort, native to Europe and western Asia but

naturalized elsewhere, is a perennial than can grow from 2 to 5 feet in height. The stems are distinctly square, and the leaves are opposite with three to five pointed lobes. The flowers are small and white-pink to purple-red in color, and they grow in clusters along the stem. The seeds are in a three-angled case. The plant prefers partial shade to full sun and moist, light, sandy soil, but it will tolerate even poor soil conditions.

MUGWORT

Botanical Name

Artemisia douglasiana (California mugwort),
   A. *frigida, A. lactiflora* (white mugwort),
   A. *ludoviciana* (western mugwort), A. *tridentata*
   (basin sagebrush), A. *vulgaris* (common mugwort)

Family

Asteraceae (Daisy Family)

Etymology

The genus name, *Artemisia*, is thought to have been given in honor of Artemis, the Greek goddess of the hunt and moon and patron to women, especially in matters of menstruation, pregnancy, labor, and menopause. The common name *mugwort* references this plant's use as a flavoring agent for alcoholic beverages (consumed in mugs), especially beer, before the use of hops.

Also Known As

Arabic: habaq ar-rahi
Cantonese: ngaai chóu
Croatian: crni pelin
Czech: cernobyl
Danish: bynke, gråbynke
Dutch: bijvoet
English: artemisia, cudweed, felon herb, mother of plants, moxa, naughty man, sagebrush, sailor's tobacco, Saint John's herb, silver sage, white sage, wombwort
Esperanto: artemezio
Estonian: harilik puju
Finnish: pujo
French: armoise commune, armoise vulgaire, herbe de Saint-Jean
German: belfuß, geissfuss, himmelkehr, mugwurz, sonnenwendgurtek
Greek: artemesia
Hebrew: artimisia
Hungarian: fekete üröm
Italian: artemisia, assenzio, erba di San Giovanni
Japanese: maguwato, yomogi
Korean: meoguweotu
Mandarin: ai cao, hao shu
Polish: bylica pospolita
Portuguese: artemísia
Romanian: pelin negru
Russian: chernobilnik, polin obiknovennya
Sanskrit: nagadamani
Serbian: crni pelen, divlji pelen
Spanish: ajeno del pais, artemisa, estafiate, romerillo, zona diri johannis
Swedish: gråbo
Thai: kot chulaalamphuaua
Turkish: misk out
Ukrainian: chornobyl
Vietnamese: ngai cuu
Yiddish: geveynlikh, polin

Parts Used

Aboveground plant (primarily), root (rarely)

Physiological Effects

Analgesic, anthelmintic, antibacterial, antifungal, anti-inflammatory, antirheumatic, antiseptic, antispasmodic, antivenomous, aromatic, astringent, bitter, carminative, cholagogue, choleretic, diaphoretic, digestive, disinfectant, diuretic, emmenagogue, expectorant, hemostatic, nervine, purgative, stomachic, uterine stimulant, vermifuge

Medicinal Uses

Mugwort warms the body, arrests bleeding, and clears toxins and parasites. Small amounts can be used to strengthen digestion and the nerves. The leaves have been found to have activity against strep and *E. coli* bacteria and also against dysentery and typhoid. Mugwort is used in the treatment of amen-orrhea, anorexia, appetite loss, arthritis, asthma, bladder stones, bronchitis, colds, cystitis, diarrhea, dysentery, dyspepsia, epilepsy, fever, flu, gallstones, gout, headache, hemorrhage, hepatitis, hysteria, irregular menstruation, jaundice, kidney stones, malaria, menopause symptoms, menorrhagia, menstrual cramps, palsy, parasites (pinworms, roundworm, scabies), rheumatism, sore throat, stomachache, and tonsillitis. It also can be used to stimulate labor and the expulsion of the placenta.

Topically, mugwort can be used as an abdominal compress to speed labor. A mugwort compress can also be used to treat boils, itching, rashes, and scabies, and a compress, poultice, or liniment can be used to treat arthritic joints, bruises, headache, insect bites, and swellings. In a gargle, mugwort relieves sore throat; in a hair rinse, it prevents hair loss, and in a footbath it warms and soothes tired feet. The crushed herb can be used as a poultice to get rid of warts.

The dried, powdered leaves are used as a snuff to relieve sinus congestion. Mugwort can also be smoked to relieve asthma symptoms or simmered for decongesting vapor inhalation. It also is used to perform moxabustion, the process of burning herbs either close to or on acupuncture points or acupuncture needles to further stimulate the points.

As a flower essence, mugwort helps users to release negative emotions and bitterness in the past. It helps those who are out of touch with reality to glean helpful information from their dreams.

Edible Uses

Although very bitter, mugwort is edible. In Europe it has been used to flavor dishes such as dumplings, salads, soups, and meats. It also is sometimes used to flavor beer, liqueurs, vermouth, and vinegars.

Eating a bit of mugwort with a meal helps counteract the digestive distress that eating fatty foods can cause.

Other Uses

Mugwort has long been credited with having magical powers and was traditionally worn as a talisman to protect a person from evil. Legend says that Saint John the Baptist wore a girdle of mugwort when he took to the wilderness. Mugwort is also sometimes used for "smudging," or burning the herb to purify an area.

A sachet filled with dried mugwort and placed in one's pillowcase inspires vivid dreams. Mugwort repels moths, cockroaches, and rodents (but if overused as an insecticide on plants can inhibit plant growth). It is sometimes smoked as a tobacco substitute. When dried, it makes excellent tinder for starting a fire.

Constituents

Iron, phosphorous, potassium, silicon, zinc, essential oils (linalool, cineole, thujone, borneol, pinene), bitter principle (absinthin), flavonoids, polysaccharides, inulin, sesquiterpene lactones (vulgarin), sitosterol, tannin, resin

Energetic Correspondences

- Flavor: bitter, pungent
- Temperature: warm
- Moisture: dry
- Polarity: yin
- Planet: Mercury/Venus/Neptune/Moon
- Element: earth/water

Contraindications

Avoid ingesting large amounts or using for extended periods, as either may adversely affect the nervous system. Avoid during pregnancy (but note that mugwort can be used to speed labor, under the guidance of a qualified health-care practitioner). Also avoid while nursing. Contact with the plant may cause contact dermatitis in some people.

Range and Appearance

Mugwort is an aromatic perennial that is native to Asia but cultivated worldwide. It can grow from 2 to 5 feet in height. The stems are grooved and hairy. The leaves are alternate, pinnate, and serrated, silvery above and tomentose below, with five to seven lobes. The flowers grow as numerous greenish yellow spikes. The plant's aroma is often described as being a cross between that of camphor and sage. In the garden mugwort requires well-drained soil, full sun to partial shade, and only moderate water; it will tolerate drought.

MUIRA PUAMA

Botanical Name

Ptychopetalum olacoides, P. uncinatum

Family

Olaceae (Olive Family)

Etymology

The etymology of the Latin and common names is uncertain. The common name is pronounced *Mo-ra poo-AH-ma*.

Also Known As

English: marapama, marapuama, potency wood
German: potenholz
Spanish: raiz del macho

Parts Used

Inner bark, root

Physiological Effects

Adaptogen, analgesic, androgenic, antidepressant, antioxidant, antirheumatic, aphrodisiac, astringent, hypotensive, nervous system stimulant, tonic

Medicinal Uses

Muira puama has been a premier remedy, especially as an aphrodisiac, for centuries in South America. It has an arousing effect, both physically and psychologically, on both men and women and is believed to increase testosterone production. It can be used to treat depression, diarrhea, dysentery, erectile dysfunction, fatigue, hair loss, hookworm infestation, hypertension, infertility, low sperm count, low libido, memory loss, menstrual cramps, neuromuscular problems, pain, paralysis, rheumatism, and sexual debility.

Natives of South America apply the cooled tea to their genitals as a sexual stimulant. They also use muira puama as a gargle to relieve sore throat and in baths to treat beriberi and improve circulation in cases of paralysis. A wash prepared from the plant can be applied to the scalp to prevent hair loss.

Edible Uses

None known

Other Uses

None known

Constituents

Fatty acids (behenic acid), alkaloid (muirapuamine), coumarin, phytosterols (beta-sitosterol), essential oils (beta-carophyllene, alpha-humulene), triterpenes (lupeol), tannin

Energetic Correspondences

- Flavor: sweet, pungent
- Temperature: warm
- Moisture: dry
- Polarity: yang
- Planet: Mars
- Element: fire

Contraindications

Muira puama is generally regarded as safe. Some people may find that it causes insomnia if taken before bedtime.

Range and Appearance

Muira puama is a small tree native to the rain forests of South America. It grows to about 16 feet in height and has a bark that is slightly pink in color. Its small white flowers have a fragrance reminiscent of that of jasmine.

MULLEIN

Botanical Name

Verbascum densiflorum, V. phlomoides, V. thapsus

Family

Scrophulariaceae (Figwort Family)

Etymology

The genus name, *Verbascum,* derives from the Latin *barbascum,* "with beard." The species name, *thapsus,* is that of an ancient town in what is now Tunisia. The common name *mullein* derives from the Middle English *moleyne,* "soft."

Also Known As

English: Aaron's rod, beggar's blanket, big taper, big tobacco, candlewick, graveyard dust, hag's taper, Indian toilet paper, Jacob's staff, Jupiter's staff, Our Lady's flannel, torches, velvet dock, witch's candle

Finnish: ukontulikukka

French: molène

German: kleinblütige königskerze

Greek: aflego

Italian: barbasito

Portuguse: barbasco, verbasco

Spanish: gordolobo comun, guardalobo

Swedish: kungsljus

Parts Used

Leaf, flower (without the calyx), root (rarely)

Physiological Effects

Leaf: alterative, anodyne, antibacterial, antihistimine, anti-inflammatory, antiseptic, antispasmodic, antiviral, astringent, demulcent, diuretic, emollient, expectorant, pectoral, vulnerary, yin tonic

Flower: analgesic, anti-inflammatory, antispasmodic, demulcent, emollient, mucilaginous, nervine, sedative

Root: diuretic

Medicinal Uses

Mullein leaf and flower nourish yin, stimulate and cleanse the lungs and lymphs, liquefy phlegm, relax the bronchioles, resolve swelling, relax spasms, and deter infection. They are often recommended for intense coughs that wear down the villi of the lungs. The flower is more demulcent than the leaf, and the leaf more astringent than the flower.

The leaf is used in the treatment of asthma, bronchitis, catarrh, colds, congestion, coughs, cystitis, diarrhea, dysentery, dyspenea, eczema, emphysema, flu, hay fever, kidney infection, laryngitis, lung weakness, mumps, pharyngitis, pleurisy, rheumatism, scrofula, shortness of breath, swollen glands, tonsillitis, tuberculosis, tumors, and whooping cough.

The flower is used in the treatment of flu, laryngitis, and pharyngitis. A drop or two of the flower-infused oil, slightly warmed, can be administered to the ears to relieve the pain of and combat ear infection.

The root is used in the treatment of incontinence.

Topically, the mucilaginous mullein leaf is used as a healing compress in cases of acne, boils, bruises, earache, eczema, glandular inflammation, hemorrhoids, mastitis, mumps, rheumatic joints, and tumors. It also can be used as a bath herb to ease rheumatic joints or smoked to treat asthma. The root can be applied topically to relieve toothache; the juice of the root can be applied topically to remove warts.

As a flower essence, mullein helps users get in touch with their conscience and inner voice, helping them become more true to themselves. It promotes teamwork and moral strength.

Edible Uses

Mullein is not generally considered edible, aside from as tea. As tea, mullein leaf has a mild, pleasant, sweet, though slightly bitter flavor. Be sure to strain the tea through a very fine strainer to remove the irritating hairs found on the leaves.

Other Uses

The leaves of mullein can be fed to animals to treat cough. The tall stalks were once dipped in tallow and lit as torches, while the leaves can be rolled and tied with thread and used as wicks in oil lamps. The soft mullein leaves have long been used by children as doll blankets. A yellow dye is made from the flower. In folkloric tradition mullein is carried to inspire courage, to prevent wild animals from attacking, and to attract love.

Constituents

Leaf: carotene, choline, calcium, magnesium, sulfur, resin, saponins, glycoside (aucubin), flavonoids (hesperidin, verbascoside), mucilage, tannins

Flower: polysaccharides (d-glactose, arabinose, manose), flavonoids (apignein, luteolin, kampferol, rutin), sterols, mucilage
Root: polysaccharides

Energetic Correspondences

- Flavor: sweet, slightly bitter
- Temperature: cool
- Moisture: moist
- Polarity: yin
- Planet: Saturn
- Element: fire/water

Contraindications

Mullein is generally regarded as safe, though the leaf contains coumarin and rotenone, which in the past have drawn expressions of concern from the U.S. Food and Drug Administration. The seeds of the plant should not be consumed, as they are somewhat toxic.

Range and Appearance

There are some three hundred species of mullein native to Eurasia and North Africa; several are now naturalized in North America. This biennial plant can reach 7 feet in height. In its first year, it forms a basal rosette of large, pointed leaves with woolly hairs. The second year, a long, unbranched stalk usually forms and produces a spike of yellow hermaphroditic flowers and alternate, elliptical stem leaves. The hairiness of mullein enables it to survive in hot, dry conditions, and it is often found in waste areas and ditches.

In the garden, mullein thrives in full sun and well-drained soil, with low to moderate amounts of water.

MYRRH

Botanical Name

Commiphora myrrha (syn. *C. molmol*)

Family

Burseraceae (Torchwood Family)

Etymology

The genus name, *Commiphora*, derives from the Greek *kommi*, "gum," and *phoros*, "carrier." The species name and common name derive from the Arabic *mur*, "bitter."

Also Known As

English: gum tree, harabol myrrh, karan
Finnish: mirhami
French: myrrhe
German: myrrhe
Italian: mirra
Japanese: motsuyaku
Korean: molyak
Mandarin: mò yào
Sanskrit: bola
Somali: bissa bol, molmol
Spanish: mirra
Swedish: afrikansk myrra, myrra

Part Used

Resin

Physiological Effects

Alterative, analgesic, antibacterial, anticatarrhal, antifungal, anti-inflammatory, antimicrobial, antiseptic, astringent, carminative, diaphoretic, diuretic, emmenagogue, expectorant, immune stimulant, rejuvenative, stimulant, stomachic, vermifuge, vulnerary

Medicinal Uses

Myrrh increases the motility of white blood cells and normalizes mucous membrane activity, which helps the body fight infection. It also promotes tissue granulation and combats blood stagnation. It is used in the treatment of amenorrhea, arthritis, asthma, bronchitis, candida, catarrh, coughs, dental problems, dysentery, dysmenorrhea, impetigo, laryngitis, pharyngitis, rheumatoid arthritis, sinusitis, sore throat, staph infection, tonsillitis, uterine tumors, and yeast infection.

Topically, myrrh can be made into a salve to treat acne, boils, impetigo, infected wounds, sores (especially those caused by pressure from prosthetic limbs), and staph infection or a liniment to treat boils, bruises, and pain. As a chest rub it helps combat respiratory infections. It is a premier herb for dental problems and can be prepared as a tooth powder, paste, or tincture to combat cavities, gingivitis, pyorrhea, and toothache. It also can be prepared as a mouthwash to treat halitosis, tonsillitis, mouth sores, and thrush.

Edible Uses

Myrrh is not generally considered edible. It was used as a wine preservative in ancient times and is still used today to make the Italian alcoholic beverage Fernet Branca.

Other Uses

Myrrh is famous as one of the gifts of the Magi to the infant Christ, along with frankincense and gold. Incense from ancient Egypt, known as kyphi, contained myrrh and is said to have been used by Moses in making holy oil to anoint priests. Burning myrrh is used to enhance meditation, dispel negative energy, elevate vibrations, heal emotional wounds, sanctify objects such as holy books, amulets and bibles. Myrrh is commonly used in perfumery and is also burned as incense, in which it repels mosquitoes and is said to promote peace, enhance meditation, dispel negative energy, and heal emotional wounds.

Energetic Correspondences

- Flavor: bitter
- Temperature: hot
- Moisture: dry
- Polarity: yin
- Planet: Moon/Saturn
- Element: water

Constituents

Gums (arabinose, galactose, xylose), resin (commiphoric acid, myrrhin, myrrhic acid), essential oils (limonene, eugenol, furanosesquiterpenes, pinene), sterols

Contraindications

Use myrrh internally only in small amounts and only for short periods of time, as the resins can be difficult for the body to eliminate. Avoid during pregnancy, as myrrh can stimulate the uterus. Large amounts can be overly laxative.

Range and Appearance

Myrrh is native to northeastern Africa, where it grows as a large shrub or small tree in harsh desert conditions, with hot sun and little water. The plant's leaves are obovate. The branches are spiny, and a pale yellow oil exudes from the tree when its dull gray bark is cut.

NEEM

Botanical Name

Azadirachta indica (formerly *Melia azadirachta*)

Family

Meliaceae (Mahogany Family)

Etymology

The genus name, *Asadirachta*, derives from the ancient Sanskrit *arishta*, "health bestower." The species name, *indica*, indicates that the plant is native to India. The common name *neem* derives from the Sanskrit name for the plant, *nimba*.

Also Known As

Arabic: nim, sherish
Cambodian: sdao
Cantonese: lian shu
English: bead tree, chinaberry tree, Indian cedar, Indian lilac, margosa, village pharmacy
French: azadirachta de l'Inde
German: niembaum
Hindi: balnimb, neem, nind
Kiswahili: mwarubaini ("forty cures")
Laotian: kadao
Mandarin: lian zao zi
Nepali: nim
Persian: azad dirakht ("the free tree")
Portuguese: margosan
Sanskrit: nimba, nimbacarishtha ("reliever of sickness")

Swahili: mkilifi, mwarubaini kamili
Tamil: veppam
Thai: cha-tang
Vietnamese: sàu dàu

Parts Used

Bark, leaf, seed

Physiological Effects

Alterative, antibacterial, anthelmintic, antiemetic antifungal, anti-inflammatory, antiseptic, antiviral, astringent (bark), bitter, emmenagogue (leaf), febrifuge, hypoglycemic, immune stimulant, pediculocide, vermifuge

Medicinal Uses

Neem is one of the most appreciated trees in the Indian culture. Hindu legend says that when sacred nectar was being flown from earth to the heavens for the use of the gods, a few drops of nectar fell on the neem tree, which besowed upon it its numerous healing virtues. The Hindu goddess Kali is said to dwell in the tree.

Neem improves circulation and combats a wide range of pathogens. The leaves are used in the treatment of arrhythmia, arthritis, cancer, convalesence, cough, diabetes, digestive disorders, eczema, fever, high cholesterol, jaundice, malaria, nausea, obesity, parasites, rheumatism, smallpox, syphillis, tumors, ulcers, and worms.

Neem leaf can be used as a bath herb to treat chicken pox, rash, and wounds or as a salve, lotion, or soap to treat acne, athlete's foot, and ringworm. The juice from the leaves can be applied topically to treat boils and eczema. Neem oil, extracted from the leaves and seeds, has strong insecticidal and antiseptic properties and can be used to get rid of lice and scabies and to repel mosquitoes and other pests. The seed is very moisturizing and is often used in medicinal soaps to treat skin ailments. The bark is often used topically to heal skin infections, gum disease, and dental problems; a decoction of the bark can be applied topically to treat hemorrhoids.

As a flower essence, neem enhances intuition and concentration and helps users to be less judgmental.

Edible Uses

Neem bark, leaf, and seed are not generally considered edible. The fresh or dried flowers can be eaten, however, and are sometimes used as decorative condiments.

Other Uses

Neem oil is used as a pesticide and fungicide that kills bacteria and over 200 types of insects and fungi but is harmless to honeybees and vertebraes. The leaves can be placed in grain bins, beds, books, cupboards, suitcases, and closets to repel bugs. The dried plant can be burned as a fumigating incense. In cosmetics neem acts a preservative, as well as benefiting many skin conditions. The seeds of neem are being investigated as a possible male and female contraceptive.

Neem wood is used in woodworking. A gum that exudes from the bark is used to dye silk.

Constituents

Leaf: mahmoodin, flavonoids, meliacins, triterpenoids, phytosterols (campesterol, stigmasterol, beta-sitosterol), omega-3 fatty acids, omega-6 fatty acids, omega-9 fatty acids (azdirachtin), nimbidin tannins
Bark: arginine, glutamic acid, methionine, tryptophan, nimbinin, gallic acid, epicatechin, polysaccharides
Seed: oleic acid, stearic acid, palmitic acid, linoleic acid

Energetic Correspondences

- Flavor: bitter, pungent
- Temperature: cool
- Moisture: moist
- Polarity: yin
- Planet: Saturn
- Element: earth

Contraindications

Neem should not be given to infants, the elderly, or the infirm. In healthy adults neem is considered safe; however, long-term internal use may result in anemia, weakness, appetite loss, and weight loss.

Range and Appearance

Native to the Indian subcontinent and now widely grown in tropics around the world, neem is a fast-growing evergreen tree that reaches a height of about 25 feet. It can tolerate poor soil, extreme heat (but not cold), and drought, but in times of drought it will shed most of its leaves. The leaves are alternate and pinnate; they are reddish brown when young, becoming dark green when mature. The tree bears small, sweet-scented white flowers that bloom in drooping panicles. The olive-shaped fruit has a bitter, yellowish pulp in which one to three seeds are found.

NETTLE

Botanical Name

Urtica dioica, U. urens

Family

Urticaceae (Nettle Family)

Etymology

The genus name, *Urtica*, is Latin, meaning "I burn." The species name *dioica* is Latin for "two dwellings" or "two houses," in reference to the plant being dioecious, or bearing male and female flowers on different plants. The common name *nettles* is thought to derive from the Anglo-Saxon *noedl*, "needle," in reference to either the use of nettles as a textile fiber or their sharp prickles. *Nettles* may also derive from the Latin *nassa*, "net," in reference to the plant's strong stems being woven into fishing nets.

Also Known As

Bulgarian: kopriva
Danish: nælde, brændenælde
Dutch: braunetel
English: big sting nettle, devil's leaf, devil's
   plaything, ettle, hidgy-pidgy, hoky-poky, Indian
   spinach, ortiga, seven-minute itch, stinging nettle,
   tanging nettle, true nettle
Finnish: nokkonen
French: ortie
German: brennessel
Greek: analypse arabic, horreig, sorbei
Hebrew: sirpad
Hindi: bichu
Italian: ortica
Norwegian: nesle
Philipino: buluhan
Polish: pokrzywa
Russian: krapiva
Sanskrit: bichu
Spanish: ortiga
Swedish: brännässla, nässla

Part Used

Aboveground plant

Physiological Effects

Adrenal tonic, alterative, antiallergenic, anticatarrhal, antihistamine, anti-inflammatory, antioxidant, anthelmintic (seed), antirheumatic, antiscorbutic, antiseptic (leaf and seed), astringent, blood tonic, carminative, cholagogue, circulatory stimulant, decongestant, depurative, diuretic, endocrine tonic (seed), expectorant, febrifuge, galactagogue, hemostatic, hypoglycemic, kidney tonic, lithotriptic, mucolytic, nervine, nutritive, parturient, pectoral, rejuvenative (seed), thyroid tonic (seed), tonic (leaf, root, seed), styptic, uterine tonic, vermifuge (seed)

Medicinal Uses

This is an herb that improves just about everything! My friend David Hoffmann, author of *The Holistic Herbal*, says, "When in doubt, use nettles."

Nettle improves the body's resistance to pollens, molds, and environmental pollutants. It stabilizes mast cell walls, which stops the cycle of mucous membrane hyperactivity, and it nourishes and tones the veins, improves veins' elasticity, reduces inflammation, and helps prevent blood clots. It also helps curb the appetite, cleanses toxins from the body, and energizes, making it a motivating ally for those who seek to stay on a healthy diet. Drinking nettle tea before and after surgery helps build the blood, promotes healthy blood clotting, speeds recovery, and helps the patient reclaim his or her energy.

Nettle is used in the treatment of acne, amenorrhea (due to blood or kidney deficiency), anemia, arthritis, asthma, atherosclerosis, boils, bronchitis, candida, catarrh, cellulite, cystitis, diabetes, dysentery, eczema, edema, food allergies, hay fever, headache, hemorrhage, hemorrhoids, hives, hypoglycemia, infertility (men and women), jaundice, kidney stones, leukemia, lumbago, menorrhagia, mononucleosis, nephritis, night sweats, obesity, pleurisy, postpartum hemorrhage, premature gray hair, psoriasis, rheumatism, rickets, sciatica, sinusitis, tuberculosis, varicose veins, and vitiligo. It is also an excellent herb to encourage convalescence.

The nettle plant's individual parts have some targeted uses. Nettle leaf and root in particular are known to tone and firm tissues, muscles, arteries, and skin. Taken internally, they decrease uric acid buildup and increase circulation to the skin's surface. The leaf can be used to prevent hair loss, while the root is used in the treatment of prostatits.

Nettle seed both detoxifies and improves the ability of the liver and kidneys to cleanse the blood. Because of this, it is an antidote to poisonous plants and also is useful in cases of spider, bee, dog, and snakebites. It is also used in the treatment of erectile dysfunction, goiter, and hypothyroidism, and it can be used to prevent hair loss.

Nettle is also used for the practice known as urtication, in which one intentionally stings oneself with the plant. This practice, which dates back at least two thousand years, induces a rush of blood to the stung area, producing a counterirritation that reduces inflammation and provides temporary pain relief. Urtication energizes the nerves, muscles, capillaries, and local lymphatic system and causes the body to secrete antihistamines. It can help relieve the pain of arthritis, coldness in the extremities, gout, lumbago, muscular weakness, multiple sclerosis, neuritis, palsy, rheumatism, sciatica, and tendonitis (chronic).

Topically, nettle can be used as a hair rinse to treat dandruff and hair loss, a cleanser for oily skin, a sitz bath for hemorrhoids, a wash for sunburn, a douche for vaginitis, and an enema for detoxification. Compresses prepared with nettle tea can be used to treat arthritic joints, burns, chilblains, eczema, gout, heat rash, insect bites, mastitis, neuralgia, rash, sciatica, tendonitis, varicose veins, and wounds.

As a flower essence, nettles is recommended in times of anger or emotional coldness that can lead to spitefulness and cruelty. It encourages fearlessness in people who feel isolated or have been "stung" by others, helping them regain the ability to connect with others by expressing their anger. It also helps users to release stress and reestablish harmony and unity within themselves.

Edible Uses

Nettles could be described as a superfood, being extremely nutritive, even more so than spinach. Nettle greens can be substituted for cooked spinach, beet greens, chard, or turnip greens in any recipe. Before they can be consumed, however, the sting must be deactivated. Cooking the nettles will do so, as will pureeing the nettles or drying and powdering them.

Nettle beer and wine are favorites of many homebrew aficionados. Fresh nettle juice can be used to curdle cheese, thereby replacing rennet and making a vegetarian-friendly cheese. The juice is also a super tonic beverage.

When stored with fruit, dried nettles can make the fruits last longer, be more resistant to mold, and maintain their flavor better. Nettle leaves can also be wrapped around apples, pears, root vegetables, and moist cheeses to deter pests and aid in their preservation.

Other Uses

Nettles have been used to make paper, rope, fiber, and even a dark green dye. They have many uses in the garden. When used to water plants in the garden, nettle tea stimulates their growth and makes them more resistant to bugs. Plants growing close to nettles tend to have more potent levels of volatile oils. And when added to the compost pile, nettle hastens the breakdown of organic materials.

Constituents

Protein, beta-carotene, xanthophylls, vitamin B, vitamin C, vitamin E, vitamin K, flavonoids (quercitin, rutin, kaempferol, rhamnetin), calcium, chromium, iron, silica, betaine, mucilage, tannin, chromium, silica, chlorophyll, albuminoids, agglutinin, amines (histamine, acetylcholine, serotonin, 5-hydroxyaliphatic acid), hydroxycoumarins, mucilage, saponins (lignin, sitosterol), glycosides, tannin

Energetic Correspondences

- Flavor: salty, slightly bitter
- Temperature: cool
- Moisture: dry
- Polarity: yang
- Planet: Mars
- Element: fire

Contraindications

All fifty species of the genus *Urtica* can be used medicinally, but stick with the *urens* and *dioica* species unless you have consulted with local herb authorities on the safety of local varieties.

Nettle is not known as stinging nettle for nothing; avoid touching or eating the fresh plant unless it is very young and/or you are very brave. Touching the fresh plant can cause a burning rash. Wearing gloves when collecting can help prevent this, but the hairs in large plants may still pierce through. A nettle sting can be soothed with a poultice of yellow dock or plantain or even the juice of the nettle plant itself (but good luck obtaining this without getting many more stings). However, you can learn to love the sting. I admit to collecting nettles barehanded with a pair of scissors and a paper bag. The arthritis I was developing twenty years ago has now become a thing of the past—and I attribute its disappearance to nettle stings.

Eating raw nettles can cause digestive disturbances, mouth and lip irritation, and urinary problems; however, these side effects are rare when the plant is puréed before ingestion and practically nonexistent when the plant is dried.

When used appropriately nettle is considered safe, even over an extended period of time, although those with overly cold, yin-deficient conditions should not use nettle for prolonged periods. Only the aboveground portions of young plants should be consumed, as older plants can be irritating to the kidneys and may cause digestive disturbances.

Range and Appearance

Nettles grow just about everywhere, from waste areas and roadsides to gardens, grasslands, and moist woods. This perennial herb has erect, somewhat branching stems and can grow to a height of 3 to 10 feet. The coarsely serrated, veined, opposite leaves are heart shaped at their base, pointed at their tips, darker on their tops than underneath, and covered with thousands of stiff, stinging hairs. The tiny green flowers are minute and inconspicuous. Nettles is dioecious, meaning that male and female flowers are borne on different plants.

In the garden, nettle spreads widely and quickly. Where once I had a single plant given to me by a kind German lady, I now have at least a thousand. Nettle can adapt to light conditions ranging from full sun to full shade, loves soil that is high in organic matter, and enjoys moderate to high watering.

NUTMEG

Botanical Name

Myristica fragrans

Family

Myristaceae (Nutmeg Family)

Etymology

The genus name, *Myristica,* derives from the Greek *myron,* meaning "ointment" or "balm," which is possibly related to the Hebrew name for myrrh, *mor,* a reference to the aromatic qualities of this plant. The species name, *fragrans,* derives from the Latin *fragrare,* "fragrant." The common name *nutmeg* derives from the Latin *nux,* "nut." The common name *mace,* which refers to the spice composed of the dried outer covering of a nutmeg kernel, has its roots in its medieval Latin name, *macis.*

Also Known As

Arabic: jouza at-teeb
Armenian: meshgengouz

Cantonese: dauh kau syuh

Czech: muskátovy

Danish: muskatnød

Dutch: nootmuskaat

English: mace

Esperanto: muskato

Estonian: muskaatpähkel

Finnish: muskottipähkinä

French: muscadier, macis (mace), noix de
muscade (mace)

German: muskatblüte (mace), muskatnußss,
mukatnussbaum

Greek: Moschokarido

Hindi: jaiphal, taifal

Hungarian: szercsendió

Icelandic: múskat

Indonesian: pala

Italian: macis, moscata, moscatom, noce moscata

Japanese: natamegu, nikuzuku

Korean: neotumek

Mandarin: rou dou kou

Nepali: jaiphal

Norwegian: muskatnøtt

Polish: muszkat

Portuguese: noz-moscada

Romanian: nucsoara

Russian: oreykh muskatny

Sanskrit: jatiphala

Spanish: nuez moscada

Swedish: muskotnöt, muskotblomma (mace)

Thai: chan thet

Tibetan: zati, dza to

Turkish: hindistancevizi

Ukrainian: muskatnyj horikh

Vietnamese: dau khau

Yiddish: mushkat

Parts Used

Kernel, aril (outer covering, known as mace)

Physiological Effects

Antiemetic, anti-inflammatory, antispasmodic, aphro-disiac, aromatic, astringent, carminative, circulatory stimulant, euphoric, hallucinogen (in large doses), stimulant, stomachic

Medicinal Uses

Nutmeg stimulates brain activity and circulation and relaxes muscles. It contains an essential oil, called myristicin, that was one of the original ingredients in the "love drug" Ecstasy. Nutmeg is used to treat bronchial irritations, colic, Crohn's disease, delirium tremens, diarrhea (especially that which occurs first thing in the morning), digestive tract infection, dysentery, eczema, flatulence, gastroenteritis, halitosis, hypothermia, indigestion, insomnia, muscle spasms, nausea, rheumatism, smoker's cough, and vomiting.

The essential oil of nutmeg is often added to massage oils to treat muscular pain. It is said to help prevent scar formation, and it can be applied as a numbing agent to a toothache until dental assistance is available. The essential oil is sometimes added to salves to treat eczema, rheumatism, and ringworm or as a hair rinse to stimulate hair growth.

Edible Uses

Both nutmeg and mace are common culinary spices. Nutmeg is best when grated fresh onto food. It is known to make alcoholic beverages even more intoxicating.

Other Uses

Nutmeg has long been used in magical traditions to attrract love and prosperity. It can be burned as an incense, and the essential oil is often an ingredient in perfumes, soaps, toothpastes, and massage oils. Nutmeg is also sometimes added to smoking mixtures and snuff.

Nutmeg Status

Ancient Arab traders first introduced Europeans to nutmeg. It was so rare and so expensive that in the fourteenth century a pound of nutmeg could be traded for three sheep, two calves, and half a cow. Over the next few hundred years, wealthy ladies and gentlemen would bring their own nutmegs and fancy graters to restaurants to flavor their food and wine as a status symbol.

Constituents

Essential oils (borneol, camphene, pinene, linalool, myristicin, safrole, eugenol), oleic acid, palmitic acid, lauric acid, linnoleic acid; the aril (known as mace) has higher levels of myristicin than the kernel

Energetic Correspondences

- Flavor: pungent
- Temperature: warm
- Moisture: dry
- Polarity: yang
- Planet: Sun/Jupiter/Moon
- Element: fire/air

Contraindications

Large amounts of nutmeg can cause feelings similar to those of a hangover. They also can cause nausea, thirst, anxiety, hallucinations, disorientation, tachycardia, and even convulsions. Ingesting two whole nutmegs can cause death. Do not use more than 3 grams of either nutmeg or mace in one day. Avoid therapeutic dosages during pregnancy and while nursing. Avoid large doses in cases of epilepsy or psychiatric disorders.

Range and Appearance

Native to the Indonesian Molucca Islands, nutmeg is not technically a nut but a single seed contained by a yellow fleshy fruit. Mace is the arillus, a thin, leathery, orangish red membrane between the kernel and pulp of the fruit. The nutmeg tree is an evergreen that can grow to 70 feet in height. It has smooth, greyish brown bark and oblong, brownish leaves. The tree thrives in hot, humid climates with well-drained soil and partial shade.

OAT

Botanical Name

Avena fatua (wild oat), *A. sativa* (cultivated oat)

Family

Poaceae (Grass Family)

Etymology

The genus name, *Avena,* is Latin for "nourishing." The common name *oat* derives from the Old English term for the grain, *āte.*

Also Known As

English: dousar, haver
Finnish: kaura
French: avoine
German: gälbelshaber, hafer, howen
Italian: avena
Japanese: ma-karasu-mugi
Russian: oves
Spanish: avena
Swedish: havre, vanlig havre, vipphavre

Parts Used

Seed (unripe), stem (also known as oatstraw)

Physiological Effects

Alterative, antidepressant, antispasmodic, aphrodisiac, blood tonic, brain tonic, chi tonic, demulcent, diaphoretic, diuretic, emollient, endocrine tonic, febrifuge, laxative, mood elevator, nervine, nervous system tonic, nutritive, rejuvenative, reproductive tonic, restorative

Medicinal Uses

With its high silicon content, oat helps nourish the skin, nails, teeth, bones, and hair. It also builds the blood, relaxes the nerves, and strengthens the nervous system, making tactile sensations more pleasurable. It even supports the elasticity of blood vessels. Its seed and stem are used in the treatment of addiction, alcoholism, anxiety, attention deficit disorder, bone cancer, broken bones, colds (chronic), constipation, convalescence, convulsions, Crohn's disease, debility, depression, diabetes, dyspepsia, emotional distress, erectile dysfunction, exhaustion, gout, headache (stress related), hemorrhoids, incontinence, infertility (male and female), insomnia, low libido, lupus, menopause symptoms, multiple sclerosis, nervous breakdown, nervousness, osteoporosis, paralysis, post-traumatic stress, rheumatism, rickets, schizophrenia, sciatica, shingles, stress, ulcers, varicose veins, and withdrawal symptoms (from tobacco, drugs, or alcohol). It is also used to facilitate recovery from childbirth. When consumed regularly, oats can lower cholesterol levels.

Topically, oat can be used as a bath herb, lotion, salve, or poultice to soften skin and relieve the itchiness of eczema, hives, rheumatism, and neuralgia. As a compress, oat can help heal stitches and relieve the pain of kidney stones.

As a flower essence, oat is helpful for those who are filled with uncertainty and dissatisfaction and are unable to find their life's direction.

Edible Uses

The oat grain is a common food staple and is high in protein. It has a light, mild, creamy flavor. The grain can also be sprouted. An edible oil can be pressed from the seed. The seeds are sometimes roasted and used as a coffee substitute.

Oat tea has a pleasant, mild, slightly sweet flavor. A tea made from oat seed or straw mixed with nettles is a particularly mineral-rich brew.

Other Uses

Oat husks are not only used to stuff bedding but are said to have a sedative effect. The straw can be used to make thatching, paper, and mulch. The hulls are also used to make construction boards and filters in the brewing industry. The hulls of oats are used in the production of furfural, a chemical used to make many industrial products such as nylon, glues, rubber tread, and lubricating oils.

Oatstraw tea can be sprayed in the garden to inhibit striped cucumber beetle infestation.

Constituents

Beta-carotene, B vitamins, calcium, iron, magnesium, manganese, potassium, selenium, silicon, zinc histamine, lysine, methionine, lipids, saponins, flavonoids, vanilloside, starch, gluten, alkaloids (trigonelline, avenine), phytosterols (b-sitosterol)

Energetic Correspondences

- Flavor: sweet
- Temperature: warm
- Moisture: moist
- Polarity: yin
- Planet: Mercury/Mars/Jupiter/Moon/Pluto/Venus
- Element: earth

Contraindications

Those with gluten allergies should use oats with caution.

Range and Appearance

Oat, native to Europe, Asia, and northern Africa but naturalized in North America, is an annual grass that grows freely in the wild along roadsides and in disturbed areas. It also is cultivated as a field crop. Its hollow stems grow to about 4 feet in height. The leaves are long, broad, and slightly hairy. Two or three florets form small, elliptical, drooping spikelets in loose, open panicles on horizontal branches; the flowers are hermaphroditic.

In the garden, oats enjoy full sun, soil that is rich in organic matter, and moderate amounts of water; they will tolerate drought. Planted en masse, they will prevent soil erosion.

When wildcrafting, avoid collecting fuzzy or blackish oat grains, which may be contaminated with ergot.

OLIVE

Botanical Name

Olea europaea

Family

Oleaceae (Olive Family)

Etymology

The genus name, *Oleum,* is Latin for "oil." The species name, *europaea,* denotes the plant's European origin. The common name *olive* derives from the Greek name for the tree, *elaia.*

Also Known As

Afrikaans: olienhout
Arabic: zaytun

Armenian: jiteni, zeytoon

Bulgarian: maslina

Cantonese: gaam láam

Croatian: maslina

Czech: oliva

Danish: oliven

Dutch: olijf

English: oliva, tree of life

Esperanto: olivo

Finnish: öljypuu

French: olivier

German: echter ölbaum

Greek: elia

Hebrew: zayit

Hungarian: olíva

Icelandic: ólífa

Italian: olivo

Japanese: oribu

Korean: ollibu

Lituanian: alyvos

Mandarin: gan lan shu

Polish: oliwka

Portuguese: azeitona, oliveira

Russian: oliva

Serbian: maslina

Spanish: olivo

Swahili: zeituni

Swedish: oliv

Thai: ma kok

Turkish: zeytin

Ukrainian: olyva

Yiddish: masline

Zulu: umquma

Parts Used

Leaf, oil of fruit

Physiological Effects

Leaf: antibacterial, antifungal, anti-inflammatory, antioxidant, antiparasitic, antiseptic, antispasmodic, antiviral, astringent, cholagogue, diuretic, febrifuge, hypotensive, immune stimulant, tonic, vasodilator

Oil of fruit: antioxidant, antiseptic, demulcent, emollient, laxative, nutritive, tonic

Medicinal Uses

Oleuropein, a phenolic compound found in the leaf and fruit (and also in the roots and bark), protects not only the tree but also, when ingested, the human body. The effect of this compound in dissolving the outer lining of pathogenic microbes is so potent that it must be removed before olive fruits can be fermented or the process will be inhibited.

The leaf increases the number and activity of phagocytes and interferes with viral infection by inactivating the virus, preventing the virus from shedding its coat, budding, or assembling at the cell membrane. It can also directly penetrate an infected host and inhibit viral replication. The leaf relaxes and dilates peripheral blood vessels and protects the body against hardening of the arteries. It is reported to kill off many pathogens including cryptosporidia, giardia, pinworm, malaria protozoa, roundworm, and tapeworm. It also helps lower blood sugar levels and helps the body better eliminate uric acid.

The leaf can be used in the treatment of AIDS, anthrax, botulism, bronchitis, candida, chicken pox, chlamydia, cholera, chronic fatigue syndrome, colds, cystitis, diabetes, dysentery, edema, Epstein-Barr virus, fever, fibromyalgia, flu, gonorrhea, heartbeat irregularities, hepatitis, herpes, HIV, hypertension, leprosy, Lyme disease, malaria, measles, mumps, New Castle disease, parasites, pinworm, pneumonia, polio, psoriasis, rheumatoid arthritis, shingles, sinusitis, small pox, staph infection, syphilis, tuberculosis, typhoid, tumors, ulcer, whooping cough, and yellow fever.

Olive oil reduces levels of digestive acids, increases bile secretions, soothes mucous membranes, and relieves congestion in the lymph system and lungs. It helps dissolve cholesterol deposits, lowers levels of low-density lipoproteins (LDL, or "bad" cholesterol), and increases blood flow. It can be used to help prevent heart disease and in the treatment of gallstones, gout, and ulcers.

Topically, the leaf can be prepared as a wash, compress, or poultice to treat athlete's foot, crabs, lice, scabies, ringworm, and wounds. It also can be prepared as a douche to treat yeast infection or nose drops to treat respiratory infection.

Olive oil can be used topically to treat burns, cradle cap, dry skin, inflammation, and wounds. The oil is also included in enemas to treat constipation and in ear drops to treat earaches and infection.

As a flower essence, olive helps relieve mental and physical exhaustion. It is helpful during convalescence and in times of excessive worry or overwork. It can help users through times of conflict and crisis, such as divorce, and for those who have lost interest in what had been an enjoyable life.

Edible Uses

Olive leaf is not generally considered edible, but the olive oil most certainly is. The oil is very nutritive. Extra-virgin olive oil is considered the highest quality, being of the first pressing of the fruits. Virgin olive oil comes from the second pressing. Subsequent pressings of the olive pulp and seeds use solvents and high heat, and the resulting oil is marketed as "pure" olive oil. However, this oil may contain traces of the solvents used in the pressing, and because it has been exposed to high temperatures, the oil may not be of the best flavor. In general, olive oil should not be heated to a high temperature, or its flavor will deteriorate.

The olives themselves are also edible. Raw, unripe olives are extremely bitter. They are often cured in lye, salt, or vinegar before being eaten.

Other Uses

Olive has been a symbol of peace since ancient times; the olive branch is still used as a symbol of peace for the United Nations. Olive oil has long been used in oil lamps. It is often included in cosmetic creams and lotions for its emollient properties. It is often used as a carrier for essential oils that need to be diluted before being applied, and it is considered a nutritive even when applied topically. Olive wood is esteemed in woodworking.

Constituents

Leaf: calcium elenolate, flavonoids (apigenin, hesperidin, luteolin, rutin, chrysoeriol, quercitin, kaempferol), phenolic compound (oleuropein), oleasterol, vauquesline

Oil of fruit: protein, polyphenols, fatty acids (linoleic acid, linolenic acid, oleic acid, eicosenic acid, palmitic acid, stearic acid, arachidic acid), phytosterin, enzymes, triterpenes (ursolic acid, oleanolic acid), oleuropein, bitter principle, lecithin

Energetic Correspondences

- Flavor: leaf—bitter; oil of fruit—sweet, pungent
- Temperature: leaf—cold; oil of fruit—hot
- Moisture: leaf—dry; oil of fruit—moist
- Polarity: yang
- Planet: Sun/Venus/Jupiter
- Element: fire

Contraindications

Olive leaf and oil are generally regarded as safe. Pathogen die-offs have been reported from olive leaf use, in which the body experiences aches, sore throat, or flulike symptoms as a result of the die-off of pathogens. Some may find olive leaf tea irritating to the stomach; consuming it soon before or after a meal will reduce this effect.

Range and Appearance

Olive trees are evergreens that can grow as tall as 20 feet, though they are often kept to a much smaller height when under cultivation. They are native to Africa, southern Europe, and western Asia. The trees can live for centuries, even for as long as two thousand years (though the average life span is three hundred to six hundred years). Though slow growing initially, they will sprout new branches if cut and have deep, hardy taproots. The bark is a pale gray-green. The leaves are lanceolate, pale green above and silvery below. The numerous flowers are white and fragrant. The small fruits are purplish black. Olive trees need a long, hot growing season, full sun, and well-drained soil and can survive dry conditions.

ORANGE

Botanical Name

Citrus x *aurantium* (bitter or Seville orange),
   C. *reticulata* (mandarin orange or tangerine),
   C. x *sinensis* (sweet orange)

Family

Rutaceae (Citrus Family)

Etymology

The genus name, *Citrus,* is the Latin name for this group of plants. The common name *orange* derives from the Sanskrit name for the fruit, *nagaranga,* which in turn derives from the Persian *naranj.*

Also Known As

Arabic: burtuqal
Armenian: narinch
Bulgarian: portokal
Cantonese: cháang
Czech: pomeranc
Danish: appelsin
Dutch: appelsien, sinaasappel
English: golden apple, sun apple
Esperanto: orango
Estonian: apelsinipuu
Finnish: appelsiini
German: apfelsine, arange
Greek: chrisomilia, portokali
Hebrew: tabuz
Hindi: narangi
Hungarian: narancs
Indonesian: jeruk
Italian: arancia
Japanee: orenji, orenzi
Korean: orenji, tungja-namu
Lithuanian: apelsinai
Mandarin: guang gan, tián chéng
Nepali : sunttala
Norwegian: appelsin
Polish: pomarancza slodka
Portuguese: laranja
Romanian: portocala
Russian: apelsin

Sanskrit: naraaruka, naranga
Serbian: naranca, pomoranca
Spanish: naranja
Swedish: apelsin
Thai: som, som kliang
Turkish: portakal
Ukrainian: apelsyn
Vietnamese: cam
Yiddish: marants

Part Used

Peel, fruit, leaf (rarely), flower (rarely)

Physiological Effects

Peel: antibacterial, antiemetic, antifungal, anti-inflammatory, antioxidant, antispasmodic, antitussive, appetite stimulant, aromatic, astringent, bitter, carminative, choleretic, cholagogue, digestive, diaphoretic, diuretic, expectorant, hypertensive, sedative, stomachic, thermogenic
Fruit: antiemetic, antiseptic, antitussive, carminative, diaphoretic, digestive, expectorant
Leaf: antispasmodic, sedative, stomachic
Flower: aromatic, sedative

Medicinal Uses

Orange peel moves chi and dries dampness. As a digestive aid, it stimulates the production of hydrochloric acid and strengthens the spleen. Its rich supply of bioflavonoids helps strengthen the capillaries and tissues of the body. It also boosts metabolism, which makes it useful in weight-loss programs. It can be used in the treatment of abscesses, belching, bloating, breast cancer, catarrh, cellulite, congestion, constipation, dyspepsia, flatulence, gallbladder congestion, hiccups, high cholesterol, indigestion, liver congestion, nausea, obesity, tumors, and uterine prolapse.

Orange flower water is used as a digestive aid. It also can be used topically in salves, lotions, and sprays to treat acne, broken capillaries, and dry and chapped skin and to stimulate new cell growth and restore the skin's acid mantle.

The essential oil of the fruit is used as an antidepressant.

As a flower essence, orange is used to relieve depression, despair, and self-pity that result from past and present abuse issues. It helps resolve conflict and brings inner joy.

Edible Uses

Everyone knows orange to be a delicious fruit, and it is used in the kitchen in ways too numerous to mention. It can also be fermented to make an alcoholic beverage such as Curacao. Orange peel is also edible, though usually only in small amounts, and it is used most often as a zesty flavoring. Orange flower water is also used as a flavoring, most often for desserts like ice cream and beverages.

Other Uses

The essential oil of the blossoms is called neroli; the essential oil of the leaves and young shoots is called petigrain; the essential oil of the peel is called orange essential oil. All three are used in perfumes, soaps, lotions, and hair-care products. Dried orange peel is often included in potpourri.

Oranges are a symbol of prosperity and good fortune. In magical traditions dried orange peel is said to attract love and prosperity.

Constituents

Carotene, vitamin B_1, vitamin C, essential oils (limonene, linalool, nerol, geraniol), flavonoids (hesperidin, zeaxanthin, cryptoxanthin), aldehydes, coumarins, bitters (naringine, aurantiamarine), synephrine

Energetic Correspondences

- Flavor: pungent, bitter (except for *C.* x *aurantium,* which is sour and bitter)
- Temperature: warm (except for *C.* x *aurantium,* which is cool)
- Moisture: dry
- Polarity: yang
- Planet: Sun/Neptune
- Element: fire

Contraindications

Use bitter orange with caution during pregnancy, as large doses may stimulate contractions. Topical use of orange peel essential oil may increase photosensitivity.

Range and Appearance

Orange trees, native to southern Asia but cultivated in many regions around the world, are small evergreens with grayish brown bark and hard yellow wood. The alternate leaves are 3 to 4 inches long, ovate, glossy, and dark green on their tops but pale underneath. The hermaphroditic, fragrant white flowers grow in small axillary cymes. The fruits are round, bright orange, and juicy. The trees require dry soil and prefer full sun, though they can survive in partial shade.

OREGANO

Botanical Name

Origanum spp., including *O. onites, O. vulgare*

Family

Lamiaceae (Mint Family)

Etymology

The genus name, *Origanum,* and common name *oregano* derive from the Greek words *oros* and *ganos,* meaning "joy of the mountain," in reference to the plant's beauty and mountainous origins.

Also Known As

Arabic: anrar, satar barri
Cantonese: ngou lahk gong
Croatian: origano
Danish: oregano
English: origanum, wild marjoram, wintersweet
Esperanto: origano
Estonian: harilik pune
Finnish: mäkimeirami
French: marjolaine sauvage, origan
German: dost, wilder majoran
Greek: rigani
Hebrew: oregano
Hungarian: oregánó

Italian: erba accuiga, origano
Japanese: hana-hakka
Norwegian: bergmynte, kung
Polish: dziki majeranek
Portuguese: orégão, orégano
Romanian: oregano
Russian: dushitsa
Serbian: origano
Spanish: orégano
Swedish: kungsmynta
Thai: origano
Turkish: kekik out
Ukrainian: materynka
Yiddish: origan

Part Used

Aboveground plant

Physiological Effects

Anti-inflammatory, antioxidant, antiseptic, antispasmodic, aromatic, carminative, cholagogue, diaphoretic, digestive, emmenagogue, expectorant, stimulant, stomachic, tonic

Medicinal Uses

Oregano is rich in essential oils that have a wide range of antiseptic properties. It improves respiratory capacity and increases circulation to the digestive tract. It is used in the treatment of asthma, bronchitis, colic, cough, delayed menses, dysmenorrhea, dyspepsia, fever, flatulence, flu, headache due to nerves, high cholesterol, indigestion, measles, motion sickness, mumps, nausea, neuralgia, pleurisy, rheumatism, and tonsillitis.

Topically, oregano can be prepared as a liniment, poultice, or compress to treat bruises, headache, joint pain, sprains, and swelling. It can be used as a bath herb or prepared as a steam inhalation to treat colds and flu and clear congestion from the lungs and sinuses. To relieve toothache, the leaves can be chewed or the diluted essential oil applied.

Edible Uses

Oregano, fresh or dried, is a common culinary herb.

It can lose much of its aromatic qualities if heated, so using it in its raw form, or adding it at the end of meal preparation, is ideal. Oregano is sometimes used to flavor beer, bitters, and vermouth. It makes a spicy tea.

Other Uses

Romans made wreaths of oregano to crown young couples, as the herb symbolizes love, honor, and happiness. The essential oil is used in perfumery and soap making; smelling it helps lift depression. In the garden the plant repels ants. In folkloric tradition, oregano is used in love spells and when carried is said to intensify love, increase prosperity, and give protection against sickness.

Constituents

Beta-carotene, vitamin C, vitamin K, calcium, iron, magnesium, manganese, essential fatty acids, essential oils (carvacrol, thymol, limonene, terpenes, borneol, terpinene, terpineol), flavonoids, tannins, bitters

Energetic Correspondences

- Flavor: pungent, bitter
- Temperature: warm
- Moisture: dry
- Polarity: yang
- Planet: Mercury
- Element: air

Contraindications

Avoid large dosages during pregnancy; using it as a culinary seasoning, however, is safe.

Range and Appearance

Oregano is a perennial (in warmer climates) native to northern Africa, Europe, and Asia but is cultivated worldwide. It bears small, opposite, oval, grayish green leaves on a square stem and can grow to about $2\frac{1}{2}$ feet tall. It produces pinkish to purple hermaphroditic flowers in erect spikes. It can grow in almost any kind of soil and thrives in dry conditions with lots of sun.

OREGON GRAPE

Botanical Name

Mahonia aquifolium (syn. *Berberis aquifolium*),
  M. nervosa (syn. *Berberis nervosa*), *M. pinnata*
  (syn. *Berberis pinnata*), *M. repens*

Family

Berberidaceae (Barberry Family)

Etymology

The genus name, *Mahonia,* was given in honor of
American horticulturalist Bernard McMahon (1775–
1816), who was a gardening mentor to Thomas
Jefferson.

Also Known As

English: barberry, holly grape, holly mahonia,
  jaundice berry, mountain grape, odostemon
Finnish: mahonia
French: mahonie
German: gewöhnliche
Italian: berberi, berbero
Spanish: yerba de sangre
Swedish: mahonia
Turkish: diken üzümü

Parts Used

Root (dried), root bark, rhizome (dried), leaf (rarely)

Physiological Effects

Alterative, antiseptic, antitumor, bitter tonic, cholagogue, digestive, diuretic, laxative, liver tonic, siliagogue, thyroid stimulant, tonic

Medicinal Uses

Oregon grape has antimicrobial properties that are
especially beneficial for the skin and intestinal tract.
It also helps dilate blood vessels and thus lowers
blood pressure. It is a traditional medicinal herb of
several Native American tribes. It is used in the treatment of acne, boils, catarrh, debility, diarrhea, dysentery, eczema, gastritis, hepatitis, herpes, malaria,
psoriasis, salmonella, shigella, and staph infection.

Topically, Oregon grape can be applied as a
compress or poultice to treat boils, itchy skin, and

wounds. The roots can be made into a gargle to
relieve sore throat.

As a flower essence, Oregon grape is used to help
transform self-criticism into acceptance and self-
love. It helps those who are ill at ease in an urban
environment to feel more comfortable.

Edible Uses

The parts used medicinally are not generally considered edible. However, the flowers are edible, as are
the berries, though usually they are deseeded first.

Other Uses

The inner bark of the stems and roots is used to make
a yellow dye, while the fruits yield a green or purple
dye and the leaves yield a green dye. In folkloric tradition, Oregon grape is carried in medicine bundles
or pouches to attract prosperity and popularity.

Constituents

Alkaloids (berberine, berbamine, canadine, hydrastine, oxycanthine, oxyberberine), 5-methoxycarpine,
tannins, resin

Energetic Correspondences

- Flavor: bitter
- Temperature: cold
- Moisture: dry
- Polarity: yin
- Planet: Mars/Saturn
- Element: earth

Contraindications

Use only the dried plant, as the fresh root and rhizome can be excessively purgative. Avoid during
pregnancy. Avoid in hyperthyroid conditions and in
cases with excessive flatulence.

Range and Appearance

Oregon grape is an evergreen herb native to western
North America. It is drought resistant and will tolerate even poor soil and shady or sunny conditions; it
is an excellent xeriscape plant. The leaves are prickly, but the stems are not. The hermaphroditic flowers
are yellow, and the berries are purplish.

OSHA

Botanical Name

Ligusticum canbyi, L. filicinum, L. grayi,
*   L. porteri, L. scoticum, L. tenuifolium*

Family

Apiaceae (Parsley Family)

Etymology

The genus name, *Ligusticum*, was given in honor of
the Italian city Liguria.

Also Known As

English: bear medicine, Canby's licorice root,
   Colorado cough root, empress of the dark forest,
   Indian root, licorice root, loveroot, mountain
   carrot, mountain ginseng, nipo, oshá, oshala,
   Porter's licorice root, Porter's lovage, Scottish
   licorice root, wild lovage
French: liveche ecossise, persil de mer (*L. scoticum*)
Jicarilla: ha'ich'idéé
Spanish: chuchupa, chuchupaste, chuchupáte,
   hierba del cochino

Part Used

Root

Physiological Effects

Alterative, analgesic, anesthetic, antibacterial, antibiotic, antifungal, antihistamine, antirheumatic,
antispasmodic, antiviral, aromatic, bitter, bronchial
dilator, carminative, circulatory stimulant, diaphoretic, diuretic, emmenagogue, expectorant, febrifuge,
hypotensive, immune stimulant, mucolytic, stomachic, vasodilator

Medicinal Uses

Osha promotes chi circulation, stimulates the lungs,
strengthens the resiliency of the alveolar sac, and
reduces mucus in the lungs. In many Native American traditions it is carried in a medicine bag around
one's neck to prevent illness. It is known to increase
respiratory capacity; in fact, Arapahoe runners
would chew the roots to increase their endurance.

It also remoistens the lungs and soothes irritated
bronchioles and sinuses. Osha is used in the treatment of allergies, altitude sickness, asthma, bronchitis, catarrh, colds, cough, emphysema, delayed
menses, fever, flatulence, flu, hay fever, headache,
herpes, indigestion, laryngitis, lung infection, pain,
placenta retention, pneumonia, rheumatism, sinus
infection, sore throat, stalled labor, stomachache,
tonsillitis, and tuberculosis.

Topically, a poultice of osha can be used to draw
out pus and to treat toothache. Applied as a tincture,
salve, or powder, osha can speed the healing of a herpes lesion. It also can be prepared as a steam inhalation to treat sinus infection and congestion or as a
gargle or spray to relieve sore throat.

Edible Uses

Osha leaves and root are edible and have a spicy,
celery-like flavor. Apache Indians traditionally boil
the root with meat.

Other Uses

Osha was considered to be a sacred plant by many
Native American peoples. Traditionally it is worn in
a medicine pouch and around the ankle to ward off
rattlesnakes. Flathead Indians would wash the roots
in a mountain stream near where they had grown to
help bring rain. The root can also be burned as
incense for purification, and it has been used to
increase psychic ability and enhance dreaming. It is
also sometimes smoked with tobacco and other
herbs in some Native American religious ceremonies.

Constituents

Silicon, essential oil (ligustilide, terpenes), lactone
glycoside, saponins, ferulic acid, phytosterols,
coumarin, flavonoids

Energetic Correspondences

• Flavor: pungent, bitter
• Temperature: warm
• Moisture: dry
• Polarity: yang
• Planet: Sun/Mars/Jupiter
• Element: fire

Contraindications

Avoid during pregnancy and in cases of blood and yin deficiency.

Range and Appearance

Osha is a hairless perennial with hollow stems that can grow to a height of 5 feet. The pinnately divided leaves are primarily basal, with several smaller leaves clasping the stalk. The hermaphroditic white flowers grow in flat umbels. The seeds have narrow wings. The plant's aroma is distinctly like that of pungent celery. *L. porteri* is native to eastern and western North America; it is often found growing among damp aspen lodgepole pine groves over 7,500 feet in altitude. Other species are native to Eurasia.

If you are collecting osha from the wild, take care not to confuse it with poison hemlock, which it resembles. Osha has not been cultivated on a large scale successfully, and wild populations are at risk of becoming endangered, so use it with respect.

PARSLEY

Botanical Name

Petroselinum crispum (syn. *P. sativum*; curly-leaved parsley), *P. latifolium* (broad-leaved parsley), *P. tuberosum* (Hamburg parsley)

Family

Apiaceae (Parsley Family)

Etymology

First-century herbalist Dioscorides named this genus *Petroselinum*, deriving the name from the Greek *petros,* "rock," and *selinon,* "celery." The common name *parsley* derives from that genus name.

Also Known As

Arabic: baqdounis
Armenian: azadkegh
Bulgarian: magdanoz
Cantonese: heong choi, yihn sai
Croatian: persin
Czech: petrzel
Danish: persille
Dutch: peterselie
English: devil's oatmeal, perceley, persil, rock parsley
Esperanto: petroselo
Estonian: petersell
Finnish: persilja
French: persil
German: petersilie
Greek: maïntano, persemolo
Hebrew: petrosilia
Hungarian: petrezselyem
Icelandic: pétursselja
Indonesian: peterseli, seledri
Italian: prezzemolo
Japanese: paseri
Korean: minari, pasulli
Mandarin: he lan qin, xiang cai
Norwegian: persille
Polish: pietruszka zwyczajna
Portuguese: salsa
Russian: petrushka
Serbian: persin
Spanish: perejil
Swedish: persilja
Thai: partasliyat, phakchi farang
Turkish: maydanoz
Ukrainian: petrushka horodnya
Vietnamese: rau mùi tây
Yiddish: petreshke

Parts Used

Leaf, root, seed

Physiological Effects

Anthelmintic, antioxidant, antirheumatic, antiseptic, antispasmodic, aperient, aphrodisiac, carminative, digestive, diuretic, emmenagogue, expectorant, galactagogue, odontalgic, ophthalmic, parturient, sedative, stomachic

Medicinal Uses

Parsley's high chlorophyll content facilitates the body's utilization of oxygen, while its essential oils increase circulation to the digestive tract. The herb also helps reduce excess fluids in the body via its action on the kidneys.

The leaves are used in the treatment of anemia, arthritis, cancer, cystitis, delayed menses, dysmenorrhea, edema, flatulence, gout, halitosis, infertility, jaundice, kidney inflammation, kidney stones, and rheumatism. They are also used to encourage convalescense. The seed is used as a galactagogue.

Topically, parsley leaf can be prepared as a poultice to treat bruises, insect bites, and sprains; as a hair rinse to reduce dandruff and graying hair; as facial steam or lotion to relieve dry skin; or as an eyewash to soothe tired eyes. They also can be rubbed on the body to repel mosquitoes. The juice can be applied topically to treat toothache.

Edible Uses

The leaves are a poplar culinary seasoning. They are best eaten fresh and raw, rather than dried or cooked. The root of *Petroselinum tuberosum* can also be eaten, raw or cooked.

Other Uses

The ancient Greeks believed that parsley sprang from the blood of Archemorus, the herald of death; soldiers avoided eating it before battle, and it was used to make wreaths for the tombs of the dead. Today, the essential oil is used in men's perfumes.

Constituents

Essential oils (apiole, myristicin, limonene, eugenol), coumarins, glycoside (apiin), flavonoids (apigenin), chlorophyll, protein, beta-carotene, B complex vitamins, vitamin C, iron, magnesium, histadine

Energetic Correspondences

• Flavor: sweet
• Temperature: neutral
• Moisture: moist
• Polarity: yang
• Planet: Mercury/Mars
• Element: air

Contraindications

Avoid large amounts during pregnancy; small amounts used for culinary seasoning are safe, however. Avoid excessive amounts of the seeds.

Range and Appearance

Parsley, a biennial native to southern Europe, thrives in full sun to partial shade and in moist soils where limestone is prevalent. The hermaphroditic, aromatic flowers grow in compound umbels. The leaves are wavy and finely divided.

PASSIONFLOWER

Botanical Name

Passiflora spp., including *P. edulis* (yellow passionflower), *P. incarnata*

Family

Passifloraceae (Passionflower Family)

Etymology

The common name *passionflower* refers not to any ability of this plant to incite passion but rather the passion of Christ. According to Jesuit missionaries who found this beautiful plant growing in South America, the blue and white color of the flower symbolizes heaven's purity. The ten white petals symbolize the ten faithful apostles (minus Peter and Judas). The filaments of the corona correlates to the crown of thorns, the five red stamens are representative of the five wounds, and the three styles of the pistils are three nails. The tendril represent the whips used on Jesus, and the pointed leaves, the spear. When the flower is only partially opened, it looks like the star seen by the Wise Men.

Also Known As

English: apricot vine, flower of the five wounds, granadilla, granadita, maracoc, maypop, passiflora, passionaria, snake tongue
French: passiflore
German: leiden christi, muttergottes-schuzchen, passionsblume, passionskraut
Hawaiian: Lilikoi (passion fruit)
Sanskrit: mukkopira

Spanish: espina de Cristo, maracuja, pasionaria
Swedish: kärsimyskukka

Parts Used

Leaf, vine, flower

Physiological Effects

Analgesic, anodyne, antibacterial, antidepressant, antifungal, anti-inflammatory, antispasmodic, antitussive, aphrodisiac, cerebral vasorelaxant, diaphoretic, diuretic, hypnotic, hypotensive, nervine, sedative

Medicinal Uses

Passionflower was an official herb of the U.S. National Formulary from 1916 to 1936. It is an aid for those who overwork, being both invigorating and soothing. It aids concentration; calms the spirit, central nervous system, liver, and heart; relaxes the nerves; slightly lowers blood pressure; increases the respiratory rate; helps slow down the breakdown of neurotransmitters; and induces rest. It aids sleep without leaving one feeling hung over the next morning, and, of course, it is not addictive.

Passionflower tea is used to treat alcoholism, anger, anxiety, asthmatic spasms, bronchitis, colic, cough, convulsions, diarrhea, depression, epilepsy, headache (due to stress), high blood pressure, hyperactivity, hysteria, insomnia, irritable bowel syndrome, irritability, menstrual cramps, migraine, muscle tension, neuralgia, nervous breakdown, pain, Parkinson's disease, PMS, restlessness, seizures, shingles, spasms, stress, tachycardia, tranquilizer addiction, whooping cough, and worry.

Topically, passionflower can be used as a compress to treat boils, bruises, burns, earache, eye inflammation or irritation, skin irritation, and toothache.

As a flower essence, passionflower helps integrate spirituality into daily life. It also helps clear emotional confusion and relieves pain and trauma.

Other Uses

The leaves and roots of some species have been used to increase the potency of consciousness-expanding substances such as ayahuasca.

> Like most foods, passion fruit has some physiologically therapeutic benefits, in this case being antiscorbutic, diuretic, and nutritive. When included in the diet, it can help get rid of a urinary tract infection, calm hyperactivity, and relax coughs. It is also considered to be a heart tonic.

Edible Uses

The flower, leaf, and vine are not generally considered edible. However, the fruit of *P. edulis*, known as passion fruit, has been a staple food for peoples of its native range for thousands of years. And a sedative chewing gum made with passionflower was patented in Romania in 1978.

Constituents

Citric acid, flavonoids (apigenin, luteolin, quercitin, rutin, chrysin), glycosides, alkaloids (harman, harmine, harmaline, harmol, harmalolsterols), sitosterol, stigmasterol, serotonin, sugars, gum

Energetic Correspondences

- Flavor: bitter
- Temperature: cool
- Moisture: dry
- Polarity: yin
- Planet: Sun/Venus/Neptune
- Element: water

Contraindications

Large doses may cause nausea and vomiting. Avoid large doses during pregnancy. Unripe fruits have some level of toxicity and should not be consumed.

Range and Appearance

There are over two hundred fruit-bearing species of *Passiflora*. They are native to the tropical rain forests of South and North America, preferring warm climates with moist soil and full sun. Though most species are vines, a few are shrubs. The leaves are palmate and trilobed, and the aromatic, hermaphroditic, large, five-petaled flowers are white, with purple- and pink-tinged centers. The edible fruit is ovoid and usually orange-yellow.

P'AU D'ARCO

Botanical Name

Tabeuia spp. (syn. *Tabebuia* spp.), including
  T. impetiginosa, T. rosea, T. serratifolia

Family

Bignoniaceae (Bignonia Family)

Etymology

The genus name, *Tabeuia,* is a native Brazilian word
meaning "ant wood," as ants live in the hollow dead
twigs. The Guarani and Tupi tribes call this tree *tajy,*
meaning "to have strength and vigor."

Also Known As

English: divine tree, taheebo, tahuari, trumpet
  bush, bow wood
Guarani: kaa jhee, tajy
Portuguese: ipe roxo, ipes
Quechua: taheebo
Spanish: lapacho, taheebo, tajibo (in Bolivia),
  tajylapacho (in Argentina)
Tupi: tajy

Part Used

Inner lining of bark (phloem)

Physiological Effects

Alterative, analgesic, antibacterial, antibiotic, antifungal, anti-inflammatory, antimutagenic, antioxidant, antiparasitic, antitumor, antiviral, aromatic,
astringent, febrifuge, immune stimulant, laxative
(mild)

Medicinal Uses

P'au d'arco was widely used as a medicinal herb during the Incan Empire, and many tribes of South
America, including the Guarani, make use of it. It is
traditionally used to increase strength and endurance. It appears to increase oxygen supply to the
body, have strong activity against a wide range of
pathogens, and increase red blood cell production.
One of its constituents, lapachol, is believed to inhib-

it the growth of tumor cells by preventing them from
metabolizing oxygen.

P'au d'arco is used in the treatment of AIDS, allergies, anemia, arthritis, asthma, boils, bronchitis, cancer,
candida, chronic fatigue, colds, colitis, constipation,
coughs, cystitis, diabetes, dysentery, eczema, fever,
flu, gastritis, gonorrhea, herpes, Hodgkin's disease,
hypertension, leukemia, lupus, lymphatic congestion, malaria, osteomyelitis, intestinal parasites,
Parkinson's disease, polyps, prostatitis, psoriasis,
rheumatism, snakebite, syphilis, trichomonas, tuberculosis, tumors, ulcers, venereal disease, yeast infection, and warts. It is also used to minimize the side
effects of medications, including hair loss, pain, and
immune dysfunction.

Topically, p'au d'arco can be used as a salve to
treat ringworm, wounds, and yeast overgrowth; as a
douche or suppository to treat yeast infection; as a
mouthwash to treat thrush; or as a foot soak to treat
athlete's foot.

Edible Uses

Not generally considered edible.

Other Uses

P'au d'arco wood is used in the construction of tools,
boats, and houses.

Constituents

Ascorbic acid, chromium, iodine, magnesium,
manganese, phosphorous, selenium, silicon, zinc,
napthaquinones (lapachol, lapachone,) alpha- and
beta-xyloidone, flavonoids (quercetin, xloidone),
carnosol, lapachenole, indoles, alkaloids (tecomine),
coenzyme Q_{10}, steroidal saponins

Energetic Correspondences

- Flavor: bitter
- Temperature: warm
- Moisture: dry
- Polarity: yin
- Planet: Saturn/Pluto
- Element: earth

Contraindications

Excess use may loosen bowels or cause nausea or vomiting. Avoid during pregnancy and while nursing. Product adulteration is common, so be sure that your source is trustworthy. Look for purple or red p'au d'arco and accept only the inner bark.

Range and Appearance

P'au d'arco is an evergreen (deciduous in colder climates) tree native to the mountainous regions of the Amazon and Andes but widely naturalized in the tropics. It can reach a height of 100 feet. The large, funnel-shaped flowers are purple, yellow, blue, magenta, or pink. The opposite leaves are ovate or lanceolate and are borne on yellow-green stems; they are usually gathered in groups of five of uneven sizes.

PENNYROYAL

Botanical Name

Hedeoma pulegioides (American pennyroyal), *Mentha pulegium* (European pennyroyal)

Family

Lamiaceae (Mint Family)

Etymology

The species names of the European and American varieties derive from the Latin *pulex,* "flea," in reference to the plants insect-repelling properties. The genus name of American pennyroyal, *Hedeoma,* derives from the Greek *hedys,* "scented." The genus name of European pennyroyal, *Mentha,* is taken from that of Minthe, in Greek mythology a nymph taken by Pluto as a lover; Pluto's jealous wife, Persephone, turned Minthe into a peppermint plant. The common name *pennyroyal* derives from an old Anglo-French name for this plant, *puliol real.*

Also Known As

English: lurk-in-the-ditch, mock pennyroyal (*Hedeoma pulegioides*), mosquito plant, organ tea, pudding grass, rub-by-the-ground, stinking balm, thickweed, tickweed
Finnish: puolanminttu
French: menthe pouliot
German: flohkraut, herminze, hirschminze, kleiner balsam, polei-minze
Italian: menta puleggio
Spanish: poleo, poleo chino
Swedish: polejmynta

Part Used

Aboveground plant

Physiological Effects

Abortifacient, antispasmodic, antiseptic, aromatic, carminative, diaphoretic, emmenagogue, expectorant, nervine, parturient, refrigerant, rubefacient, stimulant, stomachic, sudorific, uterine vasodilator

Medicinal Uses

Pennyroyal was an official herb in the United States Pharmacopoeia from 1831 to 1916. It fights infection, increases circulation to the uterus, and promotes tissue healing. When used as a digestive aid, it stimulates digestive secretions. It can be used to treat amenorrhea, colds, colic, convulsions, cough, delayed labor, delayed menses, dysmenorrhea, dyspepsia, fever, flatulence, flu, headache, hysteria, indigestion, measles, nausea, nervousness, placenta retention, stress, and whooping cough.

Topically, pennyroyal can be used as a wash to treat chicken pox, diaper rash, hives, itching skin, measles, mumps, poison ivy or oak, psoriasis, scabies, and shingles. It also can be prepared as a soak to treat gout or itchy skin or as a compress or liniment to relieve the symptoms of arthritis and rheumatism. As a bath herb it has a stimulating effect and can help relieve the symptoms of rheumatism; in a footbath it helps bring on menses that are delayed.

As a flower essence, pennyroyal clears blockages from the throat chakra and helps users to better speak out. It also assists in mending the damage from indulgence in addictions.

Edible Uses

Pennyroyal is not generally considered edible, though the tea is refreshing and is sometimes used as a culinary flavoring.

Other Uses

In ancient Greece pennyroyal was believed to purify bad water; in the Middle Ages it was used as a strewing herb.

Pennyroyal is an excellent bug repellent. The plant is rubbed on or the diluted essential oil dabbed onto the skin, providing protection against ants, chiggers, fleas, flies, gnats, mosquitoes, and ticks. The essential oil is sometimes used in dog and cat shampoos and flea collars to repel these pests. Smudging (burning the dried herb) or sprinkling the dried plant around is another method of repelling insects. The dried herb is also sometimes included in sachets to repel moths from stored clothing and is sometimes used in cleaning products.

Constituents

Beta-carotene, essential oils (pulegone, ketone, puylegone, isopulegone, menthol, pinene, limonene, piperitone, thymol), flavonoid glycosides (diosmin, herperidin), bitters, tannins

Energetic Correspondences

- Flavor: pungent, bitter
- Temperature: warm
- Moisture: dry
- Polarity: yang
- Planet: Mars/Pluto/Venus
- Element: fire

Contraindications

Although pennyroyal has abortifacient properties, it is not recommended as an abortifacient, because it is not reliable for this purpose, and using it can cause fetal damage or the placenta to implant dangerously low. Several deaths of young women who ingested the essential oil of pennyroyal as an abortifacient have been reported; of course, using any essential oil internally in quantities of more than a drop or two can be dangerous.

Excessive use of pennyroyal can irritate the kidneys or bladder. Avoid large doses of pennyroyal in cases of kidney disease or heavy menstrual bleeding. Large doses may cause dizziness and lethargy. Topi-

cal use may cause an allergic reaction on those with especially sensitive skin. American pennyroyal is higher in pulegone than the European variety and is considered more toxic.

Range and Appearance

European pennyroyal is a perennial that grows to 2 feet in height. The small leaves are opposite, ovate, serrate, and fuzzy to the touch. The flowers are lavender hued and grow from the leaf axils. The plant is often found in the wild in moist areas. It can tolerate full sun or shade and spreads readily.

American pennyroyal is an annual that grows from 6 to 18 inches in height. The leaves are opposite and lance shaped and can be toothed or entire. The two-lipped, hermaphroditic, bluish flowers have three short and two long teeth and grow from the leaf axils. The plant is often found in the wild in sunny locations with moderately fertile soil.

PEONY

Botanical Name

Paeonia albiflora, P. lactiflora (Chinese peony),
    P. officinalis, P. rubra (red peony), *P. suffruticosa*
    (tree peony)

Family

Paeoniaceae (Peony Family)

Etymology

Peony's common and genus names derive from that of Paeon, the Greek physician to the gods.

Also Known As

Mandarin: bai shao yao (*P. albiflora*), chì sháo
    yao (*P. rubra*), mu dan pi (*P. suffruticosa*)
English: bar-cher, king of flowers, moutan
    (*P. suffruticosa*)
Japanese: byakushaku (*P. albiflora*), sekishaku
    (*P. rubra*)
Korean: chôkchak (*P. rubra*), paekchak
    (*P. albiflora*)

Parts Used

Root

Physiological Effects

Alterative, analgesic, anodyne, antibacterial, anti-inflammatory, antiseptic, antispasmodic, astringent, blood tonic, cardiotonic, carminative, diuretic, emmenagogue, expectorant, febrifuge, hypotensive, immune stimulant, laxative, liver tonic, nervine, pectoral, sedative, tonic, vasodilator, yin tonic

Medicinal Uses

Since the days of Hippocrates, peony has been recommended as a remedy for epilepsy. Peony root helps clear heat, increases circulation, and clears blood congestion following traumatic injury. It also helps improve blood flow to the uterus. It is used in the treatment of amenorrhea, anemia, boils, dysmenorrhea, eczema, epilepsy, fever, hypertension, infertility (female; *P. suffruticosa*), pain, vertigo, and whooping cough.

Topically, a wash or poultice prepared from the root of the peony can be used to treat hemorrhoids and varicosities.

As a flower essence, peony helps tense, fearful people who are prone to nightmares. It can appease unconscious fears in those who are prone to cycles of darkness relating to the lunar phases.

Edible Uses

The root is edible and is usually cooked in soups. The flower petals can be eaten as a vegetable, while the seeds can be used as a culinary spice. The stems are edible and are part of a classic Chinese soup, called Four Things Soup, that is considered a women's tonic.

Other Uses

In folkloric tradition, peony is used to keep away evil spirits and to prevent nightmares.

Constituents

Monoterpene glycosides (paeoniflorin, albiflorin), asparagin, benzoic acid, triterpenoids, sitosterol

Energetic Correspondences

- Flavor: bitter, sour
- Temperature: cold (red peonies are considered less cold than white peonies)
- Moisture: neutral
- Polarity: yang
- Planet: Sun
- Element: fire

Contraindications

Avoid during pregnancy, as the plant can stimulate uterine contractions.

Range and Appearance

Peonies are ornamental perennials famed for their aromatic hermaphroditic flowers, which may not appear until the plant's fourth or fifth year. The plants prefer moderately alkaline soil, whether dry or moist, and partial shade to full sun. Many peonies can live fifty years or longer.

PEPPER

Botanical Name

Piper nigrum

Family

Piperaceae (Pepper Family)

Etymology

The common name *pepper* and genus name *Piper* derive from the Greek word for the plant, *peperi*, which in turn derives from the Sanskrit *pippali*, a name for long pepper. *Nigra*, the species name, is Latin for "black."

Also Known As

Arabic: fulfil aswad
Armenian: pghoegh
Bulgarian: piper
Cantonese: hàk wùh jìu, wùh jìu
Croatian: biber, crni papar, papar
Czech: pepr

Danish: peber
Dutch: zwarte peper
English: black pepper
Esperanto: nigra pipro
Estonian: must pipar
Finnish: mustapippuri
French: poivre noir
German: schwarzerpfeffer
Greek: piperi mauro
Hebrew: pilpel shahor
Hindi: gol mirch, gulki, kali mirch
Hungarian: feketebors
Icelandic: swartur pipar
Indonesian: merica hitam
Italian: pepe
Japanese: burakku-peppa, kosho
Korean: huchu, pullaek pepeo
Lithuanian: juodieji pipirai
Mandarin: hei hu jiao, hú jiao
Norwegian: pepper
Polish: czarny pieprz
Portuguese: pimenta-negra
Romanian: piper negru
Russian: chyornyj pyerets
Sanskrit: krishnan, marich
Serbian: biber crni, papar
Spanish: pimenta negra
Swahili: peremende, pilipili
Swedish: psvarteppar
Thai: prik thai
Tibetan: fowarilbu, pho ba ril bu
Turkish: kara biber
Ukrainian: perets chornyj
Vietnamese: cây tiêu, tiêu den
Yiddish: shvartser fefer

Part Used

Fruit (dried, unripe)

Physiological Effects

Antibacterial, antimucoid, antioxidant, antiseptic, aromatic, carminative, circulatory stimulant, diaphoretic, digestive, diuretic, rubefacient, sialagogue, stimulant, stomachic

Medicinal Uses

Pepper warms the body, improves circulation, and prevents the proliferation of pathogens. It is believed that eating lots of pepper will make one less desirable to mosquitoes. When pepper is added to food in moderation, it stimulates the production of both saliva and digestive secretions, including hydrochloric acid. Pepper is used in the treatment of arthritis, colic, diarrhea, flatulence, headache, indigestion, nausea, poor circulation, rheumatism, stomachache, and vertigo. In eastern Africa, pepper is sometimes used as an abortifacient, for which purpose it is consumed in excess quantities.

Topically, pepper can be prepared as a wash to deter ringworm and lice.

Edible Uses

Pepper has been considered a precious spice since ancient times. Attila the Hun is said to have demanded a ransom of three thousand pounds of pepper during his siege of Rome in the year 408. Pepper was an important early trade item, and the quest for this spice prompted much world exploration; Columbus, in fact, was hoping to find pepper in the East Indies when he bumped into North America. Currently pepper accounts for more than one-fourth of the world's spice trade.

Commercial black, green, and white peppers are all from the same plant, *Piper nigrum*. Black pepper is the unripe but fully grown berry. White pepper, a milder version, is the mature fruit that has been soaked and peeled. Green pepper is the young, unripe fruit.

Other Uses

Pepper essential oil is used in perfumery and is added to massage oils for its stimulating and toning properties. Pepper can be prepared as a spray to repel ants, boll weevils, flies, roaches, moths, and silverfish. In folklore tradition, pepper is reputed to repel negative energy.

Constituents

Essential oils (beta-bisabolene, camphene, eugenol, carvone, phellandrene, myristicin, pinene, limonene, safrole), resin, alkaloids (piperine, piperidine, chavicine), protein, chromium

Energetic Correspondences

- Flavor: pungent
- Temperature: hot
- Moisture: dry
- Polarity: yang
- Planet: Mars
- Element: fire

Contraindications

Overuse may cause oversecretion of digestive juices, leading to a burning sensation in the digestive tract. Large amounts may elevate blood pressure.

Range and Appearance

Black pepper is a perennial vine native to southern India. The leaves are thick, green, and ovate in shape. The species is dioecious, bearing male and female flowers on different plants; the flowers are tiny and white. The berrylike, aromatic, pungent fruits are borne on short, hanging spikes. They are green when unripe and become red at maturity. Black pepper grows in almost all types of soil but prefers soils that are loose and well-drained, in a humid climate with much rainfall and partial shade.

PEYOTE

Botanical Name

Lophophora diffusa, L. williamsii

Family

Cactaceae (Cactus Family)

Also Known As

English: buttons, cactus pudding, divine plant, dry whiskey, hikuli, mescal button, pellote, peyotl, white mule
Spanish: tuna de la tierra

Etymology

The genus name *Lophophora* derives from the Greek *lophos,* "crest," in reference to the crests or trichemes on each tubercle. The common name *peyote* is derived from the Aztec *peyotl,* "caterpillar's cocoon," in reference to the fuzzy nature of the plant, with its white, woolly hairs. The name of its principle alkaloid, mescaline, comes from that of the Mescalero Apache, from whose dwellings extraction samples were taken.

Part Used

Crown, consisting of disc-shaped buttons

Physiological Effects

Antibiotic, antiseptic, antispasmodic, bitter, cerebral stimulant, emetic, entheogen, hallucinogen, liver cleanser, lymphatic cleanser, nervous system stimulant

Medicinal Uses

With its antibiotic effects, peyote aids wound healing and prevents infection; indeed, it has been found to have activity against eighteen penicillin-resistant strains of *Staphylococcus aureus*. Peyote also increases body temperature, heart rate, and blood pressure and cleanses the liver. In some Native American traditions, it is used to relieve cramps and childbirth pain and to increase fertility. It is also used to restore physical strength.

As a medicine plant, peyote is used to treat arteriosclerosis, arthritis, blindness, cancer, cough, depression, diabetes, drug addiction, dysmenorrhea, fever, flu, grief, headache (related to the nerves), hysteria, hypochondria, infertility, intestinal problems, paralysis, pleurisy, pneumonia, restlessness, rheumatism pain, staphylococcus, tuberculosis, venereal disease, and vision problems. The peyote buttons are generally eaten or made into a tea.

Topically, peyote can be prepared as a poultice to treat burns, fractures, gum infection, insect stings, joint pain, nerve and muscle pain, snakebite, sores, and slow-healing wounds. It also can be prepared as a gargle to relieve sore throat. However, since peyote has in recent times come to be in very short supply, these topical uses are seldom employed.

Edible Uses

Peyote produces a small pink fruit that is delicious. The Huichol eat the woolly hairs of the buttons, calling them "eyebrows."

Other Uses

Peyote is documented as having been in use for more than four thousand years in Mesoamerica. It is most well known for its use as an entheogen, or a psychoactive used for religious purposes. Thanks to its alkaloid mescaline, peyote can produce amazing visions and insights, and it has long been used in Native American shamanic traditions, both historical and current. *Lophophora williamsii* has greater psychoactive properties than *L. diffusa*.

Constituents

Vitamin C, phenethylamine, alkaloids (mescaline, lophorine, pellotine, anhalonidine)

Energetic Correspondences

- Flavor: bitter
- Temperature: cool
- Moisture: dry
- Polarity: yin
- Planet: Neptune/Saturn
- Element: earth

Contraindications

Peyote often causes nausea and vomiting (though this can be part of its medicinal benefit) and may temporarily elevate blood pressure and body temperature, cause sweating, and stimulate salivation. In some cases it can cause frightening visions, fear, and anxiety.

Legal Issues

Peyote is illegal in many countries, including the United States, unless it is being used in a "bona fide" Native American religious ceremony.

Range and Appearance

Peyote is a small spineless cactus that grows sparsely from the southwestern United States through central Mexico. It tends to grow in silty limestone flood plains. Its flat crown grows almost level with the earth. It produces five ribs and has white woolly hairs composed of cellulose. Peyote flowers sporadically and requires hot, humid conditions to germinate, one reason why it is rare in its natural habitat. Cultivated plants can mature in six to ten years, as opposed to wild ones, which can take as much as thirty.

Peyote is in danger of becoming extinct in the wild. Loss of habitat and overharvesting have decimated its valuable population. Please use it with care.

PINE

Botanical Name

Pinus spp., including *P. contorta* (lodgepole pine), *P. nigra*, *P. pinaster*, *P. pinea*, *P. strobus* (white pine), *P. sylvestris* (Scotch pine), *P. tabuliformis*

Family

Pinaceae (Pine Family)

Etymology

The genus name *Pinea*, from which the common name *pine* derives, is the Latin name for the nuts derived from this tree.

Also Known As

Finnish: pitäneulasmänty
French: pin
German: arve, sumpfkiefer
Italian: pino
Swedish: långbladig

Parts Used

Inner bark, needles, young buds, pitch

Physiological Effects

Analgesic, anticatarrhal, antioxidant (bark), antiseptic, antispasmodic, antiviral, demulcent, diuretic, expectorant, rubefacient, stimulant, tonic

Medicinal Uses

Pine improves circulation and oxygen transport in the body and can encourage blood clots to dissolve. It is used in the treatment of acne, blood clots, bronchitis, coughs, croup, emphysema, fever, laryngitis, rheumatoid arthritis, scurvy, sinusitis, and tonsillitis.

Topically, pine can be used as a compress to treat bronchitis, nephritis, pneumonia, rheumatism, sciatica, and wounds. As a bath herb it can be used to treat arthritic pain, insomnia, muscle soreness, and nervous debility. It also can be prepared as a steam inhalation to relieve respiratory congestion. The sap is often included in ointments to treat eczema and psoriasis; it also can be used as a poultice to draw out splinters and to bring boils to a head.

The essential oil is said to normalize male hormones; it can be prepared as a steam inhalation or massage or bath oil.

As a flower essence, pine is helpful for those who are filled with guilt and self-blame and for those who are never satisfied with their success. It helps bring about true understanding and forgiveness and releases responsibility. It increases psychic awareness as well as insight and helps users learn from past mistakes.

Edible Uses

Pine nuts are a delicacy and can be eaten raw or cooked. Other parts of the tree are also edible, though not considered culinary wonders. Pine needles, which are rich in vitamin C, and the inner bark can be chewed and then spit out. In fact, in 1534, when the French explorer Jacques Cartier anchored in the Saint Lawrence, many of his crew had died of scurvy. Local Indians saved the survivors with a vitamin-C-rich tea made from pine needles.

Other Uses

Small pines are often decorated as Christmas trees, a practice that is thought to have originated in Germany in the 700s. The Iroquois believe the pine tree to symbolize a balanced life, as its shape resembles praying hands reaching for the sky. In Chinese tradition pine trees are planted at grave sites to bring positive chi to the area.

Pine is also a useful material. Pine cones make good tinder for starting a fire. Pine needles can be made into baskets, and they were once used to stuff mattresses to repel fleas and lice. The needles also yield a tan or green dye. Pine wood is a common building material; lodgepole pine, in particular, was once used for teepee poles.

Scotch pine (*Pinus sylvestris*) is used in reforestation as it matures rapidly and endures a wide range of temperatures, rainfall, and soil conditions.

Constituents

Lignan, coniferin, triterpenes, pinipricin, tannins, resin

Energetic Correspondences

- Flavor: bitter
- Temperature: warm
- Moisture: dry
- Polarity: yang
- Planet: Mars/Pluto
- Element: air/earth

Contraindications

Pine is generally regarded as very safe. Some people may experience contact dermatitis from the wood, resin, or sawdust.

Range and Appearance

Native to the northern hemisphere, pines are evergreen trees bearing long, slender, sharp-pointed needles. The trees are dioecious, meaning that male and female flowers are borne on different plants. The flowers are red and yellow and appear in clusters. The trees can tolerate poor soils and shady conditions and have low water requirements.

PIPSISSEWA

Botanical Name

Chimaphila menziesii, C. umbellata

Family

Pyrolaceae (Wintergreen Family)

Etymology

The genus name *Chimaphila* derives from the Greek *cheima,* "winter," and *phileo,* "to love," in reference to this plant being an evergreen. In the Cree language, *pipsissewa* means "breaks into small pieces," in reference to the herb's use in dissolving stones in the body.

Also Known As

English: bitter wintergreen, false wintergreen, ground holly, king's cure, prince's pine, rheumatism weed, umbellate wintergreen
French: pyrole en ombrelle
German: winterlieb
Italian: erica Americana
Ojibway: gagigebu

Parts Used

Aboveground plant

Physiological Effects

Alterative, antibacterial, anti-inflammatory, antiseptic, astringent, diaphoretic, diuretic, febrifuge, rubefacient, stimulant, tonic, urinary

Medicinal Uses

Pipsissewa is a close relative of uva-ursi but contains fewer tannins and is less irritating to the body and a stronger diuretic. It improves kidney and liver function by helping the body eliminate excess fluids. Its hydroquinone content has an antiseptic effect upon the genitourinary system. In many Native American traditions it is used to induce sweating and lower fevers. Pipsissewa is used in the treatment of arthritis, bladder stones, cystitis, gonorrhea, kidney stones, nephritis, ovarian cysts, prostatitis, rheumatism, typhus, urethritis, and urinary tract infection.

Topically, pipsessewa can be prepared as a poultice to treat blisters, rheumatic joints, sores, swelling, and tumors. It also can be made into an eyewash to soothe tired or infected eyes.

As a flower essence, pipsissewa helps users make clear decisions and lessens confusion about life choices.

Edible Uses

The leaves are edible and were once an ingredient in root beer and Pepsi. Both the stems and the roots make a pleasant wintergreen-tasting tea. In Mexico pipssisewa is an ingredient in navaitai, an alcoholic beverage made from fermented corn.

Other Uses

Pipssisewa is a good ground cover. The flowers are used in perfumery. In folkloric tradition, it is carried to attract positive energy and prosperity.

Constituents

Ursolic acid, hydroquinones (arbutin, chimophilin, ericolin), flavonoids (avicularin, kaempferol), triterpenes (ursolic acid, taraxasterol), phenols, methyl salicylate, essential oil, tannins

Energetic Correspondences

- Flavor: bitter
- Temperature: cool
- Moisture: dry
- Polarity: yin
- Planet: Moon
- Element: water

Contraindications

Pipssisewa may give urine a greenish color, which is not cause for alarm. The fresh plant may cause contact dermatitis in some people.

Range and Appearance

Pipsissewa, native to the northern hemisphere, grows in dry woodlands or sandy soils in full to partial shade. It grows from 6 inches to 2 feet in height and features shiny, bright green, toothed evergreen leaves arranged in pairs. The hermaphroditic, aromatic flowers grow in small umbels of four to eight blossoms and are white or pink in color. The flowers droop as they mature.

PLANTAIN

Botanical Name

Plantago asiatica, P. lanceolata (lance-leaf plantain), *P. major* (broad-leaf plantain), *P. media* (hoary plantain, sweet plantain)

Family

Plantaginaceae (Plantain Family)

Etymology

The genus name *Plantago,* from which the common name *plantain* derives, is an old French adaptation of the Latin word *planta,* meaning "sole of the foot," in reference to the plant's broad leaves.

Also Known As

English: cuckoo's bread, Englishman's foot, leaf of Patrick, ribwort, ripplegrass, snakebite, snakeweed, waybread, white man's footsteps

Finnish: piharatamo

French: plantain

German: breitwegerich, wegbreit

Italian: plantaggine

Japanese: shazenshi

Korean: ch'ajônja

Mandarin: che qían zi

Sanskrit: lahuriya

Swedish: groblad

Parts Used

Leaf, seed

Physiological Effects

Leaf: alterative, antibacterial, anti-inflammatory, antiseptic, antispasmodic, anthelmintic, antivenomous, astringent, expectorant, decongestant, demulcent, deobstruent, depurative, diuretic, expectorant, febrifuge, hemostatic, kidney yin tonic, ophthalmic, mucilaginous, refrigerant, restorative, vulnerary

Seed: demulcent, fiber laxative

Medicinal Uses

Plantago lanceolata is considered the most therapeutic and *P. major* the most diuretic. Plantain leaf clears heat and toxins, reduces inflammation, deters infection, promotes tissue repair, and soothes irritated mucous membranes. It is used in the treatment of AIDS, allergic rhinitis, asthma, bedwetting, blood in the urine, blood poisoning, bronchitis, catarrh, colitis, cough, cystitis, debility, diarrhea, dysentery, dysuria, earaches, eczema, fever, gastritis, hay fever, hemorrhoids, herpes, injury, irritable bowel syndrome, laryngitis, menorrhagia, neuralgia, psoriasis, scrofula, sore throat, thirst, tuberculosis, ulcers, urinary tract infection, urinary stones, and vision weakness.

The seeds have a mucilaginous effect and swell in the body, acting as a bulk laxative. They are used to lower cholesterol and to treat edema, hypertension, and infertility.

Topically, plantain is considered a supreme drawing agent in that it helps draw toxins from the body. It also is excellent for the topical healing of damaged tissue. It can be employed as a poultice or compress in the treatment of bee stings, boils, bruises, burns, eczema, hemorrhoids, insect bites and stings, mastitis, poison ivy/oak, ringworm, snakebite, splinters, sunburn, swelling, toothache, ulcers, and wounds. Plantain can also be made into a gargle to treat a sore throat or an eyewash to treat blepharitis and conjunctivitis. It can be used as a hair rinse for dandruff, a douche for leukorrhea and vaginitis, a wash for irritated eyes, and an enema for intestinal infection.

As a flower essence, plantain encourages enjoyment of life and strength in being grounded and clears negative thoughts.

Edible Uses

The young leaves are edible raw or cooked and have a pleasant "green" flavor; older leaves are also edible but should have their fibrous strands removed. The seeds are also edible; they are usually ground and used as a seasoning or thickener.

Other Uses

A fiber obtained from the plant is sometimes used in making fabric. In magical traditions, plantain is esteemed for its healing, protective, and strengthening powers.

Constituents

Leaf: vitamin C, vitamin K, tannins, flavonoid (apigenin), mucilage, allantoin, glycoside (aucubin), silicic acid, oxalic acid

Seed: B vitamins, protein, starch, oils, mucilage

Energetic Correspondences

- Flavor: sweet, salty, bitter
- Temperature: cool
- Moisture: dry (but with secondary moistening properties)
- Polarity: yin
- Planet: Venus
- Element: earth

Contraindications

Plantain is generally regarded as safe.

Range and Appearance

Plantain is a low-growing perennial widely naturalized in North America; it can be found growing everywhere from roadsides to lawns and even between the cracks in sidewalks. The five to seven leaves grow in a basal rosette and are ovate and somewhat toothed, with strong parallel fibers. _P. major_ has broad leaves, _P. lanceolata_ has narrow leaves, and _P. media_ has leaves somewhere between the widths of the other two; _P. asiatica_ is taller and wider than the other three species. The inconspicuous flowers are borne on a cylindrical spike that can be up to 15 inches tall. Later this spike becomes filled with numerous seeds.

In the garden, plantain prefers full sun to partial shade and moist soil.

PLEURISY

Botanical Name

Asclepias speciosa, A. tuberosa

Family

Asclepiadaceae (Milkweed Family)

Etymology

The genus name _Asclepias_ was given in honor of the Greek god of medicine bearing the same name. The common name _pleurisy_ refers to the plant's ability to help reduce the pain and inflammation of the disease pleurisy.

Also Known As

English: archangel, butterfly milkweed, butterfly weed, Canada root, chiggerflower, colic root, flux root, immortal, milkweed, orange swallow wort, silkweed tuber root, white root, wind root
French: ascelpiade tuberose
German: knollige schwalbenwurz, seidenpflanze
Spanish: raiz de asclepias

Part Used

Root

Physiological Effects

Anodyne, anti-inflammatory, antispasmodic, astringent, bronchial dilator, cathartic (in large amounts), carminative, diaphoretic, diuretic, emetic (in large amounts), expectorant, nervine, vasodilator

Medicinal Uses

Pleurisy root was included in the United States Pharmacopoeia from 1820 until 1905 and the National Formulary from 1916 to 1936. It helps expel phlegm from both the nasal and the bronchial passages, clears heat, and improves circulation, lymphatic drainage, and the function of the cilia. It is used to treat asthma, bronchitis, catarrh, chicken pox, colds, colic, cough, diarrhea, dysentery, eczema, emphysema, fever, flatulence, flu, measles, pleurisy, pneumonia, rheumatism, rheumatic fever, scarlet fever, tuberculosis, typhoid, and typhus.

Topically, pleurisy root can be used as a poultice to treat bruises, rheumatism, and wounds.

Edible Uses

The roots, as well as the young shoots, flowers, buds and immature seedpods, can be cooked and eaten. The plant is generally not eaten raw. The flowers can be boiled down to make a sweetener.

Other Uses

The plant's beautiful orange flowers have been made into a yellow dye. Some Native American tribes made bowstrings from the stalks. The bark yields a fiber that can be used in making string or cloth. The water-repellent seed fluff is used to make candle wicks and to stuff jackets, pillows, dollies, and even life jackets; it has even been used to mop up oil spills at sea.

Constituents

Beta-carotene, vitamin C, calcium, phosphorous, sulfur, glycosides (asclepiadin), bitters (asclepione), sterol (phytoestrogen), cardenolides, flavonoids (kaempferol, quercetin, rutin), essential oils, resin

Energetic Correspondences

- Flavor: bitter
- Temperature: cool
- Moisture: dry
- Polarity: yin
- Planet: Sun/Mercury
- Element: air

Contraindications

Avoid pleurisy root during pregnancy and in cases of heart conditions. Large doses and ingesting the uncooked plant may cause vomiting and diarrhea. The sap contains toxic glycosides and should not be consumed raw.

Range and Appearance

Pleurisy is a perennial, native to North America that can grow from 1 to 3 feet in height. The stems and leaves are hairy. The leaves are alternate and lance shaped, and they clasp the stems close to the flower. The hermaphroditic flowers are bright orange corymbs; the seed pods are long, narrow, and downy.

Pleurisy prefers light, sandy soil and full sun and will tolerate dry conditions.

Monarch butterflies feed upon pleurisy. Birds that eat these butterflies experience pleurisy's emetic effects afterward, which causes them to vomit and discourages them from eating the butterflies again.

POKE

Botanical Name

Phytolacca americana

Family

Phytolacaceae (Poke Family)

Etymology

The genus name *Phytolacca* derives from the Greek *phyton*, "plant," and the Latin *lacca*, "crimson lake," in reference to the plant's ability to yield a reddish dye. The common name *poke* is thought to derive from the Algonquian *poughkone*, a name for any plant that yields a red dye.

Also Known As

English: cancer root, coakum, pigeon berry, pokeweed, red ink plant, skoke
Finnish: kermesmarja
German: kermesbeere
Italian: fitolacca
Japanese: yoshu-yama gobo
Russian: fitalakamericana
Spanish: congora
Swedish: kermesbär

Part Used

Root

Physiological Effects

Alterative, anodyne, antifungal, anti-inflammatory, antirheumatic, antitumor, antiviral, cathartic, emetic, expectorant, hypnotic, immune stimulant, lymphatic decongestant, molluscidal, narcotic, purgative, spermicide

Medicinal Uses

Poke has a long history of being used to bolster weak immune systems. At one time it was used to treat syphilis, and in Africa today it is being investigated for its ability to control bilharzia, a parasite-caused disease contracted by bathing in water containing certain snails. It is used in the treatment of AIDS, arthritis, cancer, herpes, leukemia, liver cancer, lymphatic infection, mumps, rheumatism, swollen glands, tonsillitis, and tumors.

Topically, poke can be prepared as a poultice to treat boils, cancer of the skin or breasts, and fungal infections; as a compress to treat mastitis; as a salve or wash to treat bedsores, cancers, carbuncles, chicken pox, eczema, fungal infection, hemorrhoids, herpes, measles, psoriasis, shingles, sprains, swelling, and tonsillitis.

Edible Uses

All parts of poke are toxic, but some parts can be eaten after proper preparation. The root is not generally considered edible. However, the young shoots (less than 1 foot tall) can be peeled and eaten, as can the young leaves (from stalks less than 1 foot tall); both the shoots and the leaves should first be boiled in two changes of salted water (ten minutes for the first, five minutes for the next) to leach out any toxic components. The berries can be eaten when cooked but are toxic when raw.

Do not eat red-tinged portions of the plant, the mature leaves, the raw berries, or any other part of the plant.

Other Uses

The berries produce a red dye that can be used as an ink and to color paint. In fact, the United States Constitution was written in pokeberry ink.

Constituents

Triterpenoid saponins, alkaloid (phytolaccine), phyolaccic acid, formic acid, lectins, tannin, antiviral protein, histamines, fatty oil, resin, sugars

Energetic Correspondences

- Flavor: bitter, pungent
- Temperature: cold
- Moisture: dry
- Polarity: yang
- Planet: Mars
- Element: fire

Contraindications

Use poke only under the supervision of a qualified health-care professional. Avoid during pregnancy. All parts of the plant are toxic and may cause digestive distress, vomiting, lowered blood pressure, and depressed respiration. Overdoses can be fatal. Doses for this plant are much smaller than for other herbs. If preparing poke as a tea, one mouthful taken several times daily is sufficient; as a tincture, two to five drops twice daily is fine. Consume plenty of water when using poke as medicine.

Handle the root with gloves, as the sap can cause contact dermatitis. Dust of the dried plant may cause sneezing and eye irritation.

Range and Appearance

Poke, native to North America, thrives in most soils with plenty of moisture and full sun to partial shade. It is a large, smooth, branching herb with greenish, reddish, or purplish stems. The leaves are alternate. The hermaphroditic white flowers bloom on a long stem. Dark purple berries appear after the flowering; each berry is composed of five to twelve segments.

POLYGALA

Botanical Name

Polygala senega, P. sibirica, P. tenuifolia

Family

Polygalaceae (Milkwort Family)

Etymology

The genus name derives from the Greek *polys,* "much," and *gala,* "milk," alluding to the milky secretions of the plant as well as its effects, as some species can be used as galactagogues.

Also Known As

Cantonese: yan ji (*P. tenuifolia*), yuen ji (*P. tenuifolia*)
English: Chinese senega root (*P. tenuifolia*), milkwort, mountain flax (*P. senega*), rattlesnake root (*P. senega*), Seneca snakeroot (*P. senega*), Siberian milkwort (*P. sibirica*), snakeroot (*P. senega*), thin-leaf milkwort (*P. tenuifolia*)
German: kreuzblume (*P. tenuifolia*)

Italian: polygala (*P. tenuifolia*)
Japanese: onji (*P. tenuifolia*)
Korean: woji (*P. tenuifolia*)
Mandarin: xiao cao, xi xie yuan zhi
Russian: senega (*P. sibirica*)

Part Used

Root

Physiological Effects

Analgesic, antibacterial, anticonvulsant, antiseptic, cardiac sedative, cardiotonic, cerebral stimulant, cerebral tonic, decongestant, diaphoretic, diuretic, emmenagogue, expectorant, hypnotic, hypotensive, kidney tonic, liver stimulant, mucolytic, nervine, oxytocic parturient, restorative, sedative, sialagogue, uterine stimulant, tonic

Medicinal Uses

Polygala calms the spirit and enables the flow of chi to the heart. It also increases circulation and bodily secretions and strengthens the sinews and bones. It was used by the Seneca Indians to treat snakebite. It is used in the treatment of abscess, Alzheimer's disease, amenorrhea, anxiety, asthma, boils, bronchitis, carbuncles, catarrh, cough (lingering), dizziness, emphysema, fatigue, heart palpitations, hypertension, insomnia, mastitis, memory loss and confusion, nightmares, osteoporosis, Parkinson's disease, restlessness, seizures, spermatorrhea, stress, and whooping cough. It also can be used to bring on labor.

Topically, polygala can be prepared as a compress or poultice to treat boils and carbuncles.

Edible Uses

The roots, as well as the young leaves, can be eaten after being boiled in several changes of water.

Other Uses

In Asia, polygala is traditionally used to build strength of character and willpower and to promote vivid dreams.

Constituents

Iron, magnesium, silica, triterpenoid saponins, resin, glycosides, polygalitol, fatty acids, tenuidine, tenuifolin, onsitin, amyrin, xanthones

Energetic Correspondences

- Flavor: bitter, sweet, sour, pungent
- Temperature: warm
- Moisture: dry
- Polarity: neutral
- Planet: Mars/Uranus/Neptune
- Element: air

Contraindications

Avoid polygala during pregnancy and in cases of gastritis or ulcer. Large doses can be cathartic and emetic and should be avoided. Also avoid long-term use.

Range and Appearance

Polygala is a perennial native to China (*P. tenuifolia*), Asia (*P. sibirica*), and North America (*P. senega*). It grows to about 3 feet in height. Its leaves are alternate and linear or linear-lanceolate. The hermaphroditic flowers are purple and bloom terminally or axillarily. The seeds are flat with winged margins. The contorted root has a wintergreen-like aroma. The plant prefers light, moist, well-drained soil and partial shade to full sun.

POPPY

Botanical Name

Papaver rhoeas, P. somniferum

Family

Papaveraceae (Poppy Family)

Etymology

The genus name *Papaver,* from which the common name *poppy* derives, is the classical Latin name for the poppy plant. The species name *rhoeas* is Latin for "red," while the species name *somniferum* derives from the Latin *somnus,* "sleep," and *ferre,* "bring," in reference to the plant's sedative properties.

Also Known As

Arabic: abu-an-num, khashkhash

Armenian: megon, mekon

Bulgarian: gradinski mak, makovo

Cantonese: yìng suhk hohk

Croatian: mak

Czech: mák, mák sety'

Danish: valmue-frø

Dutch: heulbol, maankop

English: blind buff, corn poppy, field poppy, Flanders poppy, garden poppy, head waak, opium poppy, plant of joy, seed poppy

Esperanto: papavo

Estonian: magyn, moon

Finnish: unikko

French: pavot

German: mohn, schlafmohn

Greek: paparouna

Hebrew: pereg

Hindi: khas-khas, post

Hungarian: mák

Icelandic: birki, valmúafræ

Italian: papavero

Japanese: keshi, papi

Korean: apyeon, popi

Lithuanian: aguonos

Mandarin: ying su qiao

Norgegian: valmue

Polish: mak lekarski

Portuguese: dormideira, papoila

Romanian: mac

Russian: mak snotvornyj

Sanskrit: ahiphena

Serbian: mak

Spanish: ababa, adormidera, amapola real

Swedish: vallmo

Thai: ton fin

Ukrainian: mak snodijnyj

Vietnamese: cây thuôc phiên

Yiddish: mon, mondl

Part Used

Seed

Physiological Effects

Analgesic, anodyne, antispasmodic, antitussive, diaphoretic, expectorant, narcotic (mild), nutritive, sedative (mild)

Medicinal Uses

Poppies have been used for their medicinal properties since the time of ancient Mesopotamia. The seeds are a very effective calming agent and also help relax smooth muscles. They are used in the treatment of anxiety, asthma, bronchitis, coughs, diarrhea, insomnia, pneumonia, pleurisy, and tonsillitis.

Topically, the seeds can also be included in salves to soothe dry, itchy skin.

Edible Uses

Poppy seeds are a common culinary seasoning. They are tiny: over one million seeds would be needed to make one pound. The oil extracted from the seeds is used in cooking. The young leaves of the plant are also edible, while the petals of red poppies are used as a coloring for teas, wines, and medicines.

Other Uses

In ancient Greece poppy was dedicated to Nix, goddess of night, to Thanatos, god of death, and his twin brother Hypnos, god of sleep, and to Morpheus, son of Hypnos and god of dreams. The seeds were offered to the dead to assure them a good rest and peaceful sleep. The flower is used on Veterans Day as a symbol of the fallen.

The seeds make good bird food.

Opium is made by scoring the unripe seed capsule and collecting the latex that exudes, which is then roasted and fermented.

In folkloric tradition, poppy seeds are eaten and carried to promote fertility, luck, and prosperity.

Constituents

Calcium, protein, tannin, mucilage, alkaloids (papaverine, rhoeadine, rhoearubine), meconic acid, anthocyanins, essential fatty acids (linoleic acid, oleic acid, linolenic acid), essential oils (aldehydes, aliphatic hydrocarbons), morphine (*P. somniferum*), codeine (*P. somniferum*)

Energetic Correspondences

- Flavor: sour
- Temperature: cool
- Moisture: moist
- Polarity: yin
- Planet: Moon/Saturn
- Element: water

Contraindications

Poppy seed is generally considered safe, though in rare individuals it may cause an allergic reaction.

On occasion the consumption of poppy seed can result in a positive result from urine tests for opiates.

Range and Appearance

Poppy is believed to be native to western Asia, northern Africa, and Europe and is thought to have been among the earliest of cultivated plants. *Papaver rhoeas* and *P. somniferum* are both annuals. They have erect stems bearing pinnate, finely divided leaves and showy flowers with two sepals and four delicate petals. *P. rhoeas* has red flowers with a black spot at the base of each petal, while *P. somniferum* has mauve flowers. The fruits are contained in a capsule. The plant grows in full sun to partial shade, can tolerate cold, and enjoys a rich soil.

PORIA

Botanical Name

Poria cocos (formerly *Sclerotium cocos, Pachyma hoelen*)

Family

Polyporaceae (Polypor Family)

Etymology

In 1822 Swedish mycologist Frederick Adolph Wolf identified this plant as a polypor (mushroom) and gave it the genus name *Poria*. The species name, *cocos*, derives from the Spanish *coco*, "coconut," in reference to shape and size of the fungus. The common name *tuckahoe* is an Algonquin word for plants with edible roots.

Also Known As

Cantonese: fook leng
English: China root, hoelen, Indian bread, tuckahoe
Japanese: bukuryo
Korean: pongnyông
Mandarin: fú líng

Part Used

Entire plant (fungus growing underground)

Physiological Effects

Antitumor, cardiotonic, chi tonic, diuretic, expectorant, hypoglycemic, restorative, sedative, tonic

Medicinal Uses

Poria is an important herb in Asian medicine, where it is used to drain dampness in cases of health conditions related to fluid retention. It helps balance potassium and sodium levels in the body and supports the heart, spleen, and kidneys. It is widely used for children. Regular use is said to prolong life, calm the spirit, and quiet the heart. It is used in the treatment of abdominal distention, anxiety, chemotherapy side effects, chronic fatigue syndrome, diarrhea, dyspepsia, edema, fatigue, hair loss (following pregnancy), headache, heart palpitations, hepatitis, hyperactivity, insomnia, nearsightedness, polyuria, stress, tumors, and vertigo.

Edible Uses

Poria is edible and is often soaked or cooked and added to soups and stews.

Other Uses

None known

Constituents

Polysaccharides, beta-pachymanase, tetracyclic triterpenic acid (eburicolic acid), pachymic acid, ergosterol, choline, chitin, lipase, protease, lecithin, fiber (beta-glucans)

Energetic Correspondences

- Flavor: sweet
- Temperature: neutral
- Moisture: moist
- Polarity: yin
- Planet: Moon
- Element: water

Contraindications

Poria has a very low level of toxicity and is generally regarded as safe.

Range and Appearance

This mushroom tends to grow underground on the roots of decaying fig and pine trees. It has a white interior and dark brown exterior.

PRICKLY ASH

Botanical Name

Zanthoxylum americanum (northern prickly ash),
   Z. clava-herculis (southern prickly ash)

Family

Rutaceae (Rue Family)

Etymology

The genus name, *Zanthoxylum*, is derived from the Greek *zanthos* and *xylum,* "yellow wood."

Also Known As

English: angelica tree, Hercules's club, pellitory,
   suterberry, toothache tree, yellow wood
French: clavalier d'Amerique, frene epineux
German: Amerikanische stachelesche, gebholz,
   zahnwehholz
Sanskrit: tambura
Swedish: Amerikanskt pepparträd

Parts Used

Bark (primarily), berry (rarely)

Physiological Effects

Bark: alterative, analgesic, anodyne, anthelmintic, antibacterial, antidiarrheal, anti-inflammatory, anti-rheumatic, antiseptic, antispasmodic, astringent, carminative, chi tonic, circulatory stimulant, diaphoretic, diuretic, emmenagogue, febrifuge, immune stimulant, nervous system stimulant, rubefacient, sialagogue, stimulant, stomachic, tonic
Berry: alterative, antibacterial, antifungal, anti-rheumatic, antiseptic, antispasmodic, carminative, diuretic, sialagogue, stimulant

Medicinal Uses

Prickly ash bark was included in the United States Pharmacopoeia from 1820 to 1926 as a rheumatism remedy; it was used with success to treat the 1849 to 1850 outbreak of Asian cholera in the Midwest. Prickly ash bark generates warmth, improves circulation, breaks up congestion, relieves pain, and restrains infection. It prevents blood platelet aggregation and has a stimulating effect upon the entire body, including the lymphatic system and mucous membranes. In fact, it is as strong a stimulant as cayenne pepper but is slower acting and longer lasting.

Prickly ash bark is used to treat arthritis, cancer, candida, chilblains, chills, cholera, colds, cough, diarrhea, dyspepsia, dysentery, exhaustion, fever, flatulence, gout, lethargy, lumbago, paralysis (including of the mouth and tongue), Raynaud's disease, rheumatism, sickle cell anemia pain, sore throat, tuberculosis, typhoid, typhus, varicose veins, and venereal disease.

The berries promote the dispersal of congestion and are used to treat asthma, diarrhea, paralysis, poor circulation, sore throat, and tonsillitis.

Prickly ash was widely used by Native American peoples as a topical remedy to relieve rheumatism and toothache. The bark can be chewed as an herbal toothbrush or prepared as a mouthwash to prevent tooth decay. It also can be prepared as a poultice to treat back pain, pelvic inflammatory disease, rheumatism, toothache, and wounds or as a lotion to improve circulation.

Edible Uses

The bark and berries are not generally considered

edible. The seeds, however, can be cooked and eaten. In Asian cooking, the berries of a related species, *Zanthoxylum piperitum,* are roasted and called Schezwan or Chinese peppers; they are an ingredient in Chinese five-spice powder.

Other Uses

The fruits can be made into an orange-scented perfume for men that is said to attract love.

Constituents

Malic acid, essential oils (geraniol, limonene, citronellol), xanthoxylin, alkaloids (fagarine, magnoflorine, laurifoline, nitidine, chelerythrine, berberin), tannin, lignan (asarin), coumarins, phenol (xanthoxylin), fat, sugar, gum

Energetic Correspondences

- Flavor: pungent, bitter, sweet
- Temperature: hot (the berry is even more warming than the bark)
- Moisture: dry
- Polarity: yang
- Planet: Mars/Saturn
- Element: fire

Contraindications

Avoid during pregnancy, in cases of stomach or intestinal inflammation, or in conjunction with blood-thinning or blood-pressure medications. Prickly ash can produce a hot, tingling sensation in the mouth and throughout the body that is not cause for alarm.

Range and Appearance

Prickly ash is a shrub native to North America. It requires a well-drained, alkaline soil, moderate moisture, and full sun to partial shade.

Z. *americanum* grows to 10 to 12 feet in height, with alternate branches that have conical paired prickles. The leaves are alternate and pinnate, with five paired leaflets and one odd one; they have a lemonlike aroma when crushed. The greenish yellow flowers appear before the leaves and grow in small dense clusters. The reddish green berries are covered with lemon-scented dots.

Z. *clava-herculis* grow to 40 feet in height. Its bark bears prickles that look like triangular knobs, and the branches have even larger knobs. The greenish flowers also appear before the leaves.

PSYLLIUM

Botanical Name

Plantago arenaria (syn. *P. indica, P. psyllium*), *P. ovata*

Family

Plantaginaceae (Plantain Family)

Etymology

The genus name *Plantago* derives from the Latin *planta,* "sole of the foot," in reference to the broad leaves. The common name *psyllium* derives from the Greek word for flea, *psylla,* in reference to the appearance of the tiny seeds.

Also Known As

English: blonde ispaghula, blond psyllium, desert Indian wheat, flea seeds, Indian plantain, ispaghul plantain, spogel
French: graines de psyllium, plantain de l'Inde
German: indischer flohsamen, ispaghula
Hindi: ispaghula
Italian: psillio
Japanese: shazenshi
Korean: ch'ajônja
Mandarin: che qían zi
Sanskrit: snigdha-jira
Spanish: semilla de plantago
Thai: thian klet hoi

Parts Used

Seed, outer husk of seed

Physiological Effects

Aperient, demulcent, emollient, laxative

Medicinal Uses

Psyllium is valued for its mucilaginous and laxative properties. It absorbs up to ten times its weight in water. Its fibrous qualities makes it an excellent laxative, but it also provides intestinal bulk, which can stop diarrhea. Because the seeds tend to swell and create a feeling of fullness, they can help curb appetite. Psyllium is used in the treatment of acid indigestion, autointoxication, colitis (ulcerative), constipation, Crohn's disease, diabetes, diarrhea, dysentery, hemorrhoids, high cholesterol, irritable bowel syndrome, obesity, and ulcers.

Topically, psyllium can be prepared as a poultice to draw out infection, relieve toothache; it is used to treat abscesses, boils, skin irritation, and whitlows. It can also be prepared as a soothing eyewash. It is sometimes used as a binder for other herbs in poultices.

Edible Uses

The seeds and young leaves are edible. The seeds are usually ground before consumption.

Other Uses

Psyllium can be prepared as an emollient facial mask.

Constituents

Mucilage (arabinoxylan), aucubine, protein, enzymes, xylose, galactose, fatty acids (linoleic acid, oleic acid, palmitic acid), starch, fiber

Energetic Correspondences

- Flavor: sweet
- Temperature: neutral
- Moisture: moist
- Polarity: yin
- Planet: Moon
- Element: water

Contraindications

Psyllium can dilute digestive enzymes and is best taken between meals, especially before bed or first thing upon rising, rather than with food. Always drink plenty of water when using psyllium, or else it can cause, rather than relieve, constipation.

Range and Appearance

Psyllium is an annual herb native to western Asia, northern Africa, and Europe. It grows from 12 to 18 inches tall. The opposite leaves are linear or lanceolate-linear. The numerous flowers are small and white. The seeds are enclosed in capsules. The plant prefers cool, dry conditions with plenty of sunlight and well-drained, sandy loam.

RASPBERRY

Botanical Name

Rubus spp.

Family

Rosaceae (Rose Family)

Etymology

The genus name *Rubus* is Latin for "blackberry" or "bramble."

Also Known As

Danish: hindebar
Dutch: braamboss
English: bramble, hindberry
Finnish: vaapukka, vadelma, vattu
French: framboisier
German: himbeere
Italian: lampine, lampone
Japanese: ezopichigo, fukubonshi, razuberi
Korean: pokpunja
Sanskrit: gauriphal
Spanish: frambuesa, frambuesa roja
Swedish: hallon, skohshallonrosmarin

Part Used

Leaf

Raspberry Fruit

Although the fruit is not usually used medicinally, in addition to being a wonderful fruit it has many therapeutic effects on the body, with antacid, antioxidant, antiviral, aphrodisiac (when unripe), laxative (mild), parturient, and refrigerant properties.

Physiological Effects

Adrenal tonic, alterative, antacid, antiabortifacient, antiemetic, anti-inflammatory, antiseptic, antispasmodic, astringent, cardiotonic, digestive, hemostatic, hormone tonic, hypotensive, immune tonic, liver tonic, kidney tonic, mucous membrane tonic, nutritive, ophthalmic, oxytoxic, parturient, phytoestrogenic, postpartum tonic, prostate tonic, stimulant, stomachic, uterine tonic, yin tonic

Medicinal Uses

There are many, many species in the *Rubus* genus, including blackberry (see page 51), but most herbalists agree that all red raspberry plants share common uses, detailed here.

Raspberry leaf is considered a supreme tonic for pregnant women because it can tonify the uterus, nourish the mother and the growing baby, prevent miscarriage and false labor, and facilitate birth and placental delivery. When used after birthing, it can decrease uterine swelling and minimize postpartum hemorrhaging as well as increase the colostrum in the mother's milk. It also reduces inflammation and excess dampness. Its nourishing mineral content and ability to support the reproductive and nervous systems can even be of benefit in encouraging healing from sexual trauma and abuse. And though it is often regarded as an herb for women, raspberry leaf is also nourishing for men.

Raspberry leaf is used in the treatment of anemia, diarrhea (even in infants), dysentery, dysmenorrhea, hemorrhage, herpes, incontinence, infertility, laryngitis, muscle cramps, miscarriage (threat of), menorrhagia, morning sickness, mumps, nausea, overactive bladder, ovulation difficulty, prolapse of the uterus or anus, rheumatism, sore throat, stomachache, thrush, and weak vision.

Topically, raspberry leaf can be used as a mouthwash to treat canker sores, gingivitis, sore throat, and tonsillitis; as a wash or poultice to treat burns, varicosities, and wounds; as a douche to treat leukorrhea or organ prolapse; as an eyewash to reduce discharge and inflammation in the eyes; or in lotions, toners, or masks to tone and soothe oily or inflamed skin.

As a flower essence, raspberry helps release resentment, bitterness, and old emotional wounds. It helps users become more responsible for their actions.

Edible Uses

Raspberry leaf is not generally considered edible, aside from as tea, though the flowers and, of course, the fruits are edible. The fruits have less sugar than many other fruits and can be eaten raw or cooked. The young shoots can be peeled and eaten raw or cooked, like asparagus.

Raspberry leaf tea has a robust, astringent, mildly bitter flavor similar to that of green or black tea, but of course with no caffeine.

Other Uses

Raspberry leaf tea can be used as a hair rinse to condition and highlight dark hair. The leaf is sometimes included in smoking mixtures. The fruit can be made into a bluish dye. The stems yield a fiber that can be used to make paper.

Constituents

Vitamin B_1, vitamin E, calcium chloride, iron citrate, magnesium, manganese, potassium, phosphorous, potassium, selenium, sulfur, flavonoids, pectin, alkaloid (fragarine), organic acids (citric, malic, gallic, ellagic), furanones, tannins

Energetic Correspondences

- Flavor: bitter
- Temperature: neutral
- Moisture: dry
- Polarity: yin
- Planet: Venus/Mars/Jupiter
- Element: water

Contraindications

There are no known toxic levels. Once nursing is established, excess consumption of raspberry leaf should be avoided, as its astringent properties could lessen the amount of breast milk.

Range and Appearance

Raspberry bushes are native to Eurasia and North

America and can be found growing in the wild in woodland clearings, along roadsides, and in neglected fields where the soil is rich in nutrients. These biennial or perennial plants grow from 3 to 6 feet in height. The stems are bristly and thorned. The pinnately divided leaves are green on their tops and gray and velvety underneath. The small, white, roselike flowers bloom in early spring and summer; the compound fruits follow.

Raspberry bushes are easy to cultivate, and there are many guides to growing them. They prefer full sun but will tolerate partial shade and require moderate amounts of water.

RED CLOVER

Botanical Name

Trifolium pratense

Family

Fabaceae (Pea Family)

Etymology

The genus name *Trifolium* is Latin for "three leaved." The species name *pratense* is Latin for "found in the meadows." The common name *clover* derives from the Old English name for this plant, *clava*.

Also Known As

English: cow clover, honeystalks, marl grass,
   meadow honeysuckle, meadow trefoil, purple
   clover, shamrock, three-leaves grass, trefoil, trifoil
Finnish: puna-apila
French: triolet
German: rose klaver, rotklee
Italian: moscino, trifoglio dei prati
Sanskrit: trepatra
Spanish: trebol rojo
Swedish: rödklöver

Parts Used

Flower, leaf (young)

Physiological Effects

Alterative, antibacterial, anti-inflammatory, anti-spasmodic, antiseptic, antispasmodic, antitumor, antitussive, aperient, cardiotonic, deobstruent, depurative, diuretic, expectorant, galactagogue, nutritive, phytoestrogenic, sedative, vulnerary

Medicinal Uses

This blood-purifying plant has a special affinity for the skin, throat, lungs, and salivary glands. Red clover cleanses and clears toxins, nourishes and moves the blood, stimulates lymphatic movement, reduces swelling and inflammation, reduces respiratory irritation, and promotes tissue repair. It contains an isoflavone, biochanin, that exhibits anticancer properties, and it is helpful in supporting all the organs of elimination, expelling phlegm from the lungs, and improving health in general.

Red clover is used in the treatment of acne, arthritis, asthma, boils, blood clots, bronchitis, cancer (breast, lymphatic, or ovarian), chorea, cough, cystitis, cysts, diarrhea, dysentery, eczema, gout, heavy metal toxicity, hepatitis, infertility, laryngitis, leprosy, mastitis, measles, menopause symptoms (hot flashes, decrease in bone density), menstrual cramps, mononucleosis, phlebitis, phlegm, psoriasis, salivary gland congestion, scrofula, skin inflammation, syphilis, tuberculosis, tumors, ulcers, wheezing, and whooping cough.

Topically, red clover can be used as a compress, poultice, or bath herb in the treatment of athlete's foot, arthritic pain, burns, cancers, eczema, gout, insect bites, lymphatic swelling, psoriasis, tumors, and wounds. It can be prepared as eyewash for conjunctivitis, as a gargle for sore throat, as a douche for vaginitis, or as an enema for bowel inflammation.

As a flower essence, red clover helps users remain calm in the face of fear. It is soothing and calming and clears negativity that may have been taken from others.

Edible Uses

The young flowers are edible raw in small amounts. Mature flowers, leaves, and roots can be eaten when cooked; cooking makes them easier to digest and less likely to cause bloating. The seeds can be sprouted and eaten.

Red clover has a sweet, pleasant, honeylike flavor. Because it has a high mineral content, many vegan mothers give red clover tea to their children instead of milk.

Other Uses

Red clover is an important fodder plant for grazing animals and, because it fixes nitrogen, can be planted as a green manure. A yellow dye can be made from the flowers. In folkloric tradition, red clover is worn to promote prosperity, love, fidelity, and protection; eating a four-leafed clover with a lover is said to result in mutual love.

Constituents

Protein, beta-carotene, B-complex vitamins, vitamin C, calcium, chromium, copper, iron, magnesium, manganese, selenium, silicon, flavonoids, phenolic glycosides (salicylic acid), essential oil (methyl salicylate), polysaccharides, isoflavones (sitosterol, genistein, biochanin, formononetin, daidzein), salicylates, coumarins, cyanogenic glycosides

Energetic Correspondences

- Flavor: sweet, salty
- Temperature: cool
- Moisture: moist
- Polarity: yin
- Planet: Venus/Mercury
- Element: earth/water/fire/air

Contraindications

Red clover is not recommended for use during pregnancy, though it can be used prior to pregnancy as a fertility tonic. Avoid red clover for at least a week prior to surgery.

Range and Appearance

Red clover is a biennial or perennial native to Eurasia, northern Africa, and North America but widely naturalized elsewhere. It features several hairy stems rising from its root and can grow to 2 feet in height. It bears three oval leaflets; a pale V shape often appears in the middle of each leaf. The flowers are pink to red and occur in sessile spikes or heads. The hermaphroditic flowers are pale pink to dark reddish purple in color. Before being pollinated they stand erect; after having been pollinated by a bee, they turn down to indicate that such attentions are no longer needed. Red clover is prevalent in the wild and can be found growing in grassy areas ranging from lawns to roadsides. It prefers full sun to partial shade and moderate amounts of water and thrives in a wide variety of soils.

If wildcrafting, do not collect red clover in autumn, when they may have developed potentially toxic molds.

REDROOT

Botanical Name

Ceanothus americanus

Family

Rhamnaceae (Buckthorn Family)

Etymology

The genus name, *Ceanothus*, derives from the Greek *keanthos*, "spiny plant." The species name, *americanus*, refers to the plant being native to North America. The common name *redroot* refers to the red dye that the root yields.

Also Known As

English: bobea, mountainsweet, New Jersey tea, Walpole tea, wild snowball
French: céanothe
German: säckelblume
Italian: ceanoto
Turkish: zeres cayt

Parts Used

Root, root bark, leaf

Physiological Effects

Antispasmodic, astringent, expectorant, hemostatic, hypotensive, sedative

Medicinal Uses

It is excellent for encouraging the body to get rid of

catabolic waste buildup and to break up tumors and engorgements in the body. It also appears to improve blood coagulation. It is used in the treatment of asthma, bronchitis, catarrh, coughs, cysts, diarrhea, dysentery, fever, hemorrhoids, Hodgkin's disease, hypertension, lymphatic congestion, menorrhagia, nosebleed, Rocky Mountain spotted fever, sore throat, spleen enlargement, syphilis, tonsillitis, tuberculosis, tumors, ulcers (bleeding), and whooping cough.

Several Native American tribes traditionally use redroot as a poultice to treat skin cancers and lesions caused by venereal disease. It is also effective as a mouthwash and gargle to treat oral infections such as sore throat and tonsillitis.

As a flower essence redroot is helpful for those who feel guilty because they do not suffer as much as those around them. It also helps those who are over-influenced by superstition by helping them to have clearer perceptions and releases unnecessary entanglements with other people.

Edible Uses

Not generally considered edible.

Other Uses

The root yields a reddish dye, while the flowers yield a blue or green dye. All parts of the plant contain high levels of saponins; the flowers contain enough to be used to make soap. Redroot also fixes nitrogen and can be planted as a green manure.

Constituents

Emmolic acid, malic acid, oxalic acid, pyrophosphoric acid, resin, tannin, saponins

Energetic Correspondences

- Flavor: bitter
- Temperature: cool
- Moisture: dry
- Polarity: yin
- Planet: Saturn
- Element: earth

Contraindications

Redroot is considered very safe. It is mild enough to be used for extended periods of time.

Range and Appearance

Redroot is a small deciduous shrub native to eastern and central North America. It grows in dry woodland areas in well-drained soil and full sun to partial shade. Its reddish root is covered with a reddish or brownish bark and can reach up to 4 feet in length. The leaves are ovate or obovate, finely serrated, and dull green on top, with fine hairs on the bottom. The hermaphroditic flowers are small and white and occur in long, stalked clusters at the ends of the branches.

REHMANNIA

Botanical Name

Rehmannia glutinosa

Family

Scrophulariaceae (Foxglove Family)

Etymology

The genus name, *Rehmannia*, was given in honor of German physician Joseph Rehmann (1753–1831). The species name, *glutinosa*, is Latin for "very sticky."

Also Known As

English: Chinese foxglove
Japanese: jukujio (cooked), shojio (raw)
Korean: saenjihwang (raw), sukchihwang (cooked)
Mandarin: sheng dì húang (raw), shú dì húang (cooked)

Parts Used

Root

Physiological Effects

Alterative, antibacterial, anti-inflammatory, antiscorbutic, antiseptic, blood tonic (when cooked), cardiotonic, demulcent, diuretic, febrifuge (when raw), hemostatic (when cooked), hypertensive, hypoglycemic, kidney tonic (when cooked), laxative (when cooked), liver tonic (when raw), rejuvenative, yin tonic

Medicinal Uses

Traditional Asian medicine draws a distinction between the properties of the root when it is raw and when it is cooked. The raw root is used to quiet inflammation and heat. The cooked root is more of a building tonic to correct deficiency; it is used to strengthen the bones, marrow, and tendons, to nourish the eyes and ears, and as a tonic after birthing.

The cooked root is used in the treatment of anemia, diabetes, dysmenorrhea, fatigue, heart palpitations, insomnia, irregular menses, lumbago, menopausal flooding, menorrhagia, muscle weakness, night sweats, postpartum bleeding, spermatorrhea, tuberculosis, and vertigo. The raw root is used in the treatment of hepatitis. Both are used to treat high cholesterol, hypertension, rheumatoid arthritis, and senility and to support convalescence.

Edible Uses

Rehmannia root is edible raw or cooked and has a bittersweet flavor. It is often included in soups.

Other Uses

None known

Constituents

Phytosterols (beta-sitosterol, stigmasterol), glycosides, saponins, sugars (galactose, mannitol, glucose, raffinose), rehmannin, tannin

Energetic Correspondences

- Flavor: sweet, sour, bitter
- Temperature: cool
- Moisture: moist
- Polarity: raw root—yin; cooked root—yang
- Planet: Jupiter
- Element: water

Contraindications

Avoid excessive use in cases of loose stools or a very coated tongue.

Range and Appearance

Rehmannia is a perennial native to eastern Asia that grows in moist, well-drained soil in full sun to partial shade. The stems rise erect from a basal leaf rosette. The leaves are often hairy and can be toothed or lobed. The hermaphroditic flowers range in color from red to purple.

REISHI

Botanical Name

Ganoderma lucidum

Family

Polyporaceae (Polypor Family)

Etymology

The genus name *Ganoderma* derives from the Greek *ganos,* "brightness," and *derma,* "skin." The species name *lucidum* is Latin for "shining." Both refer to the plant's naturally glossy appearance.

Also Known As

Cantonese: ling zhi ("herb of spiritual potency")
English: glossy ganoderma, mushroom of
   immortality, shiny polyporus, varnished conk
French: ganoderme luisant, polypore luisant
German: glänzender lackporling, lackporling
Japanese: reishi
Norwegian: lakk-kjuke

Part Used

Fruiting body

Physiological Effects

Adaptogen, analgesic, antibacterial, anti-inflammatory, antioxidant, antitumor, antitussive, antiviral, cardiotonic, expectorant, hepatoprotective, hypotensive, immune stimulant, rejuvenative

Medicinal Uses

Reishi is considered a longevity herb in Chinese medicine and has been in use in that tradition for more than four thousand years. In the Taoist tradition reishi is said to enhance spiritual receptivity, and it is used by monks to calm the spirit and mind. It is known to normalize blood pressure and blood sugar levels, lower levels of low-density lipoproteins (LDL, or "bad" cholesterol), and inhibit histamine release and blood platelet aggregation. It also activates the phagocytosis of macrophages and stimulates interferon production and activity, thereby supporting the immune system, and inhibits the activity of staphyloccus and streptococcus.

Reishi is used in the treatment of AIDS, allergies, altitude sickness, arthritis, asthma, bronchitis, cancer, depression, diabetes, fatigue, food sensitivities, hemorrhoids, hepatitis, high cholesterol, HIV, hypertension, hypotension, insomnia, nephritis, pneumonia, rheumatoid arthritis, stroke, ulcers, and varicose veins.

Edible Uses

These mushrooms are too hard and woody to eat. They are sometimes made into a tea.

Other Uses

None known

Constituents

Vitamin B$_2$, vitamin C, adenosine, ganoderic acid S, ganoderic acid R, ganesterone, lipids, ash, protein, glucans, polysaccharides, phytosterols, coumarin

Energetic Correspondences

- Flavor: bitter
- Temperature: cool
- Moisture: dry
- Polarity: yin
- Planet: Saturn
- Element: earth

Contraindications

Reishi has a very low potential for toxicity. When pregnant or while nursing, use only under the guidance of a qualified health-care practitioner. Long-term use may cause dry mouth, dizziness, and digestive distress. Because reishi can inhibit blood clotting, it should be avoided at least one week before surgery, before childbirth, or in conjunction with blood-thinning medications.

Range and Appearance

Native to China, reishi is a fungus that grows on decaying hardwood in moist, shady conditions; these days it is more likely to be cultivated than to be found in the wild. Reishi has pores instead of gills. When young it has yellow and white coloring on its surface. The mature fruiting body ranges in color from orangish to black, but the red variety is considered most medicinal.

RHODIOLA

Botanical Name

Rhodiola rosea (syn. *Sedum roseum, Sedum rhodiola*)

Family

Crassulaceae (Stonecrop Family)

Etymology

The former genus name, *Sedum,* may be from *sedere,* Latin for "ground hugging," or perhaps from *sedare,* meaning "calming." The current genus name, *Rhodiola,* derives from the Greek *rhodon,* "red." The species name, *rosea,* derives from the Latin *rosa,* "rose," in reference to the plant's rose-scented roots and flowers.

Also Known As

English: arctic root, arctic rose, golden root, roseroot, sedum
Finnish: pohjanruusujuuri
German: rosenwurz
Italian: rhodiola
Swedish: fjällkaktus

Parts Used

Root

Physiological Effects

Adaptogen, anti-inflammatory, antioxidant, nootropic, stimulant, stomachic, tonic

Medicinal Uses

Rhodiola enhances T-cell immunity and can improve the function of neurotransmitters, including serotonin and dopamine, by inhibiting their destruction by enzymes; it has been found to increase serotonin levels in the brain by up to 30 percent. Rhodiola also increases mental and physical performance; it can shorten recovery time between athletic endeavors, such as workouts, and can improve memory and work productivity. In Siberia it is traditionally given to couples prior to marriage to help them bring forth healthy children.

Rhodiola is used in the treatment of anemia, cancer, colds, depression, erectile dysfunction, fatigue, flu, headache, high cholesterol, hysteria, insomnia, stress, nervous system disorders, pain, premature ejaculation, stress, and tuberculosis.

Edible Uses

The young leaves, shoots, and roots are edible raw. The stems can be cooked as a vegetable.

Other Uses

The roots can be distilled to make a cosmetic floral water.

Constituents

Organic acids (hydroxycinnammic acid), tricin-5-0-glycoside, tricin-7-0-glycoside, flavonoids (kaempherol, rhodiolin, rhodionin, rodiosin, tricin), rosavin, monoterpenes (rosaridin, rosiridol), salidroside, cinnamic alcohol, phenolic acids (hydroxycinnamic acid, gallic acid), beta-sitosterol

Energetic Correspondences

- Flavor: sweet, sour
- Temperature: cool
- Polarity: yin
- Moisture: moist
- Planet: Venus/Mars/Jupiter/Neptune/Pluto
- Element: water

Contraindications

Generally regarded as safe.

Range and Appearance

More than twenty species of *Rhodiola* exist, but according to screenings *R. rosea* is the most active pharmacologically. This perennial succulent grows in the high mountains of Europe, northern Asia, and northern North America. It can reach a height of 2 feet and bears yellow flowers that smell fragrantly like roses, hence the folk name *arctic rose*. The plant is dioecious, meaning that male and female flowers are borne on different plants. It thrives in well-drained soil, can tolerate drought once established, and requires lots of sun.

RHUBARB

Botanical Name

Rheum officinale (Chinese rhubarb), *R. palmatum* (turkey rhubarb)

Family

Polygonaceae (Buckwheat Family)

Etymology

The genus name *Rheum* is believed to derive from the Greek *rheo*, "to flow," in reference to the plant's purgative properties. The common name *rhubarb* is derived from the Latin *rha barbarum*, referring to the Rha River (now known as the Volga) that was inhabited by barbarians (otherwise known as anyone not Roman).

Also Known As

English: chinghai rhubarb, red ornamental rhubarb, Russian rhubarb
Finnish: rohtoraparperi (*R. officinale*)
French: rhubarbe officinale
German: chinesischer rhabarber (*R. officinale*), rhabarber (*R. officinale*)
Japanese: daio
Korean: taehwang
Mandarin: dà húang
Persian: chukri
Portuguese: ruibarbo
Sanskrit: amlavestasa, lakri

Spanish: ruibarbo
Swedish: flikrabarber

Parts Used

Root, rhizome

Physiological Effects

Alterative, anthelmintic, antibiotic, anti-inflamma-tory, antiseptic, antispasmodic, aperient (in small amounts), astringent (in small doses), bitter, chola-gogue, laxative, liver stimulant, purgative, siala-gogue, stomachic, vulnerary

Medicinal Uses

Rhubarb's anthraquinones contribute to the laxative and purgative properties of the herb, yet its tannin content helps balance those effects and even stops diarrhea. Rhubarb increases secretions throughout the digestive tract, assists in the metabolism of fats, and helps cleanse the digestive tract of stored debris. It also clears heat and infection from the body, and Chinese researchers are investigating its potential to inhibit the growth of cancer cells. Rhubarb is used in the treatment amenorrhea, blood clots, constipa-tion (when taken in large amounts), diarrhea (small amounts), dysentery, fever, hemorrhoids, high cho-lesterol, jaundice, and worms (pinworms, thread-worms). It also can be added to tonic wines as a digestive aid.

Topically, rhubarb root can be prepared as a poul-tice or compress to treat boils, burns, canker sores, carbuncles, and wounds.

As a flower essence, rhubarb is beneficial for those who talk too much and have exhibitionist qualities, often being inconsiderate of the boundaries of oth-ers. It helps users feel more whole.

Edible Uses

The stems of *R. officinale* and *R. palatum* are edible raw or cooked, just like those of garden rhubarb (*R. rhabarbarum*), the common eating variety that is one of the few perennial vegetables. The flower pouches that form before the flower opens, as well as the flowers themselves, are also edible.

Other Uses

The fresh root can be used to polish brass, thanks to its acid content.

Constituents

Anthraquinones, chrysophanol, emodin, physcion, sennidine, rheidine, palmmidine, tannins, catechin, gallic acid, rutin, phytosterol, calcium oxalate

Energetic Correspondences

- Flavor: bitter
- Temperature: cold (it is considered one of the coldest in Chinese medicine)
- Moisture: dry
- Polarity: yin
- Planet: Venus/Mars
- Element: earth

Contraindications

Rhubarb root and rhizome are best used under the guidance of a qualified health-care professional. Avoid during pregnancy, while nursing, and during menses. Don't use when the colon is already empty, or rhubarb's astringent properties may cause colon discomfort. Avoid in cases of arthritis, gout, or kid-ney or bladder stones. Use only for short periods.

When using rhubarb root as a laxative, combine it with carminative herbs such as fennel, ginger, or pep-permint to prevent gripe. Rhubarb root and rhizome may temporarily cause urine to appear yellow or red, which is not cause for alarm.

Avoid the leaves, which contain high amounts of oxalic acid and are toxic.

Range and Appearance

Native to China, rhubarb is a perennial plant with erect, hollow, jointed stems that can reach a height of 2 to 3 feet. The leaves are palmate. The white flow-ers grow in panicles on a stalk that can reach up to 10 feet in height. The root is thick and oval in shape and usually brown on the outside and yellowish inside. The plant requires moist soil, a warm climate, and plenty of sunlight.

ROOIBOS

Botanical Name

Aspalathus linearis (syn. *A. contaminatus*)

Family

Fabaceae (Pea Family)

Etymology

The genus name, *Asapalathus,* is a Greek term for heathlike shrubs. The species name, *linearis,* is Latin for "linear." The common name *rooibos* is the Afrikaans name for this plant and translates as "red bush," in reference to the plant's color.

Also Known As

Afrikaans: rooibus

English: Koopman's tea, naald tea, red bush tea, rooibosch, rooitea, rooitee, speld tea

Parts Used

Leaf, stem

Physiological Effects

Adaptogen, anti-inflammatory, antimutagenic, antioxidant, antispasmodic, antiviral, astringent, cardioprotective, carminative, diuretic, rejuvenative, tonic

Medicinal Uses

Rooibos (pronounced *roo-ih-bus*) leaves and stems are chopped and allowed to naturally ferment before they are dried. The dried herb contains over forty polyphenol compounds that exhibit antioxidant effects. It is used in the treatment of allergies (including milk allergy), anemia, asthma, colic, constipation, cramps, depression, diarrhea, eczema, hay fever, headache, hypertension, indigestion, insomnia, memory loss, nausea, nervousness, skin disorders, stomachache, ulcers, and vomiting. It is also considered a preventive for cancer and dental cavities.

Topically, rooibos can be used as a compress to relieve acne, diaper rash, eczema, and other rashes. It contains alpha-hydroxy acid, which promotes healthy skin.

Edible Uses

Rooibos is not generally considered edible, aside from as tea. The tea has a pleasant black-tea-like flavor, with citrusy overtones, yet no caffeine. Though rooibos is more expensive than other herbs, to make a good brew you need only about half as much of it as you would need of other herbs, so it's more economical than it seems. The tea, however, is used to flavor punches, custards, desserts, and sauces as it adds color.

Other Uses

None known

Constituents

Beta-carotene, vitamin C, vitamin E, calcium, copper, fluoride, iron, magnesium, manganese, potassium, sodium, zinc, superoxide dismutase, flavonoids (aspalathin, quercitin, rutin, luteolin, catechin, vitexin), caffeic acid, ferulic acid, polysaccharides (uronic acid), oligosaccharides

Energetic Correspondences

- Flavor: bitter
- Temperature: cool
- Moisture: dry
- Polarity: yin
- Planet: Saturn
- Element: earth

Contraindications

Rooibos is considered safe even for children and those suffering from cardiac and kidney problems.

Range and Appearance

Rooibos grows only in the western region of South Africa's Cape Province, mainly in the Cedar Mountains. It requires light, sandy, well-drained soil, full sun, and moderate water, though it will tolerate drought. It is a small shrub with slender stems. The branches are reddish brown, the leaves long and linear. The yellow flowers look like typical Pea Family flowers and grow in short clusters. The seedpods are downy and lanceolate and contain a tiny, hard, kidney-shaped yellow seed. Under cultivation, rooibos is grown from seed planted during the African winter. After eighteen months the plants are ready to be harvested.

ROSE

Botanical Name

Rosa spp., including *R. canina* (dog rose),
R. x *centifolia* (cabbage rose), *R.* x *damascena* (damask rose), *R. gallica* (red rose), *R. multiflora* (Japanese rose), *R. rubirinova* (rose mosqueta),
R. rubiginosa (syn. *R. eglanteria;* sweet briar),
R. rugosa

Family

Rosaceae (Rose Family)

Etymology

The genus name *Rosa,* from which the common name derives, is the Latin term for "red."

Also Known As

Arabic: ward
Armenian: vard, vart
Bulgarian: roza
Cantonese: muih gwai
Czech: ruze
Dutch: roos
English: queen of flowers
Esperanto: rozo
Estonian: roos
Finnish: ruusu
Greek: triantafillo
Hebrew: vered
Hindi: gulab
Hungarian: rózsa
Icelandic: rós
Indonesian: mawar
Italian: rosa
Japanese: rozu
Korean: roju
Mandarin: mei gwai
Nepali: gulaf

Polish: róza
Portuguese: rosa
Romanian: trandafir
Russian: roza
Sanskrit: shatapatra
Serbian: ruza
Spanish: rosa
Swahili: waridi
Swedish: ros
Thai: kulaap-on
Turkish: gülü
Vietnamese: hoa hu'ò'ng
Yiddish: royz

Parts Used

Flower, hip, seed, root

Physiological Effects

Flower: anodyne, antibacterial, antidepressant, antifungal, anti-inflammatory, antiseptic, antispasmodic, antiviral, aphrodisiac, aromatic, astringent, blood tonic, cardiotonic, carminative, decongestant, diuretic, emmenagogue, expectorant, hemostatic, hepatic, kidney tonic, laxative, refrigerant, sedative
Hip: antibacterial, anti-inflammatory, antimutagenic, antioxidant, antiviral, astringent, blood tonic, cardiotonic, digestive, diuretic (mild), emmenagogue, kidney tonic, laxative, nutritive, stimulant, tonic
Seed: diuretic, laxative
Root: astringent, carminative

Medicinal Uses

Rose flowers break up congestion, dry mucus, stop bleeding, clear heat, calm the heart, enhance positive emotions, regulate the menstrual cycles, and promote bile flow. It is used in the treatment of anger, anxiety, colic, depression, diarrhea, erectile dysfunction, hemorrhage, hepatitis, irregular menses, and leukorrhea.

Rose hips are rich in flavonoids that help strengthen the capillaries of the body. They also improve the body's assimilation of vitamin C. They are used in the treatment of atherosclerosis, bedwetting, bruising (as a chronic condition), cancer, colds, cough, diarrhea, exhaustion, flu, gingivitis, hemorrhoids, high cholesterol, hypertension, night sweats, overactive bladder, spermatorrhea, urinary tract infection, and varicose veins.

Rose flowers are a supreme bath herb, being aromatherapeutic, aphrodisiac, and great for the skin; they also are excellent in facial steams. Rose water, prepared from the flowers, can be applied topically to treat bruises, dry skin, muscle soreness, and sprains and prepared as a compress to soothe sore eyes and treat conjunctivitis.

Rose seeds are used primarily for their rich oil, which is often included in skin- and hair-care products for its softening, moisturizing properties.

Rose roots can be used topically in compresses to reduce inflammation. They also can be prepared as a gargle to soothe sore throat.

As a flower essence, rose dispels shame about sexuality and helps users fulfill their true desire and open their emotional heart.

Edible Uses

Rose petals (with the bitter whitish heel removed) can be eaten raw or as tea. They have a delicate, astringent, sweet, bitter, flowery flavor, sometimes described as that of scented rainwater, when made into tea; red roses tend to be more astringent than white ones. Rose water, prepared from the flowers, is also edible and is commonly added to desserts.

Rose hips can be eaten raw or cooked. During World War II, they were an important source of vitamin C in England. Rose hip tea, long a staple in Scandinavia, has a tart, fruity, sour, sweet flavor. Prepare the tea as an infusion; boiling the rose hips will dissipate their vitamin C content.

The young leaves and shoots are also edible, raw or cooked, if collected in the spring when they are still tender.

Other Uses

Roses are a universal symbol of beauty and love and have long been associated with the Virgin Mary. White roses symbolize an innocent love, while red roses symbolize passionate love, pink roses simple and happy love, and yellow roses friendship.

Rose hips yield an orange dye. The hips and flowers are sometimes added to potpourri and sachets for their aroma and color. The essential oil of the flower is used as a beautiful and costly perfume. Rose flowers and the oil extracted from the seeds are often included in cosmetics to soften and smooth the skin.

Constituents

Flower: malic acid, tartaric acid, quercetin, essential oils (eugenol, geraniol, citronellol, geraniol, nerol, terpenes)

Hip: carotenes, vitamins B_1 and B_2, vitamin C, vitamin E, vitamin K, flavonoids, calcium, iron, magnesium, manganese, phosphorous, potassium, selenium, silicon, sulfur, zinc, polyphenols, tannin, malic acid, pectin, vanillin

Seed: vitamin E, fatty acids (palmitic acid, stearic acid, oleic acid, linoleic acid, linolenic acid, arachidic acid)

Energetic Correspondences

- Flavor: flower—bitter, sweet; hip—sweet, sour; seed, root—bitter
- Planet: flower—Venus; hip, seed—Mars; root—Venus/Mars
- Temperature: flower, seed, root—cool (white flowers are more cooling than red ones); hip—warm
- Moisture: flower, seed—moist; hip—dry; root—dry
- Polarity: flower, seed, root—yin; hip—yang
- Element: flower, seed—water; hip—fire; root—earth

Contraindications

As with all herbs, avoid using rose flowers or hips that have been sprayed with toxic chemicals. Remove the irritating hairs from the seeds, found in the hips, before eating them; when making a tea from them, use a strainer to filter out the fine hairs.

Range and Appearance

There are at least ten thousand varieties of roses, and they are cultivated worldwide. These thorny woody shrubs or vines have flowers in varying colors and sizes. The hips are actually accessory fruits; they are ovoid, swollen looking, and red or orange in color. Roses bloom best in full sun to partial shade. They prefer well-drained, claylike soil. They need frequent watering but do not like to be standing in water.

If you've collected rose hips yourself, remove their seeds before drying them or brewing them as tea.

ROSEMARY

Botanical Name

Rosmarinus officinalis

Family

Lamiaceae (Mint Family)

Etymology

The genus and common name derive from the Latin *ros,* "dew," and *marinus,* "of the sea," in reference to the origins of the plant on the Mediterranean coast.

Also Known As

Arabic: ikleel al-jabal
Armenian: khngooni
Bulgarian: rozmarin
Cantonese: maih diht heung
Croatian: ruzmarin
Czech: rozmaryn lékarsky
Danish: rosmarin
Dutch: rosemarijn
English: old man, Our Lady's rose, sea dew
Esperanto: rosmareno
Estonian: rosmariin
Finnish: rosmariini
French: romarin, rosmarin
German: rosmarin
Greek: rozmari
Hebrew: rosmarin
Hungarian: rozmaring
Icelandic: rósmarín
Italian: ramerino, rosmarino
Lithuanian: rozmarinas
Mandarin: mi die xiang
Norwegian: rosmarin

Polish: rozmaryn
Portuguese: alacrim
Romanian: rozmarin
Russian: rozmarin
Sanskrit: rusmari
Serbian: ruzmarin
Spanish: romero, rosmario
Swedish: rosmarin
Thai: rosmari
Turkish: biberiye, hasalban
Ukrainian: rozmaryn
Vietnamese: lá hu'o'ng thao
Yiddish: rozmarin

Part Used

Aboveground plant

Physiological Effects

Anodyne, antibacterial, antidepressant, antifungal, anti-inflammatory, antimutagenic, antioxidant, antiseptic, antispasmodic, aromatic, astringent, bitter, cardiotonic, carminative, cephalic, cholagogue, choleretic, circulatory stimulant, diaphoretic, digestive, diuretic, emmenagogue, hypertensive, nervine, ophthalmic, rejuvenative, rubefacient, stimulant, stomachic, yang tonic

Medicinal Uses

Rosemary tonifies the nervous system, improves peripheral circulation, promotes warmth, invigorates the lungs, curbs infection, promotes immunity, and uplifts the spirits. Because it improves digestion, circulation, and memory, it is an excellent herb for the elderly. It is used in the treatment of Alzheimer's disease, amenorrhea, anxiety, asthma, bronchitis, cancer, cataracts, cellulite, colds, debility, delayed menses, depression, dyspepsia, epilepsy, fatigue, flatulence, gallstones, halitosis, headache, hypertension, hypotension, jaundice, memory loss, menstrual cramps, migraine, pain, palsy, poor circulation, poor vision, rheumatism, stress, and vertigo. It is also considered a cancer preventive.

Topically, rosemary can be used as a rejuvenative skin wash to prevent wrinkles and strengthen the capillaries or as a compress in cases of bruises, eczema, sprains, and rheumatism. In the bath or footbath, it rejuvenates the body and mind and also helps relieve pain and sore muscles. As a gargle, it can be used to treat sore throat, gum ailments, and canker sores and to freshen the breath. It makes a stimulating eyewash to soothe tired eyes. When included in shampoos and hair rinses, rosemary deters dandruff, graying, and hair loss.

As a flower essence, rosemary encourages users to be less forgetful and more aware, more present in their body, and more conscious. It strengthens the heart and mind and helps users receive strength from their loved ones.

Edible Uses

The young shoots, leaves, and flowers are all edible raw or cooked. They have a refreshing, pleasant, somewhat bitter-pungent piney flavor. When eaten with food they aid the digestion of fats and starches. Rosemary also has been found to be an effective food preservative, comparable with BHA and BHT.

Other Uses

Rosemary has long been considered a symbol of friendship, loyalty, and remembrance. Ancient Greek scholars would wear laurels of rosemary on their heads to help them stay sharp and to keep their memories clear when taking examinations. In some traditions brides wear a wreath of rosemary and carry it in their bridal bouquet as a symbol of their remembrance of their families and their marriage vows.

Rosemary's antiseptic aroma repels many kinds of insects, and it is one of the most traditional of incenses and sachet ingeredients. It can be placed in books to deter moths. It also can be burned in sick rooms to refresh and purify the air. The essential oil is widely used in massage oils, baths, and room sprays. A yellow-green dye can be obtained from the flowers and leaves.

Constituents

Beta-carotene, vitamin C, calcium, iron, magnesium, phosphorous, potassium, zinc, essential oils (borneol, camphor, cineole, eucalyptol, linalol, pinene, thy-mol, verbenol), tannins, flavonoids (apigenin, diosmin, heterosides, luteolin), rosmarinic acid, rosmaricine, triterpene (ursolic acid, oleanic acid), resin

Energetic Correspondences

- Flavor: pungent, bitter
- Temperature: warm
- Moisture: dry
- Polarity: yang
- Planet: sun
- Element: fire

Contraindications

Avoid therapeutic doses during pregnancy (though using rosemary moderately to season food is safe). Though rosemary is generally considered so safe that it is a common kitchen herb, extremely large doses could cause convulsions and death.

Range and Appearance

Rosemary is native to the Mediterranean region but cultivated worldwide. This small, woody, evergreen shrub can reach 3 to 6 feet in height. The small, thin leaves are about 1 inch long, dark green, thick, leathery, and lanceolate. The small, two-lipped flowers are whitish, blue, or purple.

This tender perennial grows best in full sun. It prefers well-drained soil and low to moderate amounts of water, though it can tolerate drought.

RUE

Botanical Name

Ruta chalepensis, R. graveolens

Family

Rutaceae (Citrus Family)

Etymology

The common name *rue* and the genus name *Ruta* derive from the Greek *reuo,* "to set free," in reference to the use of the plant to make one free of disease. The species name, *graveolens,* is Latin for "heavy scented." Branches of rue have been used to sprinkle holy water before High Masses, hence the common name *herb of grace.*

Also Known As

Afrikaans: binnewortel, wynruit
Arabic: sadab, taena
Bulgarian: sedefche
Cantonese: chau chóu
Croatian: ruta
Czech: routa
Danish: rude
Dutch: wijnruit
English: garden rue, herb of grace, herb of
  repentance, herby grass, mother of herbs
Estonian: ruud
Finnish: ruuta
French: herbe à la belle fille, herbe de grace,
  peganion, rue des jardins, rue domestique,
  rue fetide, rue odorante
German: braunminze, gartenraute, hexenkraut,
  raute, weinraute
Greek: peganon, rhyte
Hebrew: pegam, ruta
Hindi: satari
Hungarian: ruta
Icelandic: rúturunni
Italian: ruta
Japanese: henruda, ru
Korean: ru, ruta
Mandarin: chòu cao, yun-hsiang-ts'au
Norwegian: vinrute
Polish: ruta zwyczajna
Portuguese: arruda
Romanian: ruta
Russian: ruta dushistaya
Sanskrit: sadapaha
Serbian: ruta
Spanish: lota, lula, lura, luta, ruda, ruta
Swedish: vinruta
Thai: ru
Vietnamese: cuu ly huong
Yiddish: rute

Part Used

Aboveground plant

Physiological Effects

Abortifacient, anthelmintic, antiseptic, antispasmodic, antitussive, aperient, aromatic, bitter, carminative, cholagogue, circulatory stimulant, diaphoretic, emmenagogue, rubefacient, sedative, stimulant, stomachic

Medicinal Uses

In ancient Greece rue was an ingredient in mithridate, an antidote to a wide range of poisons. During the Middle Ages it was considered to protect one against evil; later, in the fourteenth century, it was an ingredient in Four Thieves Vinegar, a brew thought to prevent bubonic plague. Painters, engravers, and sculptors of the Renaissance, including Michelangelo and da Vinci, ate rue in the belief it would improve their vision.

Today, rue is known to increase circulation to the uterus, lungs, intestines, and stomach and to calm the nerves, ease spasms, and reduce pain. It is used to treat amenorrhea, Bell's palsy, colic, coughs (spasmodic), delayed labor, earache, epilepsy, headache, hypertension, hysteria, menstrual cramps, and multiple sclerosis. It is also used to get rid of parasites.

Thanks to its rutin content, rue can be used topically to strengthen weak capillaries. It can be prepared as an eyewash to soothe tired eyes or as a compress or poultice to treat gout, headache, joint soreness, sciatica, tendonitis, and wounds. It also can be prepared as a gargle to relieve sore throat, as a douche to treat leukorrhea, or as an oil to treat ear infection (as ear drops) or rheumatism (as a massage oil). The fresh leaves can be applied to the head as a headache remedy.

Edible Uses

Rue is edible but should not be ingested in large amounts. It has a bitter, pungent flavor and has been used as a seasoning since ancient Roman times. It is an ingredient in *grappa con ruta,* vermouth, and other alcoholic beverages.

Other Uses

Rue was a strewing herb during the Middle Ages, partly due to its ability to repel insects. Its essential oil is sometimes used in the manufacture of perfume, soaps, and lotions.

Constituents

Choline, iron, flavonoids (rutin, quercitin), pectin, essential oils (limonene, pinene, anisic acid, phenol, methylnonylketone, terpenes), hypericin, furanocoumarins (bergapten, psoralen, xanthotoxin), alkaloids (arborine, fagarine, graveoline), tannin

Energetic Correspondences

- Flavor: bitter, pungent
- Temperature: warm
- Moisture: dry
- Polarity: yang
- Planet: Mars/Sun/Saturn
- Element: fire

Contraindications

Use rue only in small doses, and take no more than one dose daily. Do not take immediately after a meal, as it may have an emetic effect. Large doses may cause photosensitivity. Avoid during pregnancy, while nursing, or in conjunction with blood-thinning medications. Although rue has abortifacient properties it is not recommended for them, as it can be very toxic and can cause vomiting, violent pain, and cerebral disturbances. The sap of the stem may cause contact dermatitis.

Do not confuse this plant with garden rue (*Galega officinalis*), which is a different plant in a different family.

Range and Appearance

Rue is a small evergreen shrub, native to eastern Europe and the Mediterranean, that grows from 2 to 3 feet tall. The blue-green leaves are compound and bi- or tripinnate. The tiny yellowish green flowers, borne in clusters, each have five wavy petals. Rue grows best in full sun and well-drained soil and requires low to moderate amounts of water.

SAFFLOWER

Botanical Name

Carthamus tinctorius

Family

Asteraceae (Daisy Family)

Etymology

The genus name *Carthamus* derives from the Arabic *kurthum*, "to dye." The species name *tinctorius* derives from the Latin *tinctura*, "dyeing." Both refer to this plant being used in dyeing. The common name *safflower* derives from the ancient Arabic name for this plant, 'asfar.

Also Known As

Arabic: asfour
Bulgarian: saflor
Cantonese: hong fa
Danish: safflor
Dutch: saffloer
English: bastard saffron, dyer's saffron, false saffron, parrot plant
Esperanto: tinktura kartamo
Finnish: saflori
French: carthame
German: saflor
Greek: knikos
Hebrew: kurtam
Hindi: kusam
Hungarian: pórsáfrány
Icelandic: litunarkollur
Italian: cartamo
Japanese: benibana, koka
Korean: honghwa
Mandarin: chuan hong hua, hong hua, huuang lan hua
Norwegian: saflor
Polish: krokosz barwierski
Portuguese: cártamo
Russian: saflor
Sanskrit: kusumbha
Serbian: bodalj

Spanish: cártamo
Swedish: safflor
Thai: kham nhong
Turkish: aspur, kartam, kirsafram
Vietnamese: cay rum
Yiddish: zeyfblum

Part Used

Flower (primarily), seed (rarely)

Physiological Effects

Flower: alterative, analgesic, antibacterial, anticoagulant, anti-inflammatory, antispasmodic, antitumor, antiviral, carminative, circulatory stimulant, diaphoretic (mild), diuretic, emmenagogue, febrifuge, laxative, parturient, purgative, sudorific, vasodilator, vermifuge, vulnerary
Seed: diuretic, purgative

Medicinal Uses

Safflower was widely used in ancient Chinese, Ayurvedic, and Greek medicine. The flower stimulates interferon production, improves coronary and cerebral microcirculation, and breaks up blood stagnation. It also relaxes and stimulates the uterus. It is used in the treatment of amenorrhea, arteriosclerosis, blood clots, coronary heart disease, constipation, delayed menses, fever, high cholesterol, hysteria, measles, miscarriage (incomplete), seizures, and tumors, and it can be a beneficial component of postsurgical care.

Topically, safflower flowers and the oil extracted from the seeds stimulate tissue regeneration, and they can be prepared as a liniment to treat bruises, inflammation, sprains, and wounds.

Edible Uses

The flower petals and seeds are edible, as are the young shoots and leaves. The oil from the seeds is a popular cooking oil; it is mild in flavor and rich in polyunsaturated fatty acids.

The flowers can be used as a food coloring and are sometimes used as a cheaper substitute or adulterant for saffron. The Hopi Indians, for example, use it to color bread.

Other Uses

Safflower can be used as a dye; it has been used to redden cosmetics such as rouge and to make a yellow and red dye for fabric. Egyptians often colored linens used to wrap mummies with safflower. The dried flowers are sometimes included in potpourri.

The oil extracted from the seeds is used for massage and is also an ingredient in hair-growth preparations in Asia. It can be made into paint, varnish, linoleum, and diesel fuel.

Constituents

Flavonoids, vitamin E, lignans, polysaccharides, arachic acid, linoleic acid, linolenic acid, palmitic acid, stearic acid

Energetic Correspondences

- Flavor: pungent, bitter
- Temperature: warm
- Moisture: moist
- Polarity: yang
- Planet: Sun/Saturn
- Element: fire

Contraindications

Avoid the flowers during pregnancy. The seeds should also be avoided; however, the purified seed oil is regarded as safe. Safflower is contraindicated in cases of peptic ulcer or hemorrhagic disorders.

Range and Appearance

Native to western Asia but widely cultivated, safflower can be an annual or biennial. It can grow to 3 feet tall and has a whitish stem. The leaves are narrowly ovate and alternate; they have spine-tipped teeth and clasp the stem. The plant bears terminal, hermaphroditic, tubular orange blossoms. It can thrive in poor soil and full sun in dry or moist conditions and even will tolerate drought.

SAFFRON

Botanical Name

Crocus sativus

Family

Iridaceae (Iris Family)

Etymology

The genus name *Crocus* derives from the Greek *krokos*, "thread," in reference to the plant's stigmas. The species name *sativus* is a Latin term denoting the plant's long history of cultivation. The common name *saffron* derives from the Arabic name for the spice of the same name, *za'faran*.

Also Known As

Arabic: azzafaran, saffer, zafraan
Armenian: kerkum
Bulgarian: shafran
Cantonese: faan huhng faa
Croatian: vrtni safrán
Czech: safrán
Danish: safran
Dutch: saffraan
English: Asian saffron, Bulgarian saffron, Greek saffron, saffron crocus, Spanish saffron, true saffron
Esperanto: safrano
Estonian: krookus
Farsi: za'afaran
Finnish: sahrami
French: safran
German: krokus, safran
Greek: safran
Hebrew: karcom
Hindi: zafraan
Icelandic: saffron
Indonesian: sapran
Italian: zafferano
Mandarin: fan hong hua
Japanese: safuran
Korean: sapuran
Norwegian: safran
Polish: krokus uprawny, szafran

Portuguese: açafrão
Romanian: sofran
Russian: shafran
Sanskrit: kumkuma
Serbian: safran
Spanish: azafrán, azafrano
Swahili: zafarani
Swedish: safran
Thai: ya faran
Turkish: safran
Ukrainian: shafran
Vietnamese: màu vàng nghê
Yiddish: zafren

Parts Used

Flower stigma

Physiological Effects

Abortifacient, alterative, anodyne, antidepressant, anti-inflammatory, antimutagenic, antioxidant, antispasmodic, aphrodisiac, appetite stimulant, carminative, diaphoretic, diuretic, emmenagogue, expectorant, sedative, stimulant, stomachic

Medicinal Uses

Saffron improves circulation, calms stress, regulates the menses, and tonifies the nervous system. It is used in the treatment of acne , asthma, chicken pox, depression, erectile dysfunction, fever, headache, infertility, jaundice, measles, neuralgia, rheumatic pain, scarlet fever, shock, and spleen enlargement.

Topically, saffron can be prepared as a compress to treat bruises, neuralgia, and rheumatism.

Edible Uses

Saffron is used as a culinary spice and food coloring. It is the world's most expensive spice, and among the most labor-intensive to produce. At least sixty thousand stigmas are required to yield just 1 pound of saffron.

Other Uses

Saffron is valued as an important dye plant; the stigmas yield a yellow dye and the petals a blue or green dye. Crocin, the constituent that yields the coloring, is so potent that only 1 gram of it can color 100 liters of water. Saffron is also sometimes used in perfumery. In Ayurvedic medicine, saffron is used to enhance love and spirituality.

> ## *Pure Saffron*
>
> Powdered saffron is frequently adulterated with the male stamens or with marigold, safflower, calendula, or turmeric. To make sure you are getting the real thing, buy the whole stigmas rather than the powder.

Constituents

Essential oils (cineole, safranal, pinene), bitter glycoside (crocin), glucoside (picrocrocin), carotenoids (carotene, lycopene, zeaxanthin), vitamins B_1 and B_2

Energetic Correspondences

- Flavor: bitter, sweet, pungent
- Temperature: neutral
- Moisture: dry
- Polarity: yang
- Planet: Sun
- Element: fire

Contraindications

Long-term use may damage the kidneys and central nervous system. Large doses may cause coughs or headache; they can be narcotic and even potentially lethal. Avoid therapeutic doses during pregnancy.

Range and Appearance

Native to western and central Asia, saffron is a small perennial that reproduces only through its corms, and not by seeds. It bears five to eleven vertical, narrow leaves. The aromatic flowers range in color from pale lilac to deep purple and have long red styles with three yellow stigmas and shorter yellow stamens. The plant does best in well-drained though poor soil in moist or dry conditions and full to partial sun.

Do not confuse saffron with *Colchicum autumnale,* also known as meadow saffron or autumn crocus, which is toxic.

SAGE

Botanical Name

Salvia officinalis

Family

Lamiaceae (Mint Family)

Etymology

The genus name *Salvia,* from which the common name derives, itself derives from the Latin *salvus,* "healthy."

Also Known As

Arabic: marameeah
Armenian: eghespak, yeghesbag
Bulgarian: chaj gradinski
Cantonese: lóuh méih chóu
Croatian: zalfija
Czech: salvej
Danish: salvie
English: garden sage, red sage, sawge
Esperanto: salvio
Estonian: salvei
Farsi: mariam goli
Finnish: salvia
French: sauge
German: salbei
Greek: alisfakia, faskomilo
Hebrew: marva
Hungarian: zsálya
Icelandic: salvía
Italian: salvia
Japanese: sarubia, sezi
Korean: seiji, selbieo
Mandarin: shu wei cao
Norwegian: salvie
Polish: szalwia lekarska
Portuguese: salva-mansa
Romanian: salvie
Russian: shalfej
Sanskrit: shati
Serbian: kadulja
Spanish: salvia

Swedish: salvia
Turkish: adaçayi
Yiddish: sholvie, shalfey

Part Used

Aboveground plant

Physiological Effects

Anaphrodisiac, antifungal, antigalactagogue, anti-inflammatory, antioxidant, antiseptic, antispasmodic, antisudorific, aromatic, astringent, brain tonic, carminative, choleretic, circulatory stimulant, emmenagogue, estrogenic, expectorant, diaphoretic, digestive, hypoglycemic, nervine, phytoestrogenic, tonic, vermifuge

Medicinal Uses

Sage's bitter principles stimulate digestive secretions, and its tannin content improves resistance to infection. Sage helps thin mucus secretions and also tends to have a drying effect; it has been used to mitigate excessive saliva production in those with Parkinson's disease. It also improves the digestion of fatty foods and acts as a natural preservative. Even just the aroma of sage helps promote mental alertness.

Sage is used in the treatment of anxiety, blood clots, colds, cystitis, depression, diarrhea, dyspepsia, fever, flatulence, flu, hot flashes, indigestion, irregular menses, memory problems, menopause symptoms, menorrhagia, migraines, night sweats, perspiration (excessive), respiratory congestion, rheumatic pain, and staphylococcus infection.

Topically, sage can be prepared as a compress or wash to treat eczema, insect bites, poison ivy or oak, psoriasis, and wounds; as a gargle to treat halitosis, laryngitis, mouth sores, sore throat, sore gums, and tonsillitis; as a bath herb to relieve skin eruptions; as a hair rinse to treat dandruff and oily scalp and to help darken gray hair; as a douche to treat leukorrhea; as a facial steam to treat oily or blemished skin; and as a mouthwash to freshen the breath.

Edible Uses

Sage leaves are a common culinary spice. They have a camphorlike, astringent flavor. They improve the digestion of fatty foods and act as a natural preservative. The leaves and flowers can be candied.

Other Uses

In folkloric tradition, sage is used to promote longevity and wisdom and to attract protection and prosperity.

Constituents

Beta-carotene, vitamins B_1, vitamin B_2, niacin, vitamin C, calcium, iron, magnesium, essential oils (thujone, borneol, cineol, camphor, pinene, salvene), bitter principle (picrosalvine), flavonoids, tannin, phenolic acids (rosmarinic, caffeic, labiatic), phytoestrogens, resin

Energetic Correspondences

- Flavor: pungent, bitter
- Temperature: warm
- Moisture: dry
- Polarity: yang
- Planet: Jupiter/Venus
- Element: air

Contraindications

Avoid large doses during pregnancy and, because it can dry up a mother's milk while nursing. Do not use therapeutically for extended periods. Those with epilepsy, high blood pressure, or kidney disease may be adversely affected by the thujone content and should avoid large doses of sage.

Range and Appearance

Sage is native to southeastern Europe but cultivated and naturalized elsewhere. A perennial, it often grows to a foot or more in height and has a squarish stem. The leaves grow in pairs and are grayish green in color, slightly hairy, and strongly veined. The purplish flowers grow in whorls.

In the garden, sage does best in full sun and well-drained soil, with low to moderate amounts of water.

SAINT JOHN'S WORT

Botanical Name

Hypericum spp., including _H. perforatum_

Family

Clusiaceae (Saint John's Wort Family)

Etymology

The genus name, _Hypericum_, derives from the Greek _hyper_, "above," and _eikon_, "picture," meaning "over an apparition," as the herb was once considered odiferous enough to cause evil spirits to depart and was hung in the entryway or over pictures in homes. The species name _perforatum_ refers to the tiny oil glands in the leaves, which look like holes.

The common name _Saint John's wort_ refers to the herb's association with blood, as a result of the bright red dye the plant releases when crushed (thanks to its hypericin content), which is linked to John the Baptist's beheading. The herb is often collected on June 24th, the feast day of John the Baptist. _Wort_ is an Old English word meaning "plant."

Also Known As

Afrikaans: johanneskruid

Dutch: St. Jan's kraut

English: amber, arnica of the nerves, goatweed, Klamath weed, rosin rose, Saint Joan's wort, Saint John's grass, terrestrial sun, tipton weed, touch-and-heal

Finnish: mäkikuisma

French: chasse-diable, herbe de Saint Jean, herbe aux piqures, millepertuis commun, millepertuis perfore

German: echtes Johanniskraut, hexenkraut, Johanniskraut, konradskraut, tausendolocherkraut, waldhopff, wundkraut

Italian: iperico, perforata

Mandarin: hung-ts'ao-lien

Russian: zveroboi

Spanish: corazoncillo, hierba de San Juan, hiperico

Swedish: johannesört

Turkish: yara out

Part Used

Flowering top

Physiological Effects

Alterative, analgesic, anodyne, antibacterial, antibiotic, antidepressant, anti-inflammatory, antioxidant, antiseptic, antispasmodic, antiviral, anxiolytic, aromatic, astringent, cholagogue, digestive, diuretic, expectorant, nerve restorative, sedative, styptic, vermifuge, vulnerary

Medicinal Uses

Saint John's wort has been used for over one thousand years to treat depression. It is an official herb in the pharmacopoeias of Czechoslovakia, Poland, Romania, and Russia.

Saint John's wort is used to treat anorexia, anxiety, attention deficit disorder, bedwetting, boils, burns, carbuncles, chronic fatigue syndrome, colds, colic, concussion, cough, depression (mild to moderate), diarrhea, dysentery, fear, fever, flu, gastritis (chronic), gout, headache, herpes, hydrocephalus, hypothyroidism, hysteria, insomnia, irritability, jaundice, menopause symptoms, nervous habits (nail biting, hair pulling, and so on), nerve injury, neuralgia, puncture wounds, rheumatism, shingles, shock, stomachache, tuberculosis, ulcers, viral infections, and worms.

Saint John's wort restores the nerves, breaks up chi stagnation, and calms and lifts the spirit. It also promotes tissue repair, deters infection, and helps relieve pain. It can help heal damaged nerves when used internally or externally. It is thought that its action results in part from its ability to block the reabsorption of serotonin and that it might also enhance the body's receptivity to light. One of its components, hypericin, increases serotonin and melatonin metabolism. Another component, hyperforin, inhibits the uptake of dopamine, serotonin, noradrenaline, gamma-aminobutyric acid (GABA), and L-glutamate, thereby allowing these neurotransmitters to persist longer in the body, which contributes to emotional stability.

Topically, Saint John's wort can be prepared as a compress to treat mastitis and skin ulcers. Oil infused from the fresh plant is a beautiful shade of red and is used to treat back pain, bruises, burns, hemorrhoids, herpes, insect bites, nerve pain, perineal tears, stomach cramps, temporomandibular joint (TMJ), swellings, sunburn, tumors, ulcers, varicose veins, and wounds. The oil or a liniment prepared from the plant can be rubbed onto the spinal cord in treatments for arthritis, electric shock, hysteria, lumbago, neuralgia, paralysis, rheumatism, and sciatica.

As a flower essence, St. John's wort helps calm those who feel fearful or paranoid, making them feel more protected and trusting. It can help relieve nightmares and fear of death and brings feelings of courage.

Saint John's wort's effects are not instantaneous. Continued use is necessary, and as many as two to six weeks may be needed before the herb's effects manifest.

Edible Uses

The young leaves and flowers are edible in small amounts. They can be eaten raw or dried and prepared as a gruel. The leaves and flowers are sometimes added to liqueurs and mead, while some bakers have found that adding a bit of Saint John's wort leaves and flowers to flour improves the quality of the bread made from it.

Other Uses

Saint John's wort yields green, yellow, red and pink dyes. Placing a sprig of the herb under your pillow on Saint John's Eve was once thought to bring special blessings and protection from death for the coming year. The dried herb can be used to make sleep sachets. In folkloric tradition, an unmarried woman who places a piece of the herb under her pillow will dream of her future husband.

Constituents

Carotene, vitamin C, choline, flavonoids (rutin, hyperin, quercitin, quercitrin, hyperoside), pectin, hypericin, hyperforin, pseudohypericin, essential oils (carophyllene, pinene, limonene, myrcene, sesquiterpenes), sitosterol, tannin, resin

Energetic Correspondences

- Flavor: bitter, sweet
- Temperature: cool
- Moisture: dry
- Polarity: yang
- Planet: Sun
- Element: fire

Contraindications

Saint John's wort should not be combined with antidepressant pharmaceuticals (for example, Celexa, Eldepryl, Marplan, Nardil, Parnate, Paxil, Prozac, or Zoloft), protease inhibitors, or organ antirejection drugs (such as cyclosporine), except under the guidance of a qualified health-care practitioner. In fact, because Saint John's wort cleanses the liver, it is best to use it with caution in conjunction with any pharmaceutical drug.

Saint John's wort is not recommended during pregnancy, while nursing, or for children under the age of two. It may cause photosensitivity, especially in fair-skinned individuals. There have been rare reports of dizziness, nausea, fatigue, and dry mouth from its use. Some people may experience contact dermatitis from the plant.

Range and Appearance

Saint John's wort is a perennial native to northern Africa, western Asia, Europe, and North America, where it thrives in dry, sunny locations. It grows to about 3 feet in height. The opposite, lanceolate leaves clasp the stems; they feature tiny, translucent oil glands that look like holes when the leaves are held up to the light. The five-petaled, hermaphroditic flowers, are golden yellow, with black dots on their margins, and appear in flat-topped clusters. Ovoid capsules follow, bearing several dark brown seeds.

SARSAPARILLA

Botanical Name

Smilax aristolochiifolia (syn. *S. medica*), *S. aspera,*
S. officinalis, S. ornata, S. papyracea, S. regelii
(Jamaican sarsaparilla)

Family

Smilacaceae (Smilax Family)

Etymology

The genus name, *Smilax,* is the classical Greek name
for this plant. The common name *sarsaparilla*
derives from the Spanish *zarza,* "bramble," and *par-
rilla,* "little vine."

Also Known As

Cantonese: gam gong tang (*S. china*), tou fuk ling
   (*S. glabra*), tu fu ling
English: bamboo brier, greenbrier, sawbrier
Finnish: sarsaparilla
French: salsepareille
German: klimme, sarsaparielle, sarsaparillawurzel,
   stechwinde
Italian: salsapariglia
Mandarin: ba qia (*S. china*), ba zi (*S. china*),
   gou gu zi (*S. china*), jin gang teng (*S. china*),
   leng fen tuan (*S. glabra*), tu fu ling (*S. glabra*),
   xian liang (*S. glabra*), zi ju ling (*S. glabra*)
Sanskrit: chopchini
Spanish: zarsaparilla

Part Used

Rhizome

Physiological Effects

Alterative, antibacterial, anti-inflammatory, antiseptic,
antitumor, antiviral, aphrodisiac, astringent, carminative, cholagogue, demulcent, depurative, diaphoretic, diuretic, emetic, febrifuge, hepatoprotective,
rejuvenative, stimulant, stomachic, sudorific, tonic

Medicinal Uses

Sarsaparilla was widely used by Native Americans as
a cough remedy. When it was first brought from

Mexico to Spain in the 1500s it was exalted as a
treatment for venereal diseases such as gonorrhea
and syphilis; perhaps this is the reason it was so very
popular with pirates. It was an official herb in the
United States Pharmacopoeia for the treatment of
venereal disease from 1820 to 1910.

Sarsaparilla contains compounds that bind to bacterial endotoxins in the digestive tract, decreasing the
risk of digestive distress. It clears toxins from the
skin, urinary tract, liver, and blood. It also soothes
the mucous membranes, increases all of the body's
metabolic processes, and facilitates the excretion of
uric acid and cleansing of the genitourinary system.

Sarsaparilla is used in the treatment of abscess,
acne, age spots, AIDS, anemia, arthritis, boils, cancer, colds, conjunctivitis, depression (menopausal),
eczema, endometriosis, erectile dysfunction, fatigue,
fever, gonorrhea, gout, heavy metal toxicity, hot
flashes, infertility, leprosy, leukorrhea, menorrhagia,
menstrual cramps, ovarian cysts, pelvic inflammatory disease, premenstrual syndrome, psoriasis, rheumatism, scrofula, skin dryness, syphilis, and urinary
tract infection.

Edible Uses

The rhizome is not generally considered edible,
though it is used to flavor soft drinks, especially
root beer, and to produce foam on drinks such as
beers and sodas. The young shoots are edible raw
or cooked, as are the tendrils of the vine.

Other Uses

A red dye is made from the ripe tendrils. In folkloric
tradition it is used to attract love and prosperity, and
it is said to excite the passions, making men more
virile and women more sensuous.

Constituents

Iron, sulfur, zinc, steroidal saponins (sarsapogenin,
smilagen, sitosterol, stigmasterol pollinastanol), glycosides, resin, fat, sugar

Energetic Correspondences

• Flavor: sweet, pungent
• Temperature: neutral

- Moisture: moist
- Polarity: yang
- Planet: Mars/Jupiter
- Element: fire

Contraindications

Avoid during pregnancy.

Range and Appearance

Sarsaparilla is native to many regions of the globe, including South and Central America, the Caribbean, and Asia. All species are climbing vines that can extend over 100 feet and are covered with stiff prickles. The leaves are oval with a rounded base or heart shaped; they are covered with a whitish film. The vine is dioecious, and the inconspicuous flowers are greenish, yellow, or bronze. The flowers are followed by bluish black or red berries. There are many species growing throughout the world, but not all have medicinal properties—look for roots with a rich orangish hue.

SASSAFRAS

Botanical Name

Sassafras albidum (syn. *S. officinale, Laurus sassafras*)

Family

Lauraceae (Laurel Family)

Etymology

The origin of the name *sassafras* is hazy. It is thought to have been given by Nicolas Monardes, a sixteenth-century Spanish botanist, as a corruption of *saxifraga,* the name of another genus of plants; there may have been an American Indian name for *sassafras* that sounded like *saxafraga* and contributed to the alteration. The species name *albidum* derives from the Latin *alba,* "white."

Also Known As

English: ague tree, cinnamon wood, fennel wood, knutze, saloop, saxifrax

Finnish: sassafras
French: bois de canelle, laurier des Iroquois
German: fenchelholz, fieberbaum
Italian: sassafrasso
Swedish: sassafras

Parts Used

Root, root bark

Physiological Effects

Alterative, anodyne, antigalactagogue, antirheumatic, antiseptic, aromatic, astringent, carminative, diaphoretic, diuretic, emmenagogue, stimulant, tonic, vasodilator

Medicinal Uses

Sassafras was one of the first exports from the United States to England. Many early American colonies were situated close to sassafras groves, as it was such a marketable crop. It was included in the United States Pharmacopoeia from 1820 to 1926.

In Appalachian and Ozark folk medicine, sassafras is considered an essential part of a springtime tonic. It improves circulation, deters infection, destroys pathogenic microorganisms, and causes the release of toxins through diaphoresis. Sassafras is used in the treatment of acne, arthritis, boils, carbuncles, catarrh, colds, diarrhea, dysentery, eczema, fever, flatulence, flu, gonorrhea, gout, herpes, hypertension, measles, nephritis, psoriasis, rheumatism, scrofula, shingles, skin eruptions, stomachache, and syphilis.

Topically, sassafras can be prepared as a poultice to relieve inflamed eyes or as a liniment to treat bruises, rheumatism, sciatica, sore muscles, and swellings. It also can be made into a wash to treat poison ivy/oak or nettle rash. The essential oil can be diluted and applied directly to relieve toothache or to get rid of head lice and other surface parasites.

Edible Uses

Sassafras tea has long been a popular beverage; during the Civil War, when black tea imports were cut off, sassafras was among the most popular replacements. Its most famous use is as a flavoring for root beer. It also can be used to improve the flavor of other teas and medicines.

The winter buds, young leaf tips, and flowers can be eaten raw or cooked. The leaves are flavorful and have a thickening effect. Dried and powdered, they are used in Cajun cooking and to make the Cajun spice blend gumbo filé.

Other Uses

The essential oil of the root bark is sometimes added as an aromatic or flavoring agent to soaps, toothpastes, mouthwashes, gums, beers, and perfumes.

Constituents

Iron, essential oils (safrole, asarone, eugenol, pinene, myristicin, thujone, anethole), alkaloids (boldine, norboldine, reticuline), sitosterol, lignan, mucilage, tannin, resin

Energetic Correspondences

- Flavor: pungent
- Temperature: warm
- Moisture: moist
- Polarity: yang
- Planet: Mars/Jupiter
- Element: fire

Contraindications

In the 1960s there arose some controversy about one of sassafras's components, safrole, which was shown to cause liver cancer in rats. The studies were done with large amounts of isolated safrole, not with sassafras bark as a whole. However, later studies found that the cause of the cancer was not safrole itself but liver enzymes acting on it, and in human studies it did not have the same effect. Interestingly enough, Cherokees used sassafras as a remedy for liver cancer. Nevertheless, there are safrole-free sassafras items available. Keep in mind that the safrole in sassafras is considered to be one-fourteenth as carcinogenic as the ethanol in beer. And safrole occurs naturally in many other common spices, such as basil, bay leaf, black pepper, cinnamon, nutmeg, mace, star anise, and sage.

Large doses of sassafras may have a narcotic effect. (In fact, MDMA, or Ecstasy, was originally synthesized from sassafras.) Use only occasionally and in moderate doses. Sassafras is not recommended during pregnancy. As it decreases lactation, nursing mothers should avoid it (unless drying up their milk supply is their purpose).

Range and Appearance

Sassafras, native to eastern North America, usually grows as a small deciduous shrub, though it can reach a height of 100 feet. It has a dark brown bark. Small, fragrant, greenish yellow flowers appear in clusters before the leaves. The leaves are alternate, bright green on top and downy below, and from 4 to 6 inches long; they are often three lobed and mitten shaped. A small blue-black oval fruit, containing one seed the size of a pea, is widely eaten by birds. The root is a lovely orangish brown. The plant has a spicy orange-vanilla fragrance.

Sassafras thrives in deciduous woodlands with moist, well-drained soil and partial shade.

SAW PALMETTO

Botanical Name

Serenoa repens (syn. *S. serrulata*)

Family

Arecaceae (Palm Family)

Etymology

The genus name, *Serenoa*, was given in honor of American botanist Sereno Watson (1826–1892). The species name, *repens*, is Latin for "creeping."

Also Known As

English: dwarf palmetto, fan palm, old man's friend, sabal
Finnish: sahapalmu
German: zwerpalme
Swedish: sågpalmetto

Part Used

Berry

Physiological Effects

Alterative, anabolic, antiandrogenic, anticatarrhal, antiestrogenic, anti-inflammatory, antiseptic, antispasmodic, aperient, aphrodisiac, decongestant, diuretic, expectorant, galactagogue, muscle-building tonic, nutritive, phytoestrogenic, rejuvenative, restorative, sedative (in small amounts), stimulant, thyroid tonic, urinary antiseptic, uterine tonic, yang tonic, yin tonic

Medicinal Uses

Saw palmetto was an official herb in the United States Pharmacopoeia from 1905 to 1926 and the National Formulary from 1926 to 1950. Its berry prevents the development of benign prostatic hyperplasia (BPH) by increasing the breakdown and elimination of dihydrotestosterone (DHT), which is thought to promote cellular growth in the prostate; the berry inhibits the production of the enzyme testosterone-5-alpha-reductase, which converts testosterone into dihydrotestosterone (DHT), and also inhibits DHT from adhering to the receptor sites. Saw palmetto berry also strengthens the reproductive organs, prevents atrophy of the genitals and bladder tissue, enhances sexual arousal, and reduces inflammation.

Saw palmetto is used in the treatment of acne (cystic), asthma, bronchitis, cancer, catarrh, colds (head colds), cough, cystitis, dysuria, epididymitis, erectile dysfunction, failure to thrive, genital atrophy, hirsuitism, HIV, incontinence, irregular menses, low libido, low sperm count, malabsorption of food, migraine, mucous-membrane inflammation, nocturia (excessive nighttime urination), polyuria, premature ejaculation, prostatitis, orchitis, sexual debility, sore throat, urinary infection, urinary hesitancy, and wasting diseases. It also can be used to encourage convalescence, enhance breast size, and possibly initiate sexual maturation when it has been slow to start.

Saw palmetto berries also can be mixed with cocoa butter and used as a bolus to treat uterine or vaginal problems.

Edible Uses

Native Americans of the southern United States, especially the Seminole, have long used the berries as a food source. They have also used them to create a fermented beverage that was considered a love tonic. Animals that eat the berries grow plump. The "hearts" at the base of the leaf stalks can be cut out and eaten raw. The bases of the terminal buds can also be prepared as a vegetable.

Other Uses

Various parts of the plant, including the leaves and stems, have been used to make roof thatching, baskets, mattresses, hats, scrub brushes, and paper.

Constituents

Carotene, calcium, phosphorous, potassium, essential oil, fatty acids (caproic, capric, lauric, oleic, palmitic, stearic, myristic), tannin, phytosterols (beta-sitosterol, campesterol, stigmasterol), polysaccharides, dextrose, resins

Energetic Correspondences

* Flavor: pungent, sweet
* Temperature: warm
* Moisture: dry
* Polarity: yang
* Planet: Mars/Pluto
* Element: fire

Contraindications

Avoid during pregnancy and while nursing, at least until further research has been done to ascertain its safety during these times. Mild gastrointestinal disturbances are a rare side effect.

Range and Appearance

Saw palmetto is a small evergreen palm native to the southeastern United States. It grows to about 6 to 10 feet in height. Its leaves have fifteen to thirty divisions, with sharp edges like a saw, that branch out in a fanlike shape, radiating from a central point. The flowers are whitish green with three to five petals. The reddish to dark purple berries resemble black olives and have a hard brown seed within.

Be careful when harvesting this plant from the wild, as its native habitat is often also habitat for diamondback rattlesnakes.

SCHIZANDRA

Botanical Name

Schisandra chinensis (syn. *Kadsura chinensis*),
  S. *sphenanthera*

Family

Schisandraceae (Magnolia Vine Family)

Etymology

The genus name, *Schisandra*, derives from the Greek
schisis, "crevice," and *andros*, "man," in reference
to the cleft on the stamen of some varieties.

Also Known As

Cantonese: ng mei ji
English: five-flavor fruit, five-taste berry, magnolia
  vine, schisandra
Finnish: palsamiköynnös
French: schisandra
German: schisandra
Japanese: gomishi
Korean: omicha
Mandarin: wu wei zi ("five-flavor fruit")
Russian: limonka
Swedish: fjärilsranka

Part Used

Berry

Physiological Effects

Adaptogen, antibacterial, antidepressant, antimutagenic, antioxidant, antitussive, aphrodisiac, astringent,
brain tonic, cholagogue, emmenagogue, expectorant,
hepatoprotective, immune tonic, kidney tonic, nervous system tonic, rejuvenative, reproductive tonic,
restorative, sedative (mild), yang tonic, yin tonic

Medicinal Uses

Schizandra was widely used by the royalty of ancient
China as a youth preserver, beautifier, and reproductive tonic. It is a supreme adaptogen; Russian pilots
of the 1940s used it to help them tolerate the low-
oxygen conditions of high altitudes, while to this day
hunters in Siberia consume schizandra berries for

energy and to help their bodies function in the harsh
conditions.

Schizandra quickens reflex time, stabilizes the
nervous system, normalizes brain function, and
improves coordination, intellect, and sensory perception. It also protects the heart, lungs, and liver,
nourishes kidney chi, and purifies the blood. Chinese
medicine calls for eating a few berries one hundred
days in a row as a tonic to improve coordination
and concentration. According to Chinese theory,
schizandra also helps build a person's defensive energy, known as *wei chi*, so he or she is better able to
resist infection. Indeed, schizandra has been shown
to stimulate the production of lymphocytes and
interferon.

Schizandra is both astringent and demulcent, having the ability to both dry and moisten as needed. It
is used to nourish the "water of the genitals," or the
fluids that help sensitize and moisturize the genitals.
Long-term use helps beautify the skin.

Schizandra berries are used in the treatment of
allergy, altitude sickness, anxiety, asthma, cerebral
ataxia, chemotherapy and radiation side effects, cirrhosis, chronic fatigue syndrome, cough (chronic),
depression, diabetes, diarrhea (chronic), dizziness,
eczema, exhaustion, headache, hearing loss, heart
palpitations, hepatitis, HIV, hives, hyperhidrosis
(excessive sweating), infertility (male and female),
insomnia, irritability, low libido, low sperm count,
lung weakness (shortness of breath, hypoxia, wheezing, susceptibility to respiratory infection), memory
loss, Ménière's disease, nephritis, neuralgia, neuras-
tenia, neuroses, night sweats, nocturnal emissions,
Parkinson's disease, polyuria, premature aging, premature ejaculation, post-traumatic stress disorder,
spermatorrhea, stress, tuberculosis, ulcers, vision
problems (astigmatism, short-sightedness), and wasting diseases. It also can facilitate athletic recovery
and improve sexual stamina.

In Asia powdered schizandra is used topically as a
warm poultice to treat skin ulcers.

Edible Uses

Schizandra berries can be eaten. They are also sometimes added to wine.

Other Uses

None known

Constituents

Vitamin C, vitamin E, manganese, phosphorous, silicon, sesquicarene, lignans (schizandrin, gomisin), schizoandrol, essential oils (citral, bisabolene, ylangene), phytosterols (stigmasterol, beta-sitosterol), mucilage, citric acid, malic acid, tartaric acid

Energetic Correspondences

- Flavor: sweet, sour, salty, pungent, bitter
- Temperature: warm
- Moisture: dry
- Polarity: yang
- Planet: Mars/Jupiter
- Element: fire

Contraindications

Avoid schizandra in cases of excess heat (such as fever), overly acidic conditions, cough, epilepsy, intracranial pressure, or in the early stages of rash. Schizandra is not recommended during pregnancy. Do not give to children under the age of two, except under the guidance of a qualified health-care practitioner.

Range and Appearance

Schizandra is a deciduous, climbing, woody, aromatic vine native to eastern Asia. It grows in woods in rich, loose soil, preferring a cool climate. The leaves are oblong, alternate, and smooth on top. The pale yellow flowers grow in axillary clusters. The fruits, which are reddish in color, occur in drooping bunches, each containing two kidney-shaped seeds.

SEA BUCKTHORN

Botanical Name

Hippophae rhamnoides

Family

Elaeagnaceae (Oleaster Family)

Etymology

The genus name, *Hippophae,* derives from the Greek *hippos,* "horse," and *phaos,* "shine," in reference to the shiny coat horses develop after feeding on this herb. The name has also been interpreted to mean "giving light to a horse," in reference to the plant's supposed power to cure equine blindness, or "shining underneath," in reference to the silvery undersides of the leaves.

Sea buckthorn was said to have been the preferred food of Pegasus, the flying horse of Greek mythology.

Also Known As

English: sallowthorn, sandthorn, sea berry,
    Siberian pineapple
Finnish: tyrni
French: argousier
German: gewöhnlicher, sanddorn
Italian: olivella spinosa
Polish: rokitnik
Russian: obelpikha
Spanish: espino armarillo
Swedish: finbär, havtorn
Tibetan: d'har-bu

Part Used

Berry (ripe), seed, leaf, twigs

Physiological Effects

Berry: analgesic, antibacterial, antibiotic, antifungal, anti-inflammatory, antioxidant, antitumor, febrifuge, hepatoprotective, nutritive, tonic
Seed: analgesic, antibacterial, antifungal, anti-inflammatory
Leaf, twigs: astringent, vermifuge

Medicinal Uses

Sea buckthorn reduces inflammation and helps protect the liver from the damaging effects of chemicals, ultraviolet light, and radiation. It is used in the treatment of angina, arthritis, cancer, chemotherapy side effects, colds, cough, exhaustion, eye ailments, high cholesterol, and ulcers. The berries inhibit the growth of staphylococcal bacteria, and their high flavonoid content promotes strong arteries. The infused oil (made from the berries, seeds, leaves, and twigs) can be consumed to treat stomach and intestinal disorders.

Topically, sea buckthorn can be applied to the skin in the form of oils, salves, balms, or lotions to treat acne, burns, dermatitis, eczema, infections, rosacea, and wrinkles. In fact, after the disaster at the nuclear power plant in Chernobyl, Russia, sea buckthorn oil was used to treat the burns of people exposed to the leaked radiation. Sea buckthorn can also be used to prevent sunburn and radiation burns; Russian cosmonauts, for example, have used this herb to protect their skin against radiation burns when in outer space.

Sea buckthorn is also sometimes added to hair products to prevent baldness and stimulate hair growth.

Edible Uses

The berries can be eaten raw, though they are very acidic and taste better when sweetened or when harvested after a frost, which decreases their astringency. They are seven times higher in vitamin C than lemons. Other parts of the plant are not generally considered edible.

Other Uses

Sea buckthorn has an extensive root system and is often planted to help prevent soil erosion and to repair areas that have been damaged by mining. The berries yield a yellow dye, while the young leaves and shoots yield a blackish brown dye. Its wood is durable and is useful as fuel and for making charcoal.

Constituents

Berry, seed: beta-carotene, lycopene, zeaxanthin, vitamin B complex (B_1, B_2, B_6, and folic acid), vitamin E, flavonoids (quercitin), essential fatty acids (omega-3, omega-6, omega-7, omega-9), quinic acid, malic acid, phytosterols (beta-sitosterol)
Leaf, twigs: tannins

Energetic Correspondences

- Flavor: sour
- Temperature: cool
- Moisture: moist
- Polarity: yin
- Planet: Moon/Mars/Jupiter/Saturn
- Element: water

Contraindications

In rare cases sea buckthorn may cause an allergic reaction.

Range and Appearance

Sea buckthorn is native to Asia and Europe and is usually found along seashores in sandy soil and full sun, often forming dense thickets. It is a thorny deciduous shrub usually between 3 and 10 feet tall and is covered with silvery brown scales. The trunk and branches are light brown. The deciduous leaves are lanceolate and narrow. The flowers are green and appear before the leaves. Orangish yellow berries appear after the flowers and remain on the shrubs throughout the winter, providing food for many animals. The shrubs are dioecious, meaning that male and female flowers are borne on different shrubs.

SELF-HEAL

Botanical Name

Prunella vulgaris

Family

Lamiaceae (Mint Family)

Etymology

The genus name, *Prunella,* is from the German *brunellen,* a common name given to the plant because it cured *die Braüne,* the mouth and throat inflammation, which we call quinsy. The species name, *vulgaris,* is Latin for "common." The common name *self-heal* refers to fact that this plant has been regarded almost as a panacea.

Also Known As

Cantonese: ha bu chou, ha gu chou

English: all-heal, blue curls, brunella, bumble bees, carpenter's herb, dragonhead, heal-all, heal-all spike, heart of the earth, Hercules's woundwort, hook heal, pimpernel, sickle herb, slough heal, summer dry herb, woundwort

Finnish: niityhumala

French: brunelle commune, brunette, herbe au charpentier, herbe Saint Quentin, petite consoude, prunelle vulgaire

German: gaucheil, gemeine brunelle, halskraut, mundfaulkraut, brunellen

Japanese: kagoso

Korean: hagoch'o

Mandarin: xia ku cao

Italian: prunella

Spanish: consuelda

Swedish: brunört

Part Used

Aboveground plant

Physiological Effects

Alterative, antibacterial, antibiotic, antimutagenic, antioxidant, antiseptic, antispasmodic, antiviral, astringent, bitter, carminative, cholagogue, diuretic, febrifuge, hemostatic, hypotensive, immune tonic, liver stimulant, stomachic, styptic, tonic, vasodilator, vermifuge, vulnerary

Medicinal Uses

Self-heal clears heat, relaxes the liver, relieves congestion, aids in detoxification, reduces inflammation, and promotes tissue repair. It contains the antitumor compound ursolic acid. The plant's resemblance to an open mouth leading to the throat may have prompted its traditional use as an herb for mouth and throat ailments. Today, self-heal is used to treat abcess, acne, bleeding, chemotherapy and radiation side effects, colds, colic, conjunctivitis, cough, diarrhea, diphtheria, dizziness, edema, epilepsy, eye redness, fever, flatulence, goiter, gout, Graves' disease, headache, heavy metal toxicity, hemorrhage, hemorrhoids, hepatitis, hypertension, hypothyroidism, injury, jaundice, laryngitis, liver weakness, lymphatic swelling, menorrhagia, pharyngitis, scrofula, sore throat, thyroid inflammation, vertigo, and wounds. It is also used to encourage convalescence.

Topically, a poultice or the fresh juice of self-heal can be applied directly to the skin to treat acne, backache, bleedings, boils, bruises, burns, cuts, sore eyes, headache, hemorrhoids, rashes, sprains and wounds. Self-heal can also be prepared as a mouthwash or gargle to treat mouth sores, gum disease, sore throat, and thrush or as a douche to treat leukorrhea.

As a flower essence self-heal helps users to gain the courage to be in good health. It aids in nutrient assimilation and promotes self-love and self-acceptance. It can be of particular benefit to those who have tried many therapies without benefit. It guides users in slowing down, gaining perspective, and evaluating their priorities.

Edible Uses

The leaves can be eaten raw or cooked. They make a refreshing sun tea.

Other Uses

An olive green dye can be made from the stems and flowers.

Constituents

Beta-carotene, vitamin B_1, vitamin C, vitamin K, zinc, flavonoids (hyperoside, rutin), pentacyclic triterpenes (betulinic acid, oleanolic acid, ursolic acid), rosmarinic acid, essential oils (camphor, cineol, pinene, linalool, myrcene), tannin

Energetic Correspondences
- Flavor: bitter, sweet, pungent
- Temperature: cold
- Moisture: dry
- Polarity: yin
- Planet: Venus/Mars
- Element: water

Contraindications

Self-heal is not recommended during pregnancy.

Range and Appearance

Self-heal is a low-growing, 6- to 12-inch-tall perennial found in Europe, Asia, northern Africa, and North America. It prefers moist soil and partial shade to full sun. Its leaves are opposite, oval to lance shaped, and borne on square stems. The flowers are purplish blue (though on occasion pink or white) and tinged with brown, have a two-lipped corolla, and occur in thick oblong spikes. Later, the plant bears a brown obovate nut. Unlike most members of the Mint Family, it has relatively no aroma.

SENNA

Botanical Name

Senna alexandrina (Alexandrian senna; syn. *Cassia senna*), *S. auriculata* (tanner's senna), *S. italica, S. marilandica* (American senna)

Family

Fabaceae (Legume Family)

Etymology

The name *senna* is taken from the plant's Arabic name, *sanā*.

Also Known As

Arabic: san, senna jebel
Finnish: senna
French: sene
German: sennesblatt
Mandarin: fan xia ye
Russian: alexandre, cassia
Sanskrit: nripadruma
Spanish: canafistula, hojasen, retama, sen, te de sena
Swedish: senna

Parts Used

Leaf, pod, seed

Physiological Effects

Cathartic, cholagogue, diuretic, febrifuge, laxative, purgative, stimulant, vermifuge

Medicinal Uses

Senna was introduced into Europe in the eleventh century by the Arabs. It was an official herb in the United States Pharmacopoeia from 1820 until 1882. It has been used as a laxative for over one thousand years. Due to its anthraquinones, senna increases bowel muscle contraction by acting as an irritant. It also increases the amount of water secreted into the lumen of the large intestine and helps to temporarily prevent fluid from being absorbed from the large intestine, thus contributing to softer stools. It also contains emodin, which has antibacterial properties. It is used to treat flatulence, constipation, fever, gout, jaundice, and worms.

Topically, senna can be prepared as a poultice made with vinegar to get rid of pimples.

Edible Uses

Senna is generally considered too bitter to eat. However, it can be mixed with dried fruits and consumed as a laxative candy.

Other Uses

The bark of tanner's senna (*S. auriculata*) is used for tanning leather in Africa. In folkloric tradition it is used in love spells.

Constituents

Calcium, sulfur, flavonoids, mannitol, anthraquinone glycosides (sennaosides, aloe-emodin), beta-sitosterol, chrysophanic acid, chrysophanol, tartaric acid, essential oil, mucilage, tannin, resin

Energetic Correspondences

- Flavor: bitter, sweet
- Temperature: hot (initially), cold (subsequently)
- Moisture: dry
- Polarity: yang
- Planet: Mercury/Mars/Saturn
- Element: air

Contraindications

Avoid senna during pregnancy, while nursing, and in children under twelve. Avoid in cases of colitis or conditions of inflammation of the digestive tract. Do not use in conjunction with cardiac glycoside pharmaceuticals, except under the guidance of a qualified health-care practitioner. The seeds have a gentler effect than the leaves and are more appropriate for the young, the elderly, and those prone to stomach cramps.

To prevent gripe, combine senna with carminative herbs such as cinnamon, cardamom, coriander seed, fennel seed, ginger, or peppermint. Overuse may cause laxative dependency, so do not use senna for more than ten days in a row. Large doses or overuse can cause bloody diarrhea, intestinal cramps, nausea, vomiting, and nephritis. Long-term use can cause dehydration and can deplete the body of electrolytes, including potassium, worsening constipation and weakening the muscles.

Senna may cause the urine to become reddish, which is no need for concern.

Range and Appearance

Senna is a deciduous shrub, reaching 4 to 6 feet in height, native to tropical Africa, India, the Red Sea region, and North America. The leaves are compound, thin, paired, and light green in color. The hermaphroditic flowers are yellow and have irregular sepals. The pods are flattened but bulge slightly over the seeds.

Senna does well in partial shade to full sun. It can tolerate drought but thrives in a moist soil.

SHEEP'S SORREL

Botanical Name

Rumex acetosella

Family

Polygonaceae (Buckwheat Family)

Etymology

The name *sorrel* is given to several plants that have an acid quality in their sap that gives them a sour flavor. The common name *oxalis* derives from the Greek *oxos*, "vinegar," in reference to the flavor of the leaves. The genus name, *Rumex,* is the ancient Latin name for members of this family. The species name, *acetosella,* is Latin for "vinegar salts."

Also Known As

English: cuckoo sorrel, dog-eared sorrel, field sorrel, meadow sorrow, oxalis, red sorrel, red-top sorrel, red weed, sourgrass
Finnish: ahosuolaheinä
French: alleluja, patience des alpes, petite oseille
German: kleiner sauerampfer, sauerklee
Italian: acetosella, scetosa
Russian: shavel
Spanish: acedera, lazan
Swedish: bergssyra

Parts Used

Aboveground plant, root

Physiological Effects

Antibacterial, anti-inflammatory, antioxidant, antiparasitic, antiscorbutic, antiseptic, antiviral, astringent, diaphoretic, diuretic, febrifuge, laxative, refrigerant, vermifuge

Medicinal Uses

Sheep's sorrel cleanses the bladder, kidneys, and liver, strengthens the heart, and enhances oxygen supply to the tissues. It is helpful in reducing fever and inflammation. In China, raw sheep's sorrel is given after birthing to cool the reproductive area and prevent infection. The herb's antioxidant properties help protect cells from free radical damage; in fact, it is an ingredient in the anticancer formula Essiac, originally an Ojibwa formula that a Canadian nurse, René Caisse (*Essiac* spelled backward), popularized.

Sheep's sorrel is used in the treatment of anemia, cancer, diarrhea, fever, scurvy, and a weakened immune system.

Topically, a poultice, a compress, or the fresh juice of sheep's sorrel can be applied directly to the skin to treat acne, bleeding, boils, cancer, nettle stings, ringworm, sores, tumors, and wounds. It can also be used as an astringent douche or enema to decrease secretions.

Edible Uses

Sheep's sorrel leaves and seeds can be eaten raw or cooked; they have a lovely tart flavor and are a wonderful addition to salads. They are sometimes used to thicken soup, and the juice from the leaves was once used to curdle milk to make cheese. The seeds can also be eaten. The root is edible if cooked.

Other Uses

A variety of dyes from dark green to gray can be derived from the roots.

Constituents

Beta-carotene, vitamin C, flavonoids (hesperidin, quercetin), anthraquinones (chrysophanol, rhein, emodin), oxalic acid, tartaric acid, potassium, phosphorous, tannins

Energetic Correspondences

- Flavor: sour
- Temperature: cool
- Moisture: moist
- Polarity: yin
- Planet: Venus
- Element: water/earth

Contraindications

Sheep's sorrel contains quite a bit of oxalic acid, which can lead to the formation of kidney stones and impair calcium absorption, so use on occasion rather than daily. Avoid excessive use in cases of gout, kidney stones, and rheumatism or in the very young or very old. Excessive use may cause stomach cramps.

Range and Appearance

Sheep's sorrel is a low-growing perennial, reaching only about 12 inches in height, that is native to northern Africa, Europe, and Asia but widely naturalized. The roots contain a reddish pigment. The leaves are from 1 to 6 inches long and often are shaped like a spear. The species is dioecious, meaning that male and female flowers are borne on different plants. The flower clusters turn reddish as they mature, but the flowers are small and inconspicuous. The seeds are shiny brown or black three-sided nutlets, much beloved by songbirds. The plant thrives in iron-rich, lime-deficient soil. It is considered an invasive species in some parts of North America.

SHEPHERD'S PURSE

Botanical Name

Capsella bursa-pastoris

Family

Brassicaceae (Mustard Family)

Etymology

The genus name, *Capsella*, derives from the Latin *capsa*, "box." The species name, *bursa-pastoris*, is Latin for "shepherd's purse," in reference to the shape of the seed pouches of the plant, which look like the old-fashioned leather pouches of European shepherds.

Also Known As

English: blind weed, case wort, life-preserving plant, lady's purse, mothers' hearts, old man's pharmacely, pepper and salt, picklooker, pickpocket, pick purse, purslet, rattle pouches, Saint James's weed, Saint James's wort, shepherds's sprout, shovelweed, toywort, ward seed, witches' pouches

Finnish: lutukka, rikkalutukka

French: bourse à pasteur, capselle, fleur de Saint Jacques

German: blutkraut, gansbross, gerwell, hirtentäshelkraut, sackelkraut

Italian: borsa di pastore

Russian: pastushya sumka

Spanish: bolsa de pastor

Swedish: lomme, lommeört

Parts Used

Aboveground plant (primarily), root (rarely)

Physiological Effects

Alterative, anti-inflammatory, antioxidant, antiscorbutic, antiseptic, antitumor, astringent, detergent, diuretic, emmenagogue, febrifuge, hemostatic, hypotensive, oxytocic, styptic, urinary antiseptic, vasoconstrictor, vulnerary

Medicinal Uses

Shepherd's purse is known to constrict blood vessels, normalize blood pressure, and stimulate the excretion of uric acid. It has long been used by midwives to aid uterine contraction during birthing and to prevent postpartum hemorrhaging. During World War I, medics used a liquid extract of the herb to staunch bleeding. Today, shepherd's purse is used in the treatment of bedwetting, cancer, catarrh, congestion, cystitis, diarrhea, dropsy, dysentery, gout, hematuria, hemorrhage, leukorrhea, malaria, menorrhagia, nosebleed, organ prolapse, poor vision, postpartum bleeding, spermatorrhea, tuberculosis, uterine bleeding, ulcer (bleeding), urinary tract inflammation, and varicose veins.

Topically, shepherd's purse can be used as a poultice to staunch bleeding, to reduce bruising or the inflammation and itchiness of poison ivy or oak, and, when applied to the wrists, to lower fever. Cotton soaked in a tea or the fresh juice of sheperd's purse can be placed in a nostril to stop a nosebleed. The herb can also be prepared as a mouthwash to treat pyorrhea.

Edible Uses

The leaves, flowers, and seeds are edible in moderate quantities, whether raw or cooked. The root, which is spicy, can be used as a substitute for ginger. The seeds have a peppery flavor and can be used as a seasoning.

Other Uses

When the seeds are placed in water, a gummy substance forms that attracts mosquitoes and kills their larvae.

Constituents

Beta-carotene, vitamin B complex, choline, vitamin C, vitamin K, calcium, iron, potassium, acetylcholine, tyramine, histamine, flavonoids (diosmin, luteolin, quercitin), malic acid, fumaric acid, saponins, organic acid (bursinic acid), mustard oil, sitosterol

Energetic Correspondences

- Flavor: pungent, sweet
- Temperature: warm
- Moisture: dry
- Polarity: yang
- Planet: Saturn
- Element: fire

Contraindications

Use shepherd's purse only in moderate doses, as large doses may be toxic. Avoid during pregnancy, except during labor, and then only under the guidance of a qualified health-care professional. Do not use in cases of kidney disease. There have been rare reports of the seeds causing contact dermatitis.

Shepherd's purse is best when used fresh. Dried plant material is much less effective, and plant material older than one year should not be bothered with.

Range and Appearance

Shepherd's purse is an annual, thought to be native to Europe but dispersed worldwide, that can grow to 2 feet in height. The plant features basal rosette leaves, which are 2 to 6 inches long, along with upper leaves that clasp the stalk and are irregular, arrow shaped, and either smooth or toothed. The small, white, four-petaled flowers are followed by flat, heart-shaped seeds that are divided into two portions, each containing multiple yellowish seeds. It can grow in full sun or semi-shade, and thrives in either dry or moist poor soil.

Birds, both wild and domesticated, are fond of the seeds.

SHIITAKE

Botanical Name

Lentinus edodes (syn. *Lentinula edodes*)

Family

Polyporaceae (Polypor Family)

Etymology

The genus name *Lentinus* derives from the Latin *lent,* "pliable," and *inus,* "resembling." The species name *edodes* is Latin for "edible." The common name *shiitake* derives from that of the Japanese shii tree (*Pasania* spp.), logs of which the mushrooms grow on.

Also Known As

English: black forest mushroom, glossagyne,
  mushroom of immortality, oak mushroom,
  Oriental black mushroom
Korean: pyogo
Mandarin: huagu, xianggu
Thai: hed hom

Part Used

Cap of fruiting body

Physiological Effects

Antioxidant, antitumor, antiviral, aphrodisiac, chi tonic, hepatoprotective, immune tonic, rejuvenative

Medicinal Uses

For thousands of years shiitake mushroom, known as "the mushroom of immortality," has been used to prevent premature aging. Shiitake stimulates the stem cells in the bone marrow to create more B and T cells, inhibits blood platelet aggregation, and aids in the production of interferon. It also helps the body get rid of excessive salt. It is used in the treatment of AIDS, allergies, anemia, arthritis, asthma, bronchitis, cancer, colds, chronic cough, environmental illness, fatigue, flu, hepatitis, high cholesterol, hypertension, rickets, and tumors. One mushroom a day is considered a therapeutic dosage.

Edible Uses

Shiitake mushrooms are edible and delicious. They are sold fresh or dried; the stems are often discarded, as they are tougher than the caps.

Other Uses

None known

Constituents

Amino acids (lysine, arginine), polysaccharide (lentinan), eritadenin, vitamin C, vitamin D, vitamin B_2, vitamin B_{12}, calcium, potassium, purines

Energetic Correspondences

- Flavor: sweet, neutral
- Temperature: neutral
- Moisture: moist
- Polarity: yang
- Planet: Jupiter
- Element: water

Contraindications

Shiitakes are considered nontoxic and generally safe. Avoid in cases of extreme weakness or diarrhea. There have been rare reports of allergic reactions affecting the throat, lungs, or skin.

Range and Appearance

Shiitake, native to China, is a light amber fungi with ragged gills. Its stem can be central or off-center. It grows on fallen broadleaved trees such as beech, chestnut, oak, maple, walnut, and mulberry. Kits that allow you to grow your own shiitakes are commonly available.

SKULLCAP

Botanical Name

Scutellaria californica, S. canescens, S. galericulata, S. lateriflora, S. pilosa, S. tuberosa, S. versicolor

Family

Lamiaceae (Mint Family)

Etymology

The genus name *Scutellaria* and common name *skullcap* derive from the Latin *scutella,* "little dish," in reference to the plant's inverted calyx cup, which looks like a helmet with its visor raised, and also somewhat like a skull. The common name *mad dog weed* resulted from the plant's use by a Dr. Vanderveer in the 1700s to treat people who had been bitten by rabid dogs.

Also Known As

English: blue pimpernel, helmet flower, hooded willow herb, hoodwort, mad dog weed, madweed, Quaker's hat

Finnish: rohtovuohennokka

French: scutellaire, toque

German: fieberkraut, helmkraut, schildkraut

Spanish: escutelaria

Part Used

Aboveground plant

Physiological Effects

Anaphrodisiac, anodyne, antibacterial, antispasmodic, antivenomous, astringent, bitter, brain tonic, cardiotonic, cerebral vasodilator, diuretic, emmenagogue, febrifuge, hypotensive, nervine, nervous system tonic, restorative, sedative, spinal cord tonic, stomachic

Medicinal Uses

Native Americans and early European settlers used skullcap as a treatment for malaria when quinine was not available. It was included in the United States Formulary from 1863 until 1916. Skullcap calms and strengthens the nerves, relaxes spasms, relieves pain, and promotes rest. It can help rebuild nerve sheaths. One of its constituents, scutellarin, is transformed in the body into scutellarein, which helps stimulate the brain to produce more endorphins.

Skullcap is used to treat addiction, alcoholism, anger, anxiety, attention deficit disorder, chorea, convulsions, delirium, dysmenorrhea, emotional upset, epilepsy, excessive libido, fear, headache, hiccups, high cholesterol, hypertension, hysteria, insomnia, multiple sclerosis, muscle cramps, nervous exhaustion, nervous stomach, neuralgia, pain, palsy, panic attacks, Parkinson's disease, premenstrual syndrome, restlessness, rheumatism, spasms, tremors, and withdrawal symptoms (from alcohol, drugs, and tobacco).

Skullcap works best when given over a period of time. It loses its properties more quickly than many herbs; herb stock that is more than a year old is not likely to have much therapeutic value.

As a flower essence, skullcap promotes relaxation and can be helpful for those who are preoccupied. It also aids in withdrawal from drugs, especially opiates.

Edible Uses

None known

Other Uses

In folkloric tradition, women wear skullcap to keep their husbands from being charmed by other women.

Constituents

B vitamins, pangamic acid, calcium, potassium, silicon, flavonoids (scutellarin), lignan, tannin, essential oil, scutellonin, bitter (scutellaine), palmitic acid, stearic acid, linoleic acid, oleic acid, phenols, tannin

Energetic Correspondences

- Flavor: bitter
- Temperature: cold
- Moisture: dry
- Polarity: yin
- Planet: Saturn/Mercury/Neptune/Pluto
- Element: water

Contraindications

Avoid during pregnancy. Large doses may cause confusion and giddiness.

Range and Appearance

Skullcap, a perennial native to North America and Eurasia, grows from 1 to 3 feet tall and has a square stem. The leaves are lance shaped, opposite, 1 to 3 inches long, and coarsely serrated. The hermaphroditic, pale blue flowers are tubular with a two-lipped, hooded corolla; they grow paired on spikelike, one-sided racemes from the leaf axils.

SLIPPERY ELM

Botanical Name

Ulmus rubra (syn. *U. fulva*)

Family

Ulmaceae (Elm Family)

Etymology

The genus name, *Ulmus,* is the ancient Latin name for this family of trees. The species name, *rubra,* is Latin for "red."

Also Known As

English: gray elm, Indian elm, moose elm, red elm, rock elm, slipweed, sweet elm
Finnish: puunajalava
French: l'orme rouge
German: ruesterrinde, ulmenrinde
Italian: olmo
Spanish: olmo

Part Used

Inner bark

Physiological Effects

Anti-inflammatory, antioxidant, antitussive, astringent (mild), demulcent, diuretic, emollient, expectorant, laxative, nutritive, pectoral, rejuvenative, restorative, vulnerary, yin tonic

Medicinal Uses

Slippery elm was an important remedy for both the Native Americans and the settlers of early America. This herb moistens, clears heat, neutralizes overly acidic conditions, and provides nourishment. It soothes and heals any part of the body it comes in contact with and is used to treat inflammation of the bladder, bowel, kidneys, lungs, and stomach. It is an ingredient in the anticancer formula Essiac, originally an Ojibwa formula that a Canadian nurse, René Caisse (*Essiac* spelled backward), popularized.

Slippery elm is used in the treatment of acid indigestion, AIDS, appendicitis, bipolar depression, bronchitis, colic, colitis, convalescence, cough, debil-

ity, diarrhea, diverticulitis, dysentery, gastritis, hemorrhoids, hoarseness, laryngitis, irritable bowel, nausea, nephritis, nervous breakdown, pharyngitis, pleurisy, pneumonia, sore throat, starvation, tuberculosis, typhoid, tumors, ulcers, underweight conditions, urinary tract inflammation, wasting diseases, and whooping cough.

Topically, slippery elm can be used as a poultice to treat abscess, bedsores, boils, burns, diaper rash, eczema, eye inflammation, gangrene, splinters, and wounds. It also can be added to enemas or suppositories to soothe irritated bowels or to lubricate dry intestines or to vaginal boluses to treat inflammation. It is so demulcent that midwives have used it as a hand lubricant when checking a baby's position in the birth canal during labor.

Edible Uses

Slippery elm bark is very nutritive. It is most often powdered before consumption, after which it can be eaten as a gruel, like oatmeal, that can be flavored with cinnamon, raisins, honey, and so on. Slippery elm is very easy to digest, and so it is especially beneficial for people who can't keep any other food down, such as those recovering from illness or undergoing chemotherapy. It can help nourish those who are wasting away, failing to thrive, and losing weight. It can be added to baby food as a nutritive and to nourish recently weaned infants or those who can't digest milk. It also is popular in lozenges designed to treat sore throat and coughs.

The leaves and immature fruits of the tree are also edible, raw or cooked.

Other Uses

Slippery elm is sometimes added to cosmetics as an emollient. Used as a binder, it holds herbal tablets together. At one time the bark was added to fats to prevent rancidity.

The inner bark is strong and fibrous and can be made into cordage for bow strings, bow drills, rope, clothing, mats, jewelry, roofing, wagon wheels, and even musical instruments. The powdered herb makes great tinder in starting fires.

Constituents

Vitamin C, calcium oxalate, chromium, iron, manganese, vanadium, zinc, mucilage (galactose, polysaccharides), starch, oligomeric procyanidins, tannins

Energetic Correspondences

- Flavor: sweet
- Temperature: neutral
- Moisture: moist
- Polarity: yin
- Planet: Moon/Venus/Saturn/Jupiter
- Element: air/water/Earth

Contraindications

Slippery elm is regarded as one of the safest herbs. When consuming slippery elm in capsule form, be sure to take in plenty of fluids, as it absorbs moisture in the body and can be dehydrating.

Range and Appearance

Slippery elm is a deciduous tree native to eastern and central North America. It usually grows between 20 and 60 feet in height. The brownish gray bark is deeply furrowed. The leaves are simple, alternate, 4 to 6 inches long, olive green on top and lighter below, toothed unequally, and covered with hairs on both sides. The rust-colored leaf buds are followed by dense clusters of sessile flowers of red anthers with purplish red stigmas that appear before the leaves have come out. The seeds are yellowish green, winged, and papery, with no hairs on the margins. The tree grows in open areas with full sun to partial shade and where the soil is moist and firm.

Elm trees, including slippery elm, have been subject to the fungus known as Dutch elm disease (*Graphium ulmi*), which is carried by a beetle and congests the trees' circulatory system. Elm trees are therefore becoming endangered, and using slippery elm in quantity can contribute to their demise. Marshmallow root can be used as a substitute in many cases.

SPIKENARD

Botanical Name

Aralia californica (California spikenard),
   A. nudicaulis (wild sarsaparilla), *A. racemosa*

Family

Araliaceae (Ginseng Family)

Etymology

The species name, *Aralia,* is a Latin term meaning "with racemes," in reference to the plant's structure. The common name *spikenard* derives from the Latin *spica nardi,* "spike of nard"; nard is a similar plant in the Valerian Family.

Also Known As

English: American spikenard, Indian spikenard, manroot, old man's root, petty morel, spiceberry, spignet
Finnish: terttuaralia
French: aralie
Spanish: espicanardo
Swedish: lundaralia

Part Used

Rhizome

Physiological Effects

Adaptogen, alterative, anti-inflammatory, antimicrobial, antirheumatic, aromatic, carminative, chi tonic, demulcent, diaphoretic, diuretic, expectorant, lung tonic, parturient, rejuvenative, stimulant, uterine tonic, tonic

Medicinal Uses

Spikenard is a traditional medicinal herb of the Cherokee, Shawnee, Ojibwa, and Micmac Indians. It helps the body adapt to change during stressful situations. It also stimulates phagocytosis and increases interferon synthesis in infected cells, thereby supporting immune-system function. It is used in the treatment of asthma, backache, cough, dysentery, eczema, flatulence, gout, hay fever, lumbago, premenstrual syndrome, rash, rheumatism, stomachache, syphilis, and whooping cough. It can also be used to ease childbirth.

Topically, spikenard can be used as a poultice, salve, or liniment to encourage the healing of boils, broken bones, burns, swellings, and wounds. It also can be made into a wash to treat rashes, and it is often included in cough syrups for its expectorant and demulcent properties.

Edible Uses

The root and tips of young shoots are edible and can be prepared like any vegetable. The leaves can be eaten raw or cooked. The berries are also edible and are often made into jelly and wine. Spikenard is sometimes included in root beers, tonic beers, and wines.

Other Uses

The outer bark can be burned as an incense. It is also sometimes worn in medicine bags to prevent disease and promote good luck.

Constituents

Choline, essential oils (falcarinone, falcarinolene), saponins, diterpenes acid, chlorogenic acid, ursolic acid, beta-sitosterol, araloside, tannin, resin

Energetic Correspondences

- Flavor: sweet, pungent
- Temperature: warm
- Moisture: moist
- Polarity: yin
- Planet: Saturn/Venus
- Element: water

Contraindications

Spikenard is not recommended during pregnancy, except during labor, and then only under the guidance of a qualified health-care practitioner.

Range and Appearance

A perennial native to North America, spikenard can grow from 3 to 10 feet in height. It has toothed, compound leaves that are very large, sometimes extending up to 3 feet in length. The leaves grow alternately from a zigzag stem, clasping it at the base.

The hermaphroditic flowers grow as umbels of small greenish white or greenish yellow blooms. Dark purple berries follow. The plant requires moist soil and full sun to partial shade.

SPILANTHES

Botanical Name

Spilanthes acmella (syn. *Blainvillea acmella*), *S. oleracea* (syn. *Acmella oleracea*)

Family

Asteraceae (Daisy Family)

Etymology

The genus name *Spilanthes* derives from the Greek *spiloma,* "stained flower," in reference to the plant's pollen staining its bright petals. The species name *oleracea* derives from the Latin *holus,* "leaf vegetable," while the species name *acmella* derives from the Greek *akme,* "point," "peak," or "sharp." The common name *para cress* refers to the Brazilian province Pará, the native range of *S. oleracea.*

Also Known As

Czech: plamatka
Danish: parakarse
Dutch: Braziliaanse cresson, huzarenknoop, paratuinkers
English: Para cress, Paraguay cress, toothache plant
Estonian: harilik nööpkakar
Finnish: parakrassi, spilantes
French: cresson de para, spilanthes des potagers
German: husarenknophblume, parakresse
Hungarian: huszárgomb
Indonesian: jotang
Italian: spilante
Japanese: kibana-oranda-senniti
Mandarin: jin chou kou
Portuguese: agrio do pará, jambúú
Russian: kress Brazilski, spilantes
Spanish: botón de oro, jambú
Swedish: parakrasse
Thai: phak krat, phak phet
Vietnamese: cúc áo

Parts Used

Aboveground plant

Physiological Effects

Antibiotic, antifungal, antiseptic, antiviral, immune stimulant, sialagogue

Medicinal Uses

Spilanthes is a close relative of echinacea. It stimulates wound healing, reduces swelling in glands, and is excellent for treating bacterial, fungal, and viral infections, in part by encouraging white blood cells to phagocytose bacteria. It has long been used by the Zulu people of Africa as a remedy against toothache. It is also used in the treatment of bacterial infection, bladder inflammation, candida, flatulence, fungal infection, gout, headache, malaria, nausea, rheumatic pain, staph infection, swollen glands, and viral infection. When consumed, spilanthes kills a gnat larvae that is responsible for tropical diseases such as dengue, elephantitis, jaundice, malaria, and worms.

Topically, spilanthes can be used as a compress or poultice to treat athlete's foot, nail fungus, ringworm, staph infection, snakebites, and toothache. It also can be used as a mouthwash to treat thrush or as a douche to treat candida.

Edible Uses

Spilanthes is edible. The leaves are spicy and are usually cooked, sometimes in several changes of water, to mellow them.

Other Uses

Spilanthes is sometimes included in toothpastes and mouthwashes for its antiseptic properties. The plant contains an oil that is toxic to fish, and Africans have been known to throw the squashed plant into a slow-moving body of water and wait for the dead fish to surface.

Constituents

Isobutylmine, isothiocyanates, spilanthol, polygodial, eudesmanolide, essential oils (limonene, thymol, germacrene, myrcene)

Energetic Correspondences

- Flavor: pungent, salty
- Temperature: warm
- Moisture: dry
- Polarity: yang
- Planet: Mars
- Element: fire

Contraindications

Spilanthes is nonpoisonous to humans, though toxic to cold-blooded organisms. Eating the plant can cause numbness in the mouth. The volatile isothiocyanates cause an intense pungent sensation in the mouth.

Range and Appearance

Spilanthes acmella is native to northern Africa, China, and the Indian subcontinent, while *S. oleracea* is native to South America. The leaves are opposite. The small yellow flowers grow on terminal stalks.

STAR ANISE

Botanical Name

Illicium verum

Family

Illiciaceae (Illicium Family)

Etymology

The genus name, *Illicium,* is Latin for "that which entices," in reference to the tree's pleasant scent. The species name, *verum,* is Latin for "true." The Cantonese name *baat gok* translates as "eight corners," in reference to the fruit pod's eight starry spikes.

Also Known As

Arabic: yansun najmi
Bulgarian: anason zvezdoviden
Cantonese: baat gok
Croatian: zvjezdasti anis
Czech: badyán
Danish: stjerne anis

Dutch: steranijs
English: badian anise, Chinese anise, Indian anise
Esperanto: stelanizo, ilicio
Estonian: harilik tähtaniisipuu
Finnish: tähtianis
French: anis de la Chine, anise étoilé, badiane
German: badian, sternanis
Greek: anison asteroeides
Hindi: anasphal, badayan
Hungarian: kínai ánizs
Icelandic: stjörnuanís
Indonesian: adas cina, bunga lawang, pe ka
Italian: anice stellato
Japanese: daiuikyo, kai-ko, kakkaku, suta-anisu
Korean: anisu-sutu
Mandarin: ba jiao
Norwegian: stjerneanis
Polish: badian
Portuguee: anis estreldo
Romanian: anason stelat, badian
Russian: badyan, zvezdchatyj anis
Serbian: zvezdasti anis
Spanish: anís estrella
Swedish: stärnanis
Thai: chan tanat paetklip, dok chan
Turkish: çin anasonu
Vietnamese: bát giác hu'o'ng
Yiddish: badyab

Parts Used

Fruit pod

Physiological Effects

Analgesic, anodyne, antibacterial, aromatic, carminative, circulatory stimulant, diuretic, expectorant (mild), stimulant

Medicinal Uses

Star anise soothes a wide range of digestive disorders. It is the source of one of the active ingredients, shikimic acid or shikimate, in the flu medicine Tamiflu. It is used in the treatment of backache, belching, bronchitis, colic, coughs, cramps, digestive distress, flatulence, flu, gastritis, halitosis, hernia, indigestion, nausea, and rheumatism.

Edible Uses

Star anise is widely used as a spice in Asian cuisine; in fact, it is one of the spices in Chinese five-spice blend. It has a pungent flavor that combines well with that of other herbs. Chewing a piece after a meal will freshen the breath.

Other Uses

Star anise bark can be burned as an incense. The seeds are sometimes added to potpourris and used to bait mice. They can also be used to make pendulums. The essential oil is used to scent hair products, perfumes, and soaps.

Constituents

Essential oils (anethole, anisaldehyde, caryophyllene, methycavicol, anisic acid, anisyl acetone, phellandrene, pinene, cineole, limonene, safrole), sugar, resin, tannin, shikimic acid

Energetic Correspondences

- Flavor: sweet, pungent
- Temperature: warm
- Moisture: dry
- Polarity: yang
- Planet: Jupiter
- Element: air

Contraindications

Star anise is generally regarded as safe. Do not confuse star anise (*Illicium verum*) with *I. religiosum* or *I. anisatum,* both of which are potentially toxic and can cause kidney, urinary tract, and digestive tract inflammation.

Range and Appearance

Native to southeast Asia, the star anise tree requires moist soil and full sun to partial shade. It reaches about 8 feet in height and can live to be more than one hundred years old. The leaves are lanceolate, while the hermaphroditic flowers are aromatic and yellow. The seed pods are shaped like eight-sided stars and usually are not produced until a tree is at least six years old.

STEVIA

Botanical Name

Stevia rebaudiana (formerly *Eupatorium rebaudianum*)

Family

Asteraceae (Daisy Family)

Etymology

Stevia takes its genus and common name from that of the fourteenth-century Spanish botanist P. J. Esteve. The origin of its species name is unknown.

Also Known As

Cantonese: tian ju
English: candy leaf, herb of Paraguay, honey leaf, sugar leaf, sweet herb, sweet leaf
Guarani: ka'a eirete, kaa jhee
German: honigkraut, süßkraut
Hungarian: jázmin pakóca
Italian: piccolo arbusto con foglia dolce, stevia
Japanese: kajahe, katakana, sutebia
Portuguese: capim doceestévia, erva doce
Sanskrit: madhu patra
Spanish: yerba dulce
Thai: satiwia

Parts Used

Leaf, flower

Physiological Effects

Antibacterial, antifungal, cardiotonic, diuretic, hypoglycemic, hypotensive, tonic, vasodilator

Medicinal Uses

Stevia helps lower uric acid levels and inhibits the growth of dental decay and bacteria and improves dental health. It is used in treatments for diabetes, fatigue, heartburn, hypertension, hypoglycemia, and obesity. Its primary use is as a nonsugar sweetener (see below).

Stevia has been found to promote rapid healing and to deter scarring when applied topically. It can be used as a poultice to treat acne, eczema, dermatitis, seborrhea, and wounds. It also can be used as a hair rinse to moisturize dry hair and prevent hair loss.

Edible Uses

Stevia has been used as a natural sweetener for centuries in South America, especially by the Guarani Indians. Stevia leaf is about thirty times sweeter than sugar, and it has only $1/300$ th the amount of calories contained in sugar. (One of its glycosides, stevioside, is 150 to 300 times sweeter than sugar.) Stevia is safe for those with candida, helps control sugar cravings, and does not disrupt blood sugar levels. Its flavor comes on slower than that of sugar, and some say it has a licorice aftertaste. In Japan, stevia accounts for about 40 percent of the sweetener market. Unlike many chemical sweeteners, stevia's flavor is stable when heated.

Other Uses

Stevia is sometimes used to flavor toothpastes and mouthwashes.

Constituents

Vitamin C, calcium, chromium, iron, magnesium, phosphorous, potassium, selenium, silicon, zinc, diterpene glycoside (stevioside, rebaudiosides), stigmasterol, beta-sitosterol

Energetic Correspondences

- Flavor: sweet
- Temperature: neutral
- Moisture: moist
- Planet: Venus
- Element: water

Contraindications

Generally considered safe. Too much stevia can leave an aftertaste.

Range and Appearance

Stevia is an annual and sometimes perennial shrub native to Brazil and Paraguay but cultivated in highland tropics elsewhere. It grows to about 3 feet in height. Its leaves are opposite and toothed, born on a wandlike, hairy stem. The flowers are white, hermaphroditic, and tubular. The plant prefers moist soil, a humid climate, and plenty of sunshine.

SYRIAN RUE

Botanical Name

Peganum harmala

Family

Nitariaceae (Nitaria Family)

Etymology

The genus name, *Peganum,* is the classical Greek name for a species of rue, which Syrian rue was thought to resemble, although the two are not related. The species name, *harmala,* derives from that of the Lebanese town Hermel.

Also Known As

Arabic: harmal
English: African rue, harmala, hoama, soma
French: harmel
German: gemeine syrische, steppenraute
Italian: ruta di Siria

Parts Used

Seed

Physiological Effects

Abortifacient, alterative, antibacterial, antitumor, antiviral, aphrodisiac, digestive, diuretic, emmenagogue, entheogen, euphoric, galactagogue, hallucinogen, intoxicant, narcotic, ophthalmic, purgative, sedative, uterine tonic, vermifuge

Medicinal Uses

Syrian rue has entheogenic and hallucinatory effects. Some scholars believe that it is the euphoric soma plant mentioned in the Rig Vedas, one of the holy books of Hinduism. It is sometimes used as an ayahuasca admixture.

Syrian rue increases heart activity yet lowers blood pressure. It also functions as a monoamine oxidase inhibitor. It is being investigated for its potential in treating mental illness and encephalitis. It is used in the treatment of depression, nervousness, Parkinson's disease, rheumatism, and worms.

Topically, Syrian rue can be prepared as a wash to treat eczema and psoriasis; as a hair rinse to treat dandruff and stop hair loss; and as a compress to treat hemorrhoids.

Edible Uses

Syrian rue is used as a seasoning in Mideastern dishes. An edible oil is made from the seeds.

Other Uses

The seeds are burned as an incense said to promote mental clarity. A red dye, sometimes used to color Turkish rugs, is made from the seeds and fruit. In Turkey the dried seed capsules are traditionally strung together and displayed in cars and homes to give protection against the "evil eye."

Energetic Correspondences

- Flavor: bitter
- Temperature: warm
- Moisture: dry
- Polarity: yang
- Planet: Mars
- Element: fire

Constituents

Indole alkaloids (harmine, harmaline, harmalol, peganine ruine), beta-carbolines

Contraindications

Avoid during pregnancy. Nausea, vomiting, and hallucinations are possible side effects.

Range and Appearance

Syrian rue is native to the Mideast and northern Africa, though it has been introduced into the American Southwest. This hardy desert shrub does best in well-drained soil and full sun; it will tolerate salty soil and moist or dry conditions. It grows less than 3 feet tall. It has finely divided leaves that are 1 to 2 inches long. The hermaphroditic, five-lobed, white flowers are followed by three-celled seed capsules that turn orangish brown when ripe.

TANSY

Botanical Name

Tanacetum vulgare (formerly *Chrysanthemum vulgare*)

Family

Asteraceae (Daisy Family)

Etymology

The genus name *Tanacetum* and common name *tansy* derive from the Greek *athanasia*, in Greek mythology the name of an immortality drink given to the youth Ganymede so that he might serve Zeus as his cupbearer for all time. The species name *vulgare* is Latin for "common."

Also Known As

English: bitter buttons, common tansy, gold
   buttons, Prince of Wale's feathers, stinking willie
Finnish: pietaryrtti
French: tanaisie
German: boerenwormkruid, gemeiner, rainfarn,
   wurmkraut
Italian: tanaceto, tanasia
Japanese: yomogi-giku
Spanish: atanasia, tanaceto
Swedish: renfana
Turkish: soglucan otu

Part Used

Flowering top

Physiological Effects

Abortifacient, anthelmintic, antiseptic, antispasmodic, aromatic, bitter, carminative, diaphoretic, emmenagogue, insecticide, vermifuge

Medicinal Uses

Tansy relieves spasms, stimulates the production of bile, and inhibits a wide range of pathogens, including fungi and bacteria. It is used in the treatment of amenorrhea, hysteria, jaundice, nausea, and worms (roundworm, threadworm).

Topically, tansy can be made into a lotion or wash to repel fleas, lice, and scabies; an astringent facial toner or steam; or a compress or poultice to treat bruises, rheumatism, sprains, sunburn, and swelling.

As a flower essence, tansy helps users to be more purposeful and straightforward. It is beneficial for those who suffer from lethargy, are unable to make decisions, may have suffered violent childhoods, and during times of chaos tend to withdraw.

Edible Uses

Tansy can be eaten in small amounts as a bitter edible spring green, raw or cooked. The flowers are sometimes used as an edible garnish. The leaves and stems produce a lemon-flavored tea.

Other Uses

Whether in the garden or dried and in the home, tansy can be used to repel a wide range of pests, including ants, aphids, bed bugs, Colorado potato beetles, fleas, moths, and mice. It was once used as a strewing herb, and dead bodies were once rubbed with tansy to prevent decay and mask odors. The young shoots yield a green dye, while the leaves and flowers produce a yellow dye. In the language of flowers it is said to symbolize immortality, as its dried flowers are long lasting. In folkloric tradition, it is said to promote longevity.

Constituents

Vitamin C, citric acid, butyric acid, oxalic acid, flavonoids (quercetin, jaceidin), essential oils (borneol, thujone, camphor), sesquiterpene lactones, pyrethinsresin, tannins

Energetic Correspondences

- Flavor: bitter, pungent
- Temperature: cool
- Moisture: dry
- Polarity: yin
- Planet: Venus
- Element: water

Contraindications

Avoid during pregnancy, as it can induce abortion. Also avoid in cases of epilepsy. Tansy is potentially toxic to the central nervous system; do not use for extended periods. Some may find that the plant causes contact dermatitis. Do not use the essential oil, which is very toxic.

Range and Appearance

Tansy is a perennial native to Asia and Europe but widely naturalized. It prefers well-drained soil and full sun and grows to about 3 feet tall. The leaves are pinnate and uniformly toothed, while the yellow ray flowers are hermaphroditic and grow in corymbs. In the garden, tansy attracts butterflies, but it also is aggressive and tends to overtake nearby areas. Thankfully, it also fixes minerals and is a beneficial, mineral-rich additive to composts.

TARRAGON

Botanical Name

Artemisia dracunculus

Family

Asteraceae (Daisy Family)

Etymology

The genus name *Artemisia* derives from that of the Greek goddess Artemis. The species name *dracunculus* is Latin for "little dragon," in reference to the belief that tarragon offered protection from dragons and snakes, and perhaps also to the serpentine shape of the root. The common name *tarragon* derives from the ancient Arabic name for this plant, *tarkhun*.

Also Known As

Arabic: tarkhun
Bulgarian: estragon, taros
Cantonese: ngaai hou
Croatian: estragon, tarkanj
Czech: estragon
Danish: esdragon
Dutch: dragon, drakebloed
English: dragon wormwood, French tarragon,
   little dragon, true tarragon
Esperanto: drakunkulo
Finnish: rakuuna
French: estragon, herbe dragonne
German: estragon
Greek: estrangon
Hebrew: taragon
Hungarian: tárkony
Icelandic: darnoncella, esdragon
Italian: targone
Japanese: esutoragon, taragon
Mandarin: ai hao
Norwegian: estragon
Polish: estragon
Portuguese: estragão
Romanian: tarhon
Russian: estragon, tarkhun
Serbian: estragon
Spanish: estragon, tarragón
Swedish: dragon, dragonört
Thai: taeragon
Turkish: tarhun
Ukrainian: ostrohin, polyn estrahon
Yiddish: estragon

Parts Used

Aboveground plant, root

Physiological Effects

Antiscorbutic, aperient, aromatic, carminative, digestive, diuretic, emmenagogue, febrifuge, galactagogue, hypnotic, odontalgic, stomachic, vermifuge

Medicinal Uses

Tarragon increases circulation to the digestive tract, thus offering relief from a wide range of digestive complaints. It is used in the treatment of arthritis, flatulence, gout, halitosis, hiccups, hyperactivity, insomnia, nausea, rheumatism, and worms.

Topically, tarragon can be prepared as an anesthetic compress or poultice to relive arthritis pain, toothache, and rheumatism pain.

Edible Uses

Tarragon leaf has a light, aniselike flavor and has long been used as a culinary spice. It is best when fresh, rather than dried, and it aids in the digestion of proteins and fats. The young shoots are also edible.

Other Uses

The essential oil is used in perfumery. The growing and dried plant is used as an insect repellent.

Constituents

Vitamin C, flavonoids (quercitin, rutin), iodine, essential oils (methyl chivacol, pinene, camphene, limonene, eugenol), tannins, coumarins

Energetic Correspondences

- Flavor: sweet, bitter
- Temperature: cool
- Moisture: dry
- Polarity: yin
- Planet: Mars
- Element: fire

Contraindications

Do not take therapeutic doses during pregnancy; culinary use, however, is fine. Use for no longer than one month continuously. In some cases the plant can cause contact dermatitis.

Range and Appearance

Tarragon is a perennial native to western Asia and North America. It grows to about $2\frac{1}{2}$ feet tall. The dark green leaves reach about 3 inches in length and are long, narrow, and pointed. The hermaphroditic flowers are lime green and aromatic. Tarragon prefers well-drained, dry soils and partial shade to full sun. It is drought tolerant.

TEA

Botanical Name

Camellia sinensis (syn. *Thea sinensis*)

Family

Theaceae (Tea Family)

Etymology

The genus name *Camellia* was given in honor of Georg Josef Kamel, a Moravian Jesuit missionary who died in 1706. The species name *sinensis* is a Latin term meaning "native to China." The common name *tea* derives from the name given the plant in the Amoy dialect of Chinese, *dé*.

Also Known As

Afrikaans: tee
Arabic: chai, shi
Armenian: te
Czech: thé
French: thé
German: teestrauch
Hindi: chai
Icelandic: te
Italian: tè
Japanese: cha
Norwegian: te
Spanish: té
Swahili: chai
Swedish: te
Tibetan: ja
Vietnamese: chè
Yiddish: tei

Parts Used

Leaf bud, young leaf

Physiological Effects

Analgesic, antibacterial, anticarcinogenic, antioxidant, antiseptic, antiviral, astringent, cardiotonic, decongestant, diaphoretic, diuretic, expectorant, hypotensive, immune stimulant, nervine, stimulant

Medicinal Uses

It is the constituent polyphenols, a type of flavonoid containing catechin and proanthocyanidins that have earned tea such a reputation for imbuing good health. Of the three most common types of tea—black, green, and oolong—green tea contains the most polyphenols, at about 15 to 30 percent by weight. About half of that is epigallocatechin gallate (EGCC). But black and oolong teas are not far behind.

Tea's polyphenols, especially EGCG, are recognized as antioxidant. They prevent free-radical damage and have even been found to lower levels of free

A Tea Course

There are more than three thousand tea varieties. They are often named for the areas in which they are grown, such as Assam or Darjeeling. Cultivation in different regions, soils, altitudes, and climates produces different flavors in tea. Teas grown at a higher altitude tend to mature more slowly and produce a lower yield, and they are considered of a higher quality. The best-quality tea uses just the tender young leaves and buds.

Green Teas

Green teas are made from unfermented leaves. Soon after the leaves are collected, they are left to wither, until their moisture is gone. The whole leaves are then steamed and rolled, resulting in grayish green balls. This process allows the herb to retain its enzymes, thus preventing it from oxidizing. Green tea is higher in essential oils than the black variety.

Dragonwell. A high-grade tea with jade green leaves and a nutlike flavor.

Gunpowder Green. Its name comes from early British colonists in China, who thought the tea resembled lead ball shots. The leaves are tightly rolled into small, ball-like pellets. This type of compaction helps protect the flavor and essential oil content of the tea. It is considered one of the most popular and highest grades and has a slightly bitter flavor. Also known as pearl tea.

Jasmine. Produced by drying tea leaves along with jasmine flowers. It is considered a semifermented tea, having the color of black tea but the flavor of green tea. It has a sweet, distinct flavor.

Sencha. A Japanese green tea made from long, green leaves and used for everyday consumption.

Young Hyson. A high-grade tea whose middle-aged leaves are either rolled or twisted.

Black Teas

Black teas are produced in India and China. Their leaves are withered and rolled and then fermented. This process breaks down the enzymes, producing a varnish like coating on the tea. The leaves are then dried. The fermentation process causes black tea to lose some of its medicinal activity, however.

Assam. Grown in northeast India. Has a full-bodied, malty, rich, strong flavor and a dark copper color.

It is used as a base to make many other tea blends, such as Irish and English breakfast blends.

Ceylon. Grown in Sri Lanka and one of the most popular of the black teas. Has a bright color and is flavorful hot or iced, with or without milk.

Darjeeling. From a mountainous region in northern India. Prepared from small, broken leaves. Considered medium strong, with a light golden color and an aftertaste that has been compared to that of almonds, fruit, and muscatel. It is often considered the champagne of teas and usually is consumed unblended.

Earl Grey. A black tea flavored with essential oil of bergamot, a citrus fruit that grows in the Mediterranean region.

Keemum. From northern China. Has a light, delicate aroma, low tannin content, and rich, deep flavor.

Lapsang Souchong. A smoky, tarry-flavored, large-leafed tea from China. Its smoky, pungent flavor comes from the leaves being smoked over pinewood fires. The smoking causes the leaves to dry more quickly than through sun drying. It is considered to be one of China's best black teas.

Oolong Teas

Oolong teas come mainly from the southeastern coasts of China and Taiwan. After being harvested, the leaves are left to wither to remove some of their moisture. They are then rolled by a machine to release their juices, followed by a partial fermenting process and oven firing. The tea's copperish color is somewhere between that of green and black teas. Oolong tea's flavor is milder than that of black tea but stronger than that of green tea. It contains the same cancer-fighting properties as green and black teas.

Formosa Oolong. A product of Taiwan. Allowed to

ferment longer than most other oolongs. Has a balanced, fruity, peachlike flavor and is usually consumed black, without any milk or sweetener. It is the most popular of the oolongs.

Pouchong. Fermented for less time than most other oolongs. Sometimes used to make jasmine tea.

Ti Kuan Yin. The name means "iron goddess of mercy" in Chinese. A highly prized oolong tea with a smooth flavor.

White Teas

Of all the teas prepared from *Camellia sinensis,* white tea undergoes the least amount of processing and so contains the highest level of antioxidants. It also is very rare and expensive. It has a sweet, subtle flavor.

radicals produced by the environmental toxin paraquat. EGCG has been found to be twenty times stronger than vitamin E in protecting brain lipids, which are very susceptible to oxidative stress.

Polyphenols are also anticarcinogenic. Surveys of Japanese tea drinkers show that those consuming four to six cups daily have lower rates of breast, esophageal, liver, lung, and skin cancers than those who consume less or none at all. Other studies support these findings, indicating that consuming green tea can reduce the occurrence of a wide range of cancers.

Green tea prevents blood platelet aggregation, the "clumping together" of blood that can lead to blood clots, heart attacks, and stroke. Tea's polyphenols, along with its vitamin C content, also help strengthen blood vessel walls. In fact, the consumption of green tea with meals has been shown to reduce the occurrence of arterial disease, while a study of six thousand Japanese women who were nondrinkers and nonsmokers over the age of 40 found that those who drank about five cups of green tea daily had a 50 percent decrease in the risk of stroke.

Whereas coffee can elevate cholesterol levels, green tea helps lower them. The catechin content of green tea helps break down cholesterol and increase its elimination through the bowels. Green tea also helps keep blood sugar levels moderate. Tea also stimulates the metabolism and is used as an aid in weight loss.

Even though caffeine gets a bad rap, it has many healthful benefits. Green tea has about 25 mg of caffeine per cup; black tea has about 35 to 40 mg. The caffeine content of green tea is about as much as that of a can of soda and one-third to half as much as that of a cup of coffee. Caffeine blocks the naturally occurring tranquilizer adenosine, so that the brain becomes stimulated. It also increases the synthesis of catecholamines, which are stimulant chemicals that relay nerve impulses in the brain. It is believed that the constituent tannins and vitamin C help moderate the effects of caffeine in tea, so that the deleterious side effects—jitteriness, irritability, and (after the effect has worn off) fatigue—are minimal compared to other caffeine sources, which may explain why Zen monks rely on green tea to help them remain alert yet calm during long periods of meditation.

The xanthines in green tea help relax bronchial spasms and can help relieve the symptoms of allergies and asthma, which can be especially useful in emergencies when other remedies are not readily available.

Green tea helps prevent dental decay by inhibiting the enzyme streptococcus mutans, which is responsible for plaque formation, and it also is a rich source of natural fluoride, which helps strengthen tooth enamel. A cup of green tea a day has been found to decrease cavities in children by half. It can also help inhibit the bacteria that cause halitosis.

Many other of tea's constituents compounds have been and are being studied. One of the widely researched components in tea is the alkaloid theanine; it is an amino acid that has been found to decrease anxiety, aid in sleep, and promote mental focus. Russian research indicates that the tannins in tea can help the body excrete strontium 90, a radioactive substance that can build up in the bones.

All in all, tea has many amazing therapeutic usages. More specificially, it is used in the treatment of allergies, arteriosclerosis, asthma, cancer, catarrh, cholera, high cholesterol, colds, congestion, coughs, depression, diarrhea, digestive tract infection, dysentery, external viral conditions (black tea), fatigue, fever, flu, hangover, hepatitis, influenza (green tea), migraines, obesity, tooth decay, typhus, and tumors.

Topically, green tea is styptic, meaning that it stops bleeding. It can be applied as a lukewarm compress or poultice to treat acne, athlete's foot, open wounds, and sunburn.

Compresses of cooled black tea can be used to reduce the inflammation of herpes, insect bites, puffy eyes, shingles, and sunburn.

Edible Uses

Tea has long been a popular beverage. The processing of and amount of essential oils and tannins in tea leaves, which varies depending on where and how the tea was cultivated, create a variety of flavor nuances. In general, green tea has a milder flavor than black tea. Drinking tea after a meal aids in the digestion of fats, reducing the risk of arterial disease.

Tea flowers are edible; they are often battered and deep fried. An oil obtained from the seeds is also edible.

Other Uses

A gray dye is made from the flowers of the plant. The wood from the tea plant is used in making walking sticks. In folkloric traditions tea is burned as an incense to attract prosperity and carried to impart strength and courage.

Constituents

Carotenoids, vitamin C, vitamin E, manganese, potassium, zinc, fluoride, xanthines alkaloids (caffeine, theanine, theophylline, theobromine), tannins (polyphenols, epigallocatechin, epicatechin, epigallocatechin gallate, proanthocyanidins), flavonoids (kaempferol, quercitin), fats, gamma-amino butyric acid, polysaccharides, alkaloids (theanine)

Energetic Correspondences

- Flavor: bitter, sweet
- Temperature: warm (black tea) or cool (green and oolong teas)
- Moisture: dry
- Polarity: yang
- Planet: sun
- Element: fire

Contraindications

Excessive use of tea may cause nervous irritability and digestive distress such as ulcers. Some believe tea to be addictive. Avoid tea in cases of hypertension and insomnia; avoid large doses during pregnancy and while nursing.

Range and Appearance

Left to their own devices, evergreen tea shrubs are capable of growing to heights of 25 to 30 feet, but when cultivated they are pruned to about 4 feet to facilitate the harvesting of the leaves. The leaves are alternate and oval or lanceolate, with short stalks. The small white or pink flowers are solitary or grouped in twos or threes, and they have five to nine petals formed in a corolla.

Tea shrubs grow best in warm, humid climates; they are native to China, India, and Indochina but are widely cultivated. Each bush produces about a quarter pound of tea leaves a year and can continue producing for twenty-five to fifty years and even up to one hundred years, especially if organically cultivated. The leaves are harvested every six to fourteen days.

TEASEL

Botanical Name

Dipsacus spp., including *D. fullonum* (common teasel), *D. japonicus*

Family

Dipsacaceae (Teasel Family)

Etymology

The genus name *Dipsacus* derives from the ancient Greek *dipsao*, "to be thirsty," in reference to the characteristic cups formed by the leaves, which hold water. The common name *teasel* derives from the Old English *tæsan*, "to tease," in reference to the use of the tops in carding wool.

Also Known As

Dutch: vollers kaarden

English: brushes and combs, church brooms, gypsy combs, tazzel, Venus basin, Venus bath, water thistle

French: chardon à bennetier, chardon à foulon

German: grote kaardebol, schuttkarde, weberkarde

Italian: cardo di venere, dissaco, scardaccione, verga da pastore

Japanese: zokudan

Korean: sokdan

Mandarin: xù dùan

Spanish: cardencha

Turkish: coban daragi

Part Used

Root

Physiological Effects

Alterative, aperient, astringent, circulatory stimulant, diaphoretic, digestive, diuretic, ophthalmic, stomachic, sudorific, tonic

Medicinal Uses

Teasel helps strengthen the stomach, improves blood circulation, and clears obstructions in the liver so they can be eliminated. It is used in the treatment of arthritis, cancer, diarrhea, jaundice, osteoporosis, rheumatism, and warts. It is also used to prevent miscarriage.

Topically, teasel can be prepared as a healing wash to treat acne, eye inflammation, itchy skin, sties, and wounds. It also can be prepared as a poultice to get rid of warts.

Edible Uses

The young leaves, can be eaten raw or cooked.

Other Uses

The tops of the teasel plant, with their downward-hooked bracteoles, have long been used to tease or card wool. A blue dye can be made from the plant.

Constituents

Inulin, bitter substances, sabioside, alkaloid (lamine), essential oil

Energetic Correspondences

- Flavor: bitter
- Temperature: warm
- Moisture: dry
- Polarity: yang
- Planet: Mars
- Element: fire

Contraindications

Generally regarded as safe.

Range and Appearance

Teasel is a bienniel or perennial herb that can grow to 6 feet tall. The opposite or whorled leaves unite at the plant's base, forming a cup around the stem. The irregular, tubular, hermaphroditic, pink or purple flowers form in dense, conelike heads at the top of the erect stems. The stems and leaf veins and margins are spiny.

Teasel prefers moist, clayey, rich soil and full sun. It attracts butterflies to the garden. In many areas, though, it is considered an invasive weed.

THYME

Botanical Name

Thymus spp., including *T. serpyllum* (wild thyme), *T. vulgaris* (garden thyme)

Family

Lamiaceae (Mint Family)

Etymology

The genus name *Thymus* and common name *thyme* are thought to derive from the Greek *thymon*, "to fumigate," in reference to the plant's use as incense.

Also Known As

Arabic: satr, zatr

Armenian: cotor, dzotor

Bulgarian: mashterka gradinska

Cantonese: baak leih heung

Croatian: timijan

Czech: tymián

Danish: timian

Dutch: tijm

Esperanto: timiano

Estonian: tüümian

Finnish: timjami

French: thym

German: thymian

Greek: thymari

Hebrew: timin, koranit

Hungarian: timián

Icelandic: timjan

Indonesian: timi

Italian: timo

Japanese: taimu

Korean: taim

Mandarin: bai li xiang

Norwegian: timian

Polish: tymianek

Portuguese: tomilho

Romanian: cimbru

Russian: timyan

Sanskrit: ipar

Serbian: timijan

Spanish: tomillo

Swedish: timjan

Thai: taymat

Turkish: dag kekigi

Ukrainian: chebrets

Yiddish: feldkiml

Part Used

Aboveground plant

Physiological Effects

Anthelmintic, antibiotic, antifungal, antimicrobial, antiseptic, antispasmodic, antitussive, aromatic, astringent, bronchial dilator, carminative, decongestant, diaphoretic, diuretic, emmenagogue, expectorant, immune tonic, rejuvenative, rubefacient, sedative (in small amounts), stimulant (in larger amounts), vermifuge, vulnerary

Medicinal Uses

Thyme helps loosen mucus, soothes inflamed mucous membranes, loosens the bronchials, and promotes tissue repair. It also strengthens the immune system and nourishes and warms the lungs, nerves, and adrenals. It is used in the treatment of alcoholism, asthma, bronchitis, colds, colic, coughs, depression, diarrhea, dysmenorrhea, dyspepsia, flatulence, flu, hangover, hay fever, headaches, herpes, hysteria, indigestion, laryngitis, pleurisy, rheumatism, shingles, sinusitis, sore throat, stomachache, tetanus, tuberculosis, whooping cough, and worms (hookworm, roundworms, threadworms).

Topically, thyme cleanses infection and increases circulation to the area to which it is applied. It can be used as a gargle or mouthwash to treat dental decay, halitosis, laryngitis, mouth sores, plaque formation, sore throat, thrush, and tonsillitis. As a compress thyme treats bronchitis, bruises, colds, congestion (in the lungs), flu, insect bites, mastitis, and wounds. It can be prepared as a soak to treat fungal infections such as athlete's foot, ringworm, and parasites such as crabs, lice, and scabies or as a douche to deter candida. Thyme tea can be used an as eyewash for sore eyes and as a hair rinse for dandruff. As a bath herb, it relieves sore muscles, arthritis, and the congestion and achiness of colds and flu.

As a flower essence, thyme supports strength, courage, and stamina. It helps users adapt to the passage of time and helps protect the mind and body from aging too quickly.

Edible Uses

Thyme is a common culinary spice and also aids in the digestion of fatty foods. Thyme-infused honey is excellent. As a tea thyme is congestion-relieving, stimulating, and aromatic.

Other Uses

Fairies are said to dance upon beds of thyme. In ancient Roman times thyme was burned to deter scorpions. It is still used for embalming. The essential oil is used in perfumery, cosmetics, and soaps.

Constituents

Vitamin B, vitamin C, chromium, manganese, essential oils (borneol, carvacrol, cymol, linalool, phenol, thymol), bitter principle, tannin, flavonoids (apigenin, luteolin), saponins, triterpenic acids

Energetic Correspondences

- Flavor: pungent, mildly bitter
- Temperature: warm
- Moisture: dry
- Polarity: yang
- Planet: Mars/Venus
- Element: fire/water

Contraindications

Avoid therapeutic doses during pregnancy.

Range and Appearance

Thyme, native to Europe, Asia, and northern Africa but widely cultivated, is a semi woody plant growing to between 6 and 8 inches in height. It has small, flat, oval leaves that range in color from gray-green to dark green. The tiny, aromatic, hermaphroditic flowers are lilac, white, or pink in color and grow in loose spikes.

Thyme prefers light, warm, well-drained, and somewhat dry soil, along with full sun. It requires little care in the garden.

TRIBULUS

Botanical Name

Tribulus cistoides, T. terrestris

Family

Zygophylaceae (Caltrop Family)

Etymology

The genus name, *Tribulus*, is a Greek term for the caltrop, a spiky weapon used against cavalry, in reference to the appearance of the plant's fruit.

Also Known As

Cantonese: baak jat lai
English: caltrop, goat's head, ground burnut,
    Jamaica feverplant, Mexican sandbur,
    puncture vine, terror of the earth, yellow vine
Japanese: byakushitsuri
Korean: paekchillyo
Mandarin: bai ji li, ci ji li
Sanskrit: gokshura, shvadamstra
Spanish: abrojo

Part Used

Fruit

Physiological Effects

Abortifacient, alterative, analgesic, anodyne, anthelmintic, antibacterial, anti-inflammatory, antiparasitic, antispasmodic, aphrodisiac, bone tonic, bronchial dilator, carminative, demulcent, diuretic, galactagogue, hepatotonic, hypotensive, kidney tonic, lithotriptic, nervine, parturient, pectoral, rejuvenative, restorative, sedative, tonic

Medicinal Uses

Tribulus is used in Ayurvedic medicine to enhance mental clarity. It is often promoted to athletes as an agent to increase muscle buildup and burn fat, though more research is needed to substantiate these claims. It is known to relieve pain, increase testosterone levels, improve the flow of liver chi, clear the lungs, stimulate circulation, and soothe the mucous membranes of the urinary tract.

Tribulus is used in the treatment of amenorrhea, anemia, arteriosclerosis, atherosclerosis, irritable bowel syndrome, Bright's disease, cancer, cystitis (chronic), diabetes, dizziness, dyspenea, dysuria, eczema, edema, erectile dysfunction, eye irritation (redness, swelling), flatulence, gonorrhea, gout, headache (related to hypertension), hemorrhoids, high cholesterol, hives, hypertension, incontinence, infertility, kidney stones, leukorrhea, low sperm count, lumbago, nocturnal emissions, nosebleeds, pain, premature ejaculation, polyuria, postpartum bleeding, psoriasis, shingles, spermatorrhea, tinnitis, uric acid buildup, urinary stones, venereal disease, vision problems, and vitiligo. It also can be used to ease labor that has been difficult and to facilitate postpartum bleeding.

Topically, tribulus-infused oil can be applied to the scalp to keep alopecia (balding) from progressing and in some cases to stimulate new hair growth. It can also be applied topically to treat psoriasis and leprosy.

Edible Uses

The immature fruits (ground into a meal) and young leaves and shoots are edible, though they are usually cooked before being consumed. They are not particularly tasty and are considered an emergency food.

Other Uses

None known

Constituents

Beta-carotene, protein, iron, vitamin C, linoleic acid, kaempferol, sapogenins (chlorogenin, diosgenin, gitogenin), essential oil, alkaloids (harmine), tribuloside, tannin

Energetic Correspondences

- Flavor: sweet, bitter
- Temperature: warm
- Moisture: dry
- Polarity: yang
- Planet: Mars
- Element: fire

Contraindications

Avoid during pregnancy, except under the guidance of a qualified health-care practitioner. Avoid in cases of dehydration or blood or chi deficiency. In rare cases tribulus may cause stomach upset, which is diminished by taking the herb with food.

Range and Appearance

Tribulus is native to Africa, Asia, Australia, and Europe but widely naturalized; it is considered an invasive weed in some parts of North America. This low-growing annual or biennial vine requires well-drained soil and full sun but can thrive in drought or desert conditions. It reaches a length of about 3 feet. The oval leaves grow opposite in evenly pinnate-compound leaflets, with five to seven pairs. It has purple and yellow hermaphroditic flowers. The fruits are made of four or five segments, each segment resembling a triangular hatchet, and are covered with sharp spines.

TURMERIC

Botanical Name

Curcuma longa

Family

Zingerberaceae (Ginger Family)

Etymology

The genus name *Curcuma* derives from the Arabic *kurkum,* "saffron," in reference to turmeric's saffronlike color. The common name *turmeric* derives from the medieval Latin *terra merita,* "deserving earth," perhaps in reference to turmeric's color resembling mineral pigments. In many languages the literal translation of the common name for this plant is simply "yellow earth."

Also Known As

Arabic: kurkum
Armenian: toormerik
Bulgarian: kurkuma
Cantonese: wòhng gèung

Croatian: kurkuma

Czech: kurkuma

Danish: gurkemege

Dutch: geelwortel, kurkuma

English: Indian saffron, yellow ginger

Esperanto: kurkumo

Estonian: kurkum

Finnish: kurkuma

French: curcuma

German: curcuma, gelbwurz, kurkuma

Greek: kitrinoriza, kourkoumas

Hawaiian: olena

Hindi: haldi

Hebrew: kurkum

Hungarian: kurkuma

Icelandic: túrmerik

Indonesian: kunyit, kunir

Italian: curcuma

Japanese: tamerikku, ukon

Korean: kang-hwanh, tumerik

Mandarin: huang jiang

Napali: besar, haldi

Norwegian: gurkemeie

Polish: kurkuma

Portuguese: curcuma

Russian: imbir zhyoltyj, kurkuma

Sanskrit: haridra, nisha, ragani

Serbian: kurkuma

Spanish: cúrcuma

Swahili: manjano

Swedish: gurkmeja

Thai: kha min, kha min chan

Tibetan: gaser, sga ser

Turkish: hint safrani, zerdecube

Ukrainian: kurkuma

Vietnamese: bôt nghêê

Part Used

Rhizome

Physiological Effects

Alterative, analgesic, antifungal, anti-inflammatory, antimutagenic, antioxidant, antimicrobial, antiseptic, aromatic, astringent, carminative, cholagogue, choleretic, circulatory stimulant, emmenagogue, hepatoprotective, hepatotonic, hypoglycemic, stimulant, stomachic, vulnerary

Medicinal Uses

Turmeric helps stabilize the body's microflora, thus inhibiting yeast overgrowth. It also sensitizes the body's cortisol receptor sites and thus is an excellent anti-inflammatory agent. It helps regulate the menses, can prevent blood clots from forming, and is restorative after childbirth. It is used in the treatment of arthritis, asthma, bloating, cancer, candida, catarrh, colds, eczema, flatulence, flu, gastritis, high cholesterol, jaundice, nausea, trauma, and uterine tumors.

Topically, turmeric can be prepared as a poultice to treat athlete's foot, bruises, eczema, psoriasis, swelling, and wounds.

Edible Uses

Dried or fresh turmeric root is a popular spice in Asian, and particularly Indian, cuisine. The root is eaten raw in southern India. Turmeric aids in the digestion of fats and protein.

It can be used in small amounts to make yellow food coloring. The fresh leaves can also be used as a flavoring.

Other Uses

In Asia turmeric is sometimes an ingredient in cosmetics. An extract from the leaf is used in sunscreens. In northern Indian traditional wedding ceremonies, turmeric is applied to the bride and groom to offer protection from "the evil eye." In Nepal, traditionally shepherds anoint their "third eye" (in the center of the forehead) with a turmeric paste before going out to work in the high mountains to bestow protection, blessings, and success. In other folkloric traditions turmeric is considered a symbol of prosperity and is used for purification.

Constituents

Curcumin, essential oils (artumerone, zingberene, borneol, turmerone), valepotriates, alkaloids, protein

Energetic Correspondences

- Flavor: pungent, sweet
- Temperature: warm
- Moisture: dry
- Polarity: yang
- Planet: Mercury/Sun/Moon
- Element: fire

Contraindications

Avoid therapeutic dosages during pregnancy (though culinary use is fine). Turmeric may cause photosensivity in some individuals. It may also cause contact dermatitis in rare cases.

Range and Appearance

Native to southern Asia, turmeric is a perennial that grows up to $1\frac{1}{2}$ feet tall. The leaves are long and bladelike. The beautiful white flowers grow in spikes. The orange root grows to about 2 feet in length. The plant requires a warm, frost-free climate, light shade, and moderate water.

USNEA

Botanical Name

Usnea spp., including *U. barbata, U. bayle,*
 U. californica, U. ceratine, U. dasypoga,
 U. diffracta, U. filipendula, U. florida, U. hirta,
 U. lobata, U. longissima, U. plicata

Family

Parmeliaceae (Usnea Family)

Etymology

The genus and common name *usnea* derives from the Arabic *usna,* "moss."

Also Known As

Cantonese: chung lo
English: beard moss, hair lichen, old man's beard, tree moss, witch's broom
Finnish: naava
French: barbe de capucin, usnee barbue
German: bart-flechte

Italian: barba di bosco
Japanese: kayu angin, saruogase
Mandarin: hai feng teng, song luo
Swedish: grå skägglav

Parts Used

Mycelia (of the thallus)

Physiological Effects

Analgesic, antibacterial, antibiotic, antifungal, anti-inflammatory, antiparasitic, antiseptic, antispasmodic, antitumor, antiviral, bronchial dilator, expectorant, febrifuge, immune stimulant, vasodilator, vulnerary

Medicinal Uses

Usnea's medicinal use dates back to ancient China, when it was used to treat infection. It is still used for that purpose today. It is believed usnea works against gram-positive bacteria thanks to its usnic acid content, which penetrates the bacteria cell walls and blocks the cells' production of adenosine triphosphate, or ATP (a nuclear peptide that functions as a cellular energy source), essentially rendering them useless. It does not, however, adversely affect human cells, since usnic acid is not able to penetrate their cell walls. In addition, unlike many other antibiotics, usnea does not kill off friendly intestinal flora.

Usnea is used in the treatment of bacterial infection, bronchitis, candida, chlamydia, colds, cough, cystitis, diarrhea, dysentery, flu, giardia, gonorrhea, hemorrhage, impetigo, infection, leukorrhea, lupus, mastitis, pleurisy, pneumonia, sinus infection, staph infection, strep throat, trichomonas, tuberculosis, and urethritis.

Topically, usnea tea, diluted tincture, or powdered herb can be applied directly to the skin to treat impetigo, ringworm, and wounds. The herb is often included in foot powders to treat athlete's foot. It can be prepared as a compress to treat eye inflammatino or mastitis, as a gargle to treat throat infection, as a nasal spray to treat sinus infection, or as a tea used as a douche or sitz bath to treat candida, chlamydia, leukorrhea, and trichomonas.

Usnea, though sometimes used as a tea, is more effective as a tincture. In a wilderness situation where tea or tincture is unavailable, usnea can simply be chewed and swallowed.

Edible Uses

Usnea is edible, though it is so bitter that it would be considered for consumption only in emergencies. It would be best when soaked in several changes of water to leach out the bitter constituents.

Other Uses

Throughout history, when fabric or animal hides were not available, people used usnea to make capes, blankets, and shoes. Today the plant is sometimes included in soaps and deodorants for its antibacterial properties. It is also sometimes used for its absorbent properties in baby diaper lining and menstrual pads. A yellow dye can be made from it.

Constituents

Vitamin C, usnic acid, barbatic acid, lobaric acid, polysaccharides, fatty acids (linoleic acid, oleic acid, arachidonic acids)

Energetic Correspondences

- Flavor: sweet, slightly bitter
- Temperature: cool
- Moisture: dry
- Polarity: yin
- Planet: Saturn/Mercury/Mars
- Element: air

Contraindications

Avoid during pregnancy. There have been rare cases of contact dermatitis from applying the herb directly to the skin.

Range and Appearance

Usnea is a gray-green lichen (part fungus, part algae) that grows primarily in cool, damp forests on the branches and trunks of apple, Douglas fir, oak, and pine trees, often in hilly regions. It can grow from a few inches to 3 feet in length and has a coarse, dry feel. It features a white, threadlike inner core, is roundish in shape, and is covered with minute hairs called papillate.

There is an usnea look-alike that does not have the same properties; it lacks the white inner core.

Usnea is a very slow-growing plant, and its populations can be decimated by overharvesting. When purchasing usnea or products made from it, make sure it was harvested ecologically.

UVA-URSI

Botanical Name

Arctostaphylos spp., including *A. alpina, A. glauca, A. manzanita, A. nevadensis, A. polifolia, A. pungens, A. rubra, A. uva-ursi*

Family

Ericaceae (Heath Family)

Etymology

The genus name, *Arctostaphylos,* is from the Greek *arcto,* meaning "bear," and *staphyles,* meaning "bunch of berries or grapes," hence the common name *bearberry.* The species name *uva-ursi* also translates as *bearberry,* deriving from the Latin *uva,* meaning "grape," and *ursi,* meaning "of the bear." The common name *manzanita* is Spanish for "little apple," as the berries look like the apples.

Also Known As

Algonquian: k'nick k'nack
Dutch: beerendruif
English: arbutus, bearberry, bear's bilberry, bear's grape, chipmunk's apples, hog cranberry, kinnikinnik, manzanita, mealberry, mountain box, mountain cranberry, sandberry, sagackhomi, upland cranberry
Finnish: sianpuola
French: arbousier, arbre aux fraises, arctostaphyle, loonier, petitbuis, busserole, raisin d'ours
German: bärentraub, harnkraut, moosebeere, sandbeere, wilder inchs, wolfsbeere
Italian: uva d'orso, uva orsina

Spanish: coralillo, gayuba, gayuba de europa,
  manzanita, pinguica, uva-ursi
Swedish: mjölon

Parts Used

Leaf (primarily), fruit (rarely)

Physiological Effects

Antifungal, antiseptic, antiviral, astringent, bladder tonic, demulcent, diuretic, genitourinary antiseptic, lithotriptic, parturient, vasoconstrictor

Medicinal Uses

Uva-ursi has been used by European herbalists to treat kidney problems since the Middle Ages. In North America, the Cheyenne and Sioux used it to promote labor contractions, and it was included in the United States Pharmacopoeia from 1820 until 1936.

Uva-ursi clears heat and toxins, reduces inflammation, stimulates kidney activity, and curbs infection. In the urinary tract arbutin, one of this herb's constituents, is converted to hydroquinine, which helps to alkalinize the urine, thereby inhibiting urinary tract infection. Uva-ursi also soothes and promotes the healing of urinary tissue.

Uva-ursi is used in the treatment of bedwetting, bladder infection, bladder stones, blood in the urine, Bright's disease, bronchitis, cystitis, diabetes, diarrhea, dysmenorrhea, dysuria, endometriosis, enuresis, gallstones, gonorrhea, herpes, incontinence, kidney infection, kidney stones, leukorrhea, nephritis, pelvic inflammatory disease, pulmonary edema, syphilis, urethritis, and urinary tract infection. It also can be used to prevent postpartum infection.

Topically, uva-ursi can be made into a compress, poultice, or wash to treat boils, bruises, burns, hives, poison ivy or oak, skin rash, sprains, thrush, and wounds. It can be used as a mouthwash to treat canker sores, thrush, and weak gums; as a hair rinse to treat dandruff; as a douche to treat vaginal infections and ulcerations; and as a sitz bath after childbirth to prevent excessive bleeding and promote tissue repair.

Edible Uses

The leaves are not generally considered edible, aside from as tea. The berries can be eaten raw or cooked. They are bland, but they do help quench thirst and stimulate saliva flow and can be used as survival food. They are best, however, when mixed with other foods such as fruits or juices.

Other Uses

Uva-ursi is used to tan leather in Scandinavia. Not coincidentally, it also can be prepared as a foot soak to help toughen the feet, which can be useful for hikers. The leaves are sometimes included in smoking mixtures. The leaves yield a yellowish brown dye. The mashed berries were once applied as a waterproofing agent on cedar baskets.

Constituents

Calcium, chromium, iron, potassium, selenium, glycosides (arbutin, ericolin), flavonoids (quercitin, myricacitrin), allantoin, tannins, ellagic acid, gallic acid, malic acid, ursolic acid, resin (ursone)

Energetic Correspondences

• Flavor: bitter, pungent
• Temperature: cold
• Moisture: dry
• Polarity: yang
• Planet: Mars/ Saturn/Venus/Pluto
• Element: earth

Contraindications

Use for ideally no longer than one week (take a one-week break and then resume, if needed). Large or frequent doses may be irritating to the stomach mucosa and could possibly cause nausea and vomiting. Long-term use may be constipating; it can be beneficial to combine it with a demulcent herb such as cornsilk, marshmallow root, or licorice. Avoid during pregnancy, as uva-ursi may decrease circulation to the uterus.

Arbutin inhibits the breakdown of insulin and should be used cautiously by those that are hypoglycemic. It can turn urine a greenish color, due to the hydroquinone, though this effect is not harmful.

Range and Appearance

Uva-ursi is a small, low-growing evergreen shrub native to Asia, Europe, and North America. It is often found growing in woodlands at elevations of up to 10,000 feet in coarse, gravelly soil. The tips of the shrub grow upright to a height of 20 inches, at the most. The stems trail, forming a carpet. The leaves are alternate, obovate, shiny on top, and paler below, and they have a leathery texture. The pale pink, bell-shaped flowers grow in terminal clusters. The fruit is a small scarlet berry with mealy pulp.

VALERIAN

Botanical Name

Valeriana spp., including *V. officinalis*

Family

Valerianaceae (Valerian Family)

Etymology

The name *valerian* is thought to derive from the Latin *valere,* "to be in health," or from the name of Valerianus, a Roman emperor. The species name *officinalis* refers to this being an official herb of the apothecaries.

Also Known As

English: all-heal, capon's tail, catwort, elfwort, garden heliotrope, herba benidicta, madcap, moonwort, phu, Saint George's herb, setwall, theriak herb, tobacco root, treacle, vandal root
Finnish: rohtovirmajuuri
French: herbe aux chats, valeriane
German: baldrian, baldrianwurzel, gemeiner baldrian, katzenwurz
Italian: amantilla, valeriana
Russian: valeriana
Sanskrit: tagara
Spanish: valeriana
Swedish: läkevänderot

Parts Used

Root, rhizome

Physiological Effects

Anodyne, anthelmintic, antibacterial, antispasmodic, aromatic, astringent, bitter, carminative, diaphoretic, diuretic, febrifuge, hypnotic, hypotensive, nervous system tonic, nervine, restorative, sedative, smooth muscle relaxant, stomachic, tonic

Medicinal Uses

Valerian is most commonly used as a sedative. During World War I this herb was given to treat shell shock and stress in civilians. In Europe today it is the most common nonprescription sedative; in Germany it is more likely to be recommended than Xanax or Valium. Valerian calms the nerves, increases blood flow to the heart, and relaxes the muscles. One of its constituents, valerenic acid, has been shown to inhibit the action of the enzyme that breaks down GABA (gamma-aminobutyric acid), thus contributing to increased levels of calming GABA in the body. Valerian is sometimes referred to as a "daytime sedative" because it can improve performance, concentration, and memory during the day as well as help one to sleep better during the night.

Valerian is used in the treatment of addiction (tobacco or tranquilizer), aggressiveness (chronic), anxiety, arthritis pain, attention deficit disorder, chorea, convulsions, cough, delirium tremens, dysmenorrhea, epilepsy, flatulence, flu, headache, hypertension (due to stress), hyperactivity, hypochondria, hysteria, inflammatory bowel disorder, insomnia, intestinal cramping, mental illness, migraine, muscle pain, nervousness, nervous breakdown, neuralgia, overeating, pain, premenstrual syndrome, restlessness during illness such as with chicken pox, shingles pain, shock, stress, tachycardia, traumatic injury, vision weakness, and worms.

Topically, valerian can be used as a poultice to relieve pain in the body or to draw out a splinter. It can be used as a wash to treat acne or in the bath to relieve rheumatic pain. It also can be made into a sachet and used in a sleep pillow.

As a flower essence, valerian calms, encourages healthy sleep, and eases physical pain. It is helpful during convalescence. For those who did not receive adequate love during childhood, it lifts the spirits and fosters inner peace.

Avoid boiling the root when making tea, which would diminish the plant's activity. Many will find the aroma of valerian unpleasant, much like that of dirty socks. Some find that making valerian tea with raisins added to the water improves the flavor.

Edible Uses

The root is a staple food of many native peoples. They can be dried and made into a flour. Some enjoy the flavor of the root, while others do not; the root of *V. edulis* is considered one of the better tasting ones.

Young valerian leaves can be eaten as a spring green. Juice can be extracted from the fresh plant. Valerian is also sometimes used in wine making.

Other Uses

Valerian is a supreme bait for rats; in fact, legend says that the Pied Piper of Hamlin used valerian to lure the rats out of the city. Some cats are even more attracted to valerian than to catnip and like to play with an old sock stuffed with it. The dried leaves and roots are sometimes mixed with tobacco and smoked. It also has sedative properties and can be sewn into sleep pillows. And at one time valerian was worn as a protective amulet against evil.

Constituents

Calcium, magnesium, manganese, phosphorous, silicon, choline, B-complex vitamins, valepotriates, iridglyycosides, valeriac acid, isovaleric acid, valerenic acid, alkaloids (valeriane, chatarine), essential oils (acetic acid, borneol, pinene, camphene), caffeic acid, beta-sitosterol, esters, tannin

Energetic Correspondences

- Flavor: pungent, bitter, slightly sweet
- Temperature: warm
- Moisture: dry
- Polarity: yang
- Planet: Venus/Sun/Mercury/Mars/Saturn
- Element: air

Contraindications

Large doses of valerian can cause depression, nausea, headache, and lethargy. Some individuals, especially those who are already overheated, may find valerian stimulating, rather than sedating. Do not use large doses for more than three weeks in a row. Avoid during pregnancy, except in very small doses. Do not give to children under the age of three. Avoid in cases of very low blood pressure or hypoglycemia; avoid long-term use in cases of depression. Use with caution if you are going to be driving, operating heavy machinery, or undertaking other activities that require fast reaction times after taking valerian. Valerian may potentiate the effects of benzodiazepine and barbiturates. Those taking sedatives, antidepressants, or anti-anxiety medications should use valerian only under the guidance of a qualified health-care professional.

Range and Appearance

Valerian is a perennial native to Eurasia and North America. There are about two hundred species worldwide. The plant grows 2 to 5 feet in height on a hollow stem. The leaves are opposite and oddly pinnate, with seven to ten in a pair. Small, pleasantly scented, hermaphroditic, pinkish white flowers bloom in compound cymose inflorescences.

In the garden valerian requires a moist soil and full sun. It stimulates earthworm activity and the growth of nearby plants.

VANILLA

Botanical Name

Vanilla planifolia, V. pompona

Family

Orchidaceae (Orchid Family)

Etymology

The genus name *Vanilla* derives from the Latin *vaina*, "sheath," "pod," or "little vagina," in reference to the suggestive shape of the flower.

Also Known As

Arabic: fanilya
Aztec: tlilxochitl
Armenian: vanil
Bulgarian: vaniliya
Cantonese: heung lan, wahn nei la
Croatian: vanilija
Czech: vanilka
Danish: vanilje
Dutch: vanille
Esperanto: vanilo
Estonian: vanillikaun
Finnish: vanilja
French: vanille
German: vanille
Greek: vanillia
Hebrew: vanil
Hungarian: vanília
Icelandic: vanilla
Indonesian: pameli
Italian: vaniglia
Japanese: banira
Korean: panilla
Mandarin: fan ni lan, xiang jiá lán
Náhuatl: tlilxochitl
Norwegian: vanilje
Polish: wanilia plaskolistna
Portuguese: baunilha
Romanian: vanilie
Serbian: vanila
Spanish: vainilla
Swedish: vanilj
Thai: wanila
Turkish: vanilya
Ukrainian: vanil
Yiddish: vanil

Part Used

Seed pod (cured)

Physiological Effects

Aphrodisiac, aromatic, carminative, digestive, febrifuge, stimulant

Medicinal Uses

The Aztecs were the first to use vanilla; among other things, they added it to their chocolate drinks. The smell of vanilla is said to be one of the closest to mother's milk; perhaps as a result, smelling or eating vanilla can have a calming effect and help awaken childhood memories.

Vanilla is well known as an aphrodisiac; its aphrodisiac qualities perhaps result from the fact that it causes urethral irritation. It is used infrequently in modern herbal medicine, but it can be helpful in cases of emotional trauma, hysteria, and low libido.

As a flower essence, vanilla is helpful for those who are overcome by negative influences, helping them remain clearheaded and feel more in control in life situations.

Edible Uses

Vanilla bean and extract are popular flavorings for a wide variety of confections, liqueurs, and even pharmaceuticals.

Other Uses

Vanilla is used to scent perfumes, cosmetics, potpourri, and smoking mixtures. It is also used in love magic.

Constituents

Vanillin, coumarins, phenols, esters, carbohydrates, sugars, fat

Energetic Correspondences

- Flavor: sweet
- Temperature: cool
- Moisture: moist
- Polarity: yin
- Planet: Venus
- Element: water

Contraindications

Excessive use may be irritating to the genitourinary tract.

Range and Appearance

Vanilla is a vine native to Central and South America, where it grows in humid, shady conditions. It yields the world's second most expensive spice (after saffron), in part because vanilla flowers must be hand pollinated within a few hours of opening, with the exception of only a few small areas in Mexico where certain species of bees and hummingbirds help out.

The vine produces short leaves, yellow to orange flowers, and long, slender, tough but pliable seed pods that contain thousands of minute black seeds and take about nine months to mature.

VERVAIN

Botanical Name

Verbena spp., including *V. hastata* (blue vervain), *V. lasiostachys* (syn. *V. prostrata*), *V. officinalis* (European vervain), *V. stricta* (hoary vervain)

Family

Verbenaceae (Vervain Family)

Etymology

Verbena, the genus name, may be a corruption of *herba veneris,* Latin for "herb of Venus." The common name *vervain* is derived from the Celtic *ferfaen,* "to drive away stone," in reference to the herb's use in treating bladder stones.

Also Known As

Cantonese: ma-pien ts'ao
English: enchanter's plant, herb of enchantment, herb of grace, herb of the cross, holy herb, holy wort, Indian hyssop, Juno's tears, pigeon grass, simpler's joy, verbena
French: herbe sacrée, verveine
German: eisenkraut, segenkraut, taubenkraut, verbene
Italian: verbena
Spanish: dormilon, moradilla, verbena azul

Parts Used

Aboveground plant (primarily), root (rarely)

Physiological Effects

Alterative, antidepressant, anti-inflammatory, antispasmodic, astringent, antitumor, aphrodisiac, astringent, bitter, cardiotonic, cholagogue, diaphoretic, digestive, diuretic, emetic (in large doses), emmenagogue, expectorant, febrifuge, galactagogue, liver stimulant, nervine, rubefacient, sedative, stomachic, sudorific, tonic, vasoconstrictor, vermifuge, vulnerary

Medicinal Uses

Vervain has been held in high regard by much of human culture for thousands of years. According to Egyptian legend, vervain represents the tears shed by Isis in mourning for the loss of Osiris. At one time it was used in ancient Egyptian and Roman sacrifices and to decorate altars. Ancient Druids considered it second only to mistletoe in importance. Ancient Romans carried it as a symbol of peace. Christians used vervain sprigs to sprinkle holy water, believing that it had grown at the base of Jesus's crucifix and was used to staunch the bleeding of his wounds. Vervain has also been used by various cultures for casting spells, for purification rituals, as an ingredient in love potions, as part of amulets for protection against illness and evil forces, and to induce visions.

Vervain has been shown to promote sweating, stimulate uterine activity, and calm the nerves, stomach, and parasympathetic nervous system. As a digestive aid, it improves nutrient assimilation. Indications are that it helps normalize the production of thyroid hormones. It is considered an excellent remedy for soothing cranky, fidgety children.

Vervain is used in the treatment of amenorrhea, anorexia, anxiety, appendicitis, asthma, cancerous growths (of the neck, scrotum, and spleen), cirrhosis, colds, cough, debility, depression, diarrhea, digestive distress, dysentery, dysmenorrhea, epilepsy, fever, gallstones, gout, Graves' disease, headache (nervous), hemorrhage, hepatitis, hyperactivity, hypothyroidism, hysteria, insomnia, irregular menses, jaundice, kidney stones, mastitis, migraine (related to the menses), neck tension, nervousness, nervous stomach, ovarian cysts, pleurisy, pneumonia, premenstrual tension, rheumatism, scrofula, seizure, stress, tuberculosis, urinary tract infection, whooping cough, and worms. It also can be used to encourage convalescence and to ease labor that has been difficult.

Topically, vervain can be used as a poultice to treat burns, bruises, hemorrhoids, and wounds or as a salve to treat eczema and neuralgia. It also can be used as a gargle to relieve sore throat, as a mouthwash to prevent cavities and to treat gum disease, as a cleansing powder to brush the teeth. It also can be dried and powdered and used as a snuff to stop nosebleed.

As a flower essence, vervain calms zealots who try to impose their will and beliefs on others, helping them to relax and allow others to lead their own lives. It is helpful for those who are argumentative and highly strung, as well as those who are overstressed and have muscle tension, headaches, and eyestrain.

Edible Uses

Vervain herb is sometimes included in liqueurs. The seeds are bitter but can be roasted and ground to make a gruel.

Other Uses

Druid women were once crowned with vervain to denote high rank. In ancient England tradition held that children who carried vervain would love learning and be joyous, and bards, singers, and poets who wore it would improve their performance. Smiths once plunged their ironwork into vervain water in the belief that it would give the iron strength.

In magical traditions, vervain is said to attract love and prosperity and is carried in medicine bags to give protection against lightning. When burned as an incense it helps dispel love that is not returned. The juice of the fresh plant can be rubbed on the body to enhance clairvoyance, make enemies friendly, attract love, and offer protection against enchantment.

Constituents

Vitamin C, potassium, sulfur, zinc, glycosides (verbenaline, verbenine), essential oil (citral), mucilage, saponins, tannins

Energetic Correspondences

- Flavor: pungent, bitter
- Temperature: cold
- Moisture: dry
- Polarity: yin
- Planet: Sun/Mercury/Venus/Saturn
- Element: earth

Contraindications

Avoid during pregnancy, except during labor. Large doses may cause vomiting.

Range and Appearance

Vervain species can be found around the globe, including Africa, Asia, Australia, Europe, and North and Central America. They are hardy perennials that range in height from low-growing creepers to plants that reach 4 feet. They require moist soil and full sun to partial shade. The leaves are toothed and opposite. The hermaphroditic, light purple flowers grow in spikes.

VIOLET

Botanical Name

Viola odorata

Family

Violaceae (Violet) Family

Etymology

The genus name *Viola,* from which the common name *violet* derives, itself derives from that of Ione (or Io), in Greek mythology a woman whom Zeus took as a lover. Zeus's wife, Hera, was jealous. To hide Ione from Hera, Zeus turned her into a white heifer. Ione wept, and Zeus turned her tears into violets to give her something wonderful to graze upon.

Also Known As

English: heartsease, sweet violet
Finnish: tuoksuorvokki
French: violette
German: veilchen

Italian: viola
Russian: fialka polevaya
Sanskrit: banafshah
Spanish: violetta
Swedish: doftviol, lukviol

Parts Used

Leaf, flower, root

Physiological Effects

Alterative, antifungal, anti-inflammatory, antiseptic, antiscorbutic, astringent, cathartic (root), demulcent, diaphoretic, discutient, diuretic, emetic (root), emollient, expectorant, febrifuge, laxative (mild), nutritive, pectoral, restorative (after surgery), purgative (root), vulnerary

Medicinal Uses

Violet clears heat, reduces swellings, and deters infection. It is used in the treatment of abscess, acne, anger, asthma, boils, bronchitis, cancer (breast, lung, digestive tract, skin, throat, tongue), carbuncles, catarrh, colds, cysts, eczema, fever, fibrocystic breast disease, grief, headache, heartbreak, laryngitis, lymphatic congestion, mastitis, mumps, pleurisy, psoriasis, sore throat, tuberculosis, tumors, ulcers, urinary tract infection, varicose veins, and whooping cough.

Topically, violet can be used as a compress or poultice to treat boils, conjunctivitis, breast cysts, cancers, and hemorrhoids. Apply a cloth soaked in violet tea to the back of the neck to treat headaches.

As a flower essence, violet helps those who feel lonely despite being surrounded by others. It increases openness, faith, and warmth and strengthens the ability to interact with others while protecting the individual.

Edible Uses

The leaves, buds, and flowers are all edible. Violet tea is most often prepared from the leaves. However, the flowers can be used to make a beautifully aromatic cold-water infusion.

Other Uses

Violets are regarded as a symbol of innocence and modesty; ancient Romans planted violets upon the graves of children. The flowers can be eaten as a breath freshener. The flowers yield a pigment that is used in making litmus paper. In folkloric traditions, violet flowers are carried to bring good fortune.

Constituents

Leaf, flower: beta-carotene, vitamin C, salicylates, saponins (highest in roots), alkaloid (violene), flavonoid (rutin), mucilage, essential oil
Root: violone

Energetic Correspondences

- Flavor: pungent, bitter, sweet
- Temperature: cool
- Moisture: moist
- Polarity: yin
- Planet: Venus/Saturn
- Element: water

Contraindications

Violet is not recommended in cold conditions such as chills. Otherwise, violet leaf tea is safe and gentle; it even can be used as a substitute for baby aspirin.

Other Violets

There are over one hundred of the *Viola* genus. Most are perennial, though there are a few annuals in the genus. Other violets used medicinally include *Viola pedata* (blue violet, bird's-foot violet), *V. tricolor* (pansy), *V. cucullata* (common blue violet), *V. orbiculata* (evergreen violet), *V. canina* (dog violet), *V. adunca* (western dog violet), *V. canadensis* (Canada violet), and *V. patrinii* and *V. yedoensis* (also wild Chinese violets), among others.

Range and Appearance

Viola odorata is native to western Asia and Europe but is widely cultivated and naturalized. This evergreen perennial grows to about 6 inches in height and has heart-shaped leaves. The flowers are cleistogamous (self-pollinating) and purple, pink, or white in color. They usually have five petals, two on the upper portion, two laterals, and one on the bottom. Though flowers appear in early spring, the true seed-producing flower is inconspicuous and appears in autumn.

In the garden, violet provides nectar for early butterflies. The plant prefers full to partial shade, soil that is rich in organic matter, and moderate to high amounts of water.

VITEX

Botanical Name

Vitex agnus-castus

Family

Verbenaceae (Vervain Family)

Etymology

The genus name *Vitex* derives from the Latin *vitilis,* "made by plaiting," in reference to the use of the flexible branches in making braided fences. In the species name, *agnus* is ancient Greek for "lamb," and *castus* is ancient Greek for "chaste" or "spotless." The common names *monk's pepper* and *chaste tree* refer to the berries' ability to reduce sexual desire.

Also Known As

Arabic: kaf marim
Bulgarian: viteks
Cantonese: sing git muih
Czech: drmek obecny
Danish: kyskhedstræ
Dutch: monnikenpeper, kuisboom
English: Abraham's balm, chaste tree, hemp tree, Indian spice, monk's pepper, sage tree
Estonian: harilik mungapipar
Finnish: munkinpippuri, siveydenpuu
French: arbre au poivre, gattilier, poivre des moines
German: Abrahamsstrauch, keuschlamm, mönchspfeffer
Greek: agnos, lygos
Hebrew: siah Avraham mazui
Hungarian: barátcserje
Italian: agnocasto
Japanese: itarianinjin-boku
Korean: italliamokhyeong
Mandarin: jing li, sheng ji mei
Polish: niepokalanek pieprzowy
Portuguese: agno casto
Romanian: lemmul lui Avram
Russian: avraamovo derevo, viteks
Serbian: rakita
Swedish: kyskheträd, munkpeppa,
Turkish: ayit, hayit
Yiddish: viteks

Part Used

Berry

Physiological Effects

Anaphrodisiac, antiandrogenic, aphrodisiac, aromatic, diaphoretic, diuretic, emmenagogue, febrifuge, galactagogue, ophthalmic, phytoprogesteronic, sedative, stomachic, vulnerary

Medicinal Uses

Vitex increases the production of progesterone, luteinizing hormones, and prolactin and inhibits the release of follicle stimulating hormone. It helps to reregulate the menstrual cycle for women coming off birth control pills. It can help normalize the menses, shortening a long cycle or lengthening a short one. It also helps normalize the functions of the pituitary gland.

Vitex is used in the treatment of amenorrhea, cysts (in the breasts, ovaries, and uterus), depression (related to menopause), dysmenorrhea, endometriosis, fibroids (in the breasts, ovaries, or uterus), infertility, herpes (related to menses), menorrhagia, migraines (related to menstrual cycle), polymenorrhea, premenstrual acne, premenstrual syndrome, and threatened miscarriage. It can also be beneficial after hysterectomy.

In order to improve hormonal problems with vitex, the herb should be taken for at least six months.

Topically, the berries can be prepared as a poultice to treat limb weakness and to help restore circulation and movement in limbs.

Edible Uses

The berries are not generally considered edible. The seeds can be ground into a peppery condiment. The aromatic leaves can also be used as a seasoning.

Other Uses

The flowers can be made into a perfume. The flexible young stems are sometimes made into baskets. The leaves, seeds, and roots yield a yellow dye.

Constituents

Essential oils (cineol, limonene, pinene, sabinene), flavonoids (casticin, isovitexin, orientin), alkaloids (vitticine), iridoglycosides (agnuside, aucubin, eurostoside)

Energetic Correspondences

- Flavor: sweet, bitter, pungent
- Temperature: neutral
- Moisture: moist
- Polarity: yin
- Planet: Venus/Mars/Moon/Pluto
- Element: air

Contraindications

Discontinue if diarrhea, nausea, or abnormal menstrual changes occur. Large doses can cause formication, a strange symptom in which one feels as if ants were crawling on one's skin.

Range and Appearance

Vitex is a deciduous shrub native to northern Africa, western Asia, and Europe. It can grow to 9 feet in height. Its aromatic leaves are large, palmate, and bluish green. The aromatic, hermaphroditic flowers are bluish and give way to blue-gray seeds.

WALNUT

Botanical Name

Juglans nigra (black walnut), *J. regia* (English walnut, Persian walnut)

Family

Juglandaceae (Walnut Family)

Etymology

The genus name, *Juglans,* derives from the Latin *jovis glans,* "Jupiter's nut," in reference to the mythological recounting of the gods dining on walnuts while on earth. The common name *walnut* derives from the Old English *wealhhnutu,* "foreign nut."

Also Known As

Cantonese: hap tou yan
Dutch: walnoot
English: walnoot
Finnish: saksanpähkinä
French: noyer royal
German: steinnuss, walnussbaum
Italian: noce
Japanese: koto
Korean: hodo
Mandarin: hú táo rén
Spanish: nogal
Swedish: valnöt
Turkish: ceviz ag

Parts Used

Leaf, dried inner bark, green hull of nut, nut

Physiological Effects

Leaf: alterative, anthelmintic, antifungal, anti-inflammatory, antiseptic, antiviral, astringent, detergent
Inner bark: alterative, anthelmintic, antifungal, antiseptic, antiviral, astringent, cathartic, detergent, laxative, purgative
Green hull: anthelmintic, antifungal, antiseptic, antiviral, astringent, detergent, laxative, sudorific, vermifuge
Nut: anti-inflammatory, bronchial dilator, kidney tonic, yang tonic

Medicinal Uses

Walnut leaves, bark, and hull have an astringent effect, drying damp, mucousy conditions, stopping bleeding, cleansing the bowels, and getting rid of parasites. They also help oxygenate the blood. Ellagic acid, a constituent found in the leaf and inner bark, has been shown to stimulate the central nervous system and has been used to help people recover from electric shock.

Walnut leaf is used in the treatment of diarrhea, dysentery, and eczema. The bark is used in the treatment of chronic constipation. The hull is used in the treatment of AIDS, athlete's foot, bone weakness, cancer, candida, hypothyroidism, impetigo, parasites, ringworm, scrofula, syphilis, and worms.

The highly nutritive nut is a kidney yang tonic and contains moisturizing oils. It is used in the treatment of constipation, cough, erectile dysfunction, high cholesterol, tuberculosis, and wheezing.

Topically, the leaf, bark, or hull can be prepared as a wash, compress, or poultice to treat athlete's foot, eczema, impetigo, herpes, ringworm, scabies, tooth weakness, and wounds. A salve made from the green hulls is excellent for getting rid of fungal problems like athlete's foot, jock itch, and ringworm. Walnut leaf can be made into a facial wash to reduce enlarged pores, a hair rinse to get rid of dandruff and to darken graying hair, or a gargle to treat tonsillitis.

As a flower essence, walnut is useful for times of transition, such as job changes, moving, puberty, or menopause, and offers protection from overstimulation from outside forces. It can help users break free from existing habits and establish new healthy patterns.

Edible Uses

The nuts can be eaten raw, toasted, or pickled. The oil extracted from the nuts is often used in cooking. The dry green hulls are sometimes used to make liqueur. A delicious syrup, similar to maple syrup, is made from the sap of the tree.

Other Uses

The leaves can be crushed and rubbed on the body to repel insects. They also can be simply scattered in a room to repel flies, and walnut leaf tea can be spritzed around living spaces to prevent bed bugs. The roots, hull, and leaves produce a black dye that is sometimes used in hair coloring.

Walnut oil is used to make soaps and nondrying paint. The wood has long been used in construction and woodworking.

In folkloric traditions, walnuts are carried as a charm for fertility.

Constituents

Leaf: napthquinones (juglone), tannins, ellagic acid, gallic acid, flavonoids, inositol, essential oils
Inner bark: calcium, iodine, silica, juglone, ellagic acid, tannins
Green hull: iodine, juglone
Nut: beta-carotene, vitamin B_2, essential fatty acids (linoleic acid, linolenic acid), vitamin C, manganese, phosphorous, serotonin

Energetic Correspondences

- Flavor: leaf, green hull, inner bark—bitter, astringent; nut—sweet
- Temperature: leaf, green hull, inner bark—cold; nut—warm
- Moisture: leaf, green hull, inner bark—dry; nut—moist
- Polarity: yang
- Planet: Sun/Mercury/Venus/Saturn
- Element: fire

Contraindications

Avoid walnut leaf, inner bark, and green hull during pregnancy; the nut is safe. The nut has caused mouth sores in sensitive individuals. The green hulls and leaves have been known to cause contact dermatitis. The inner bark should be dried for one year before use, as the fresh bark can cause intestinal gripe.

Range and Appearance

Walnut is a deciduous hardwood tree that can reach a height of 30 to 80 feet. The leaves are alternate and pinnate, composed of seven or eight pairs of leaflets, each 2 to 3 inches long, oblong-lanceolate in shape, and rounded at the bases. The plant is monoecious, meaning that male and female flowers grow on the same tree; the flowers are greenish. The fruit may be single or grouped, green when immature and brown when ripe. *Juglans nigra* and *J. cinerea* are native to North America; *J. regia* is native to Asia and southeastern Europe but widely naturalized.

Walnut trees can be found growing in moist, fertile soils with lots of sun. They tend to repel other plants and trees from growing too close to them.

WHITE OAK

Botanical Name

Quercus alba

Family

Fagaceae (Beech Family)

Etymology

The genus name, *Quercus*, is thought to derive from the Celtic *quer*, "fine," and *cuez*, "tree." The species name, *alba*, is Latin for "white."

Also Known As

English: acorn tree, cups and ladles, Jove's nuts, king of trees, Quebec oak, royal protector, tanner's bark

French: bouvre, chene

German: eiche, eichenrinde, weisseiche

Italian: quercia, querciloa, rovere

Russian: dub

Sanskrit: majuphul

Spanish: encino, roble

Turkish: pelud mesesi

Parts Used

Inner bark, gall (growth produced by fungus or insect)

Physiological Effects

Inner bark: anthelmintic, anti-inflammatory, antiseptic, antivenomous, astringent, expectorant, febrifuge, hemostatic, lithotriptic, styptic, tonic, vermifuge

Gall: astringent

Medicinal Uses

Oak inner bark, which was included in the United States Pharmacopoeia from 1820 until 1916, helps dry dampness, heals damaged tissues, and can slow or stop both external and internal bleeding. Its high tannin content is responsible for a wide range of its activity; the tannins bind with protein in the tissues, thus making them impermeable to infection. Oak bark tea can be used to treat anal prolapse, blood in the urine, cancer, catarrh, cholera, diarrhea, dysentery, fever, gallstones, hemorrhage, kidney stones, night sweats, uterine prolapse, and varicose veins.

Oak bark is excellent as a gargle to treat sore throat and tonsillitis, as a mouthwash to treat bleeding gums, or as a tooth powder to treat receding gums, loose teeth, and pyorrhea. Topically, it can be used as a compress or wash to treat burns, bruises, capillary weakness, cuts, eczema, hemorrhoids, poison ivy/oak, ringworm, toothache, and varicose veins. It also can be applied as a poultice to stop bleeding. Oak bark can be prepared as an enema, suppository, or sitz bath to treat hemorrhoids or as a douche to treat leukorrhea. Powdered, it can be used as a snuff to stop nosebleeds. The tea can also be used as a hair rinse to treat dandruff.

Oak galls are used in the treatment of cholera, diarrhea, and dysentery. They can be applied topically as a compress in the treatment of hemorrhoids.

As a flower essence, oak can relieve despair and despondency, offering assistance to those who have doubts about their ability to accomplish their goals. It supports strong, reliable people who shoulder their burdens without complaint, though they may have taken on too much. Consider oak flower essence when perseverance leads to exhaustion and ill health causes limitations.

Edible Uses

The inner bark and galls are not generally considered edible. The tree's acorns are edible and contain high levels of carbohydrates, protein, and fat. The best come from white oaks, and they are usually soaked in water for at least 24 hours to leach out the tannins and then ground into a meal, which can be added to soups and cereals. Acorns can also be roasted as a coffee substitute.

Other Uses

Tannic acid from oak is used in tanning leather. The tree's hardwood timber is a favorite building material, which has led to many oak forests being cut down. The bark produces a purplish dye, while the galls produce a brown dye. A mulch of the dried leaves repels slugs and grubs. The young stems of the tree can be used as chewing sticks for cleaning and massaging the gums and teeth.

In magical traditions, acorns are worn in a medicine bag around the neck as a protection, fertility, and longevity charm.

Constituents

Phosphorous, potassium, sulfur, tannins (phlobatannin, ellagitannins, gallic acid), flavonoids (quercitrin, quercetrol); the galls have higher concentrations of tannins than the bark

Energetic Correspondences

- Flavor: pungent, bitter
- Temperature: cool
- Moisture: dry
- Polarity: yang
- Planet: Jupiter/Sun
- Element: fire

Contraindications

Oak galls are extremely astringent; use only in small quantities. Use oak bark for no longer than a month continuously.

Range and Appearance

White oak is native to North America. This decidous tree can reach up to 100 feet in height and features a wide-spread, irregular crown of foliage and gray-brown bark. The leaves have seven to ten rounded, fingerlike lobes and are whitish underneath, with prominent veins. The tree is monoecious, bearing both male (staminate) and female (pistillate) flowers. The male flowers are yellow-green and borne in catkins, while the female flowers are reddish green and borne in small, single spikes. The acorns are often not produced until a tree is at least twenty years old.

Oak galls, also known as oak apples, are rounded growths that occur most often in small shoots and twigs. They result from gall wasps laying eggs in the twigs of the trees. The wasps that lay the eggs and the larvae that hatch from them secrete chemicals that cause abnormal growth and cell division in the host tree, resulting in the growth of a gall around each larva. The larva feed upon the gall tissue as they develop, and when they mature, they bore a hole through it and escape as wasps. The galls are best collected when their tannin content is highest, in early fall when they are flecked with red.

WILD CARROT

Botanical Name

Daucus carota

Family

Apiaceae (Parsley Family)

Etymology

The genus name *Daucus* is thought to derive from the ancient Greek *daukos,* a name for members of the Umbelliferae family. The species and common name are thought to derive from the Greek name for the plant, *karoton.*

Also Known As

English: bee's nest, bird's nest, philtron, Queen Anne's lace
Finnish: porkkana
French: carotte
German: möhre, mohrükarotte
Italian: carota
Spanish: zanahoria
Swedish: morot, vildmorot

Parts Used

Seed, root, leaf

Physiological Effects

Seed: abortifacient, anthelmintic, astringent, carminative, contraceptive, deobstruent, diuretic, emmenagogue, galactagogue, lithotriptic, ophthalmic
Root: anthelmintic, antibacterial, astringent, carminative, deobstruent, diuretic, galactagogue, lithotriptic, liver tonic, ophthalmic, urinary antiseptic
Leaf: anthelmintic, astringent, carminative, deobstruent, diuretic, galactagogue, lithotriptic, ophthalmic

Medicinal Uses

The seed, root, and leaf of carrot strengthen the stomach, spleen, liver, and lungs. They are used in the treatment of bladder stones, cystitis, gallstones, gout, indigestion, jaundice, kidney stones, and parasites (threadworms). The seed in particular is also used in the treatment of edema, flatulence, hangover, and delayed menses, while the flower is used in the treatment of diabetes. Carrot root juice is an excellent remedy to cleanse the liver, but it should be first diluted with water, as it is very sweet.

The seed works to make pregnancy difficult by making the endometrium slick, so that the egg can't implant; one teaspoon daily is the dosage to inhibit implantation.

As a flower essence, wild carrot brings insight and groundedness, helps dispel persistent negative thoughts, and eases worry and anxiety. It is of particular benefit to those who tend to close their eyes to reality.

Edible Uses

The root of wild carrot is, like that of its cultivated relative, edible. It can be eaten fresh or cooked or dried and roasted and used as a coffee substitute. The young fresh tops are also edible, as are the flowers. The seed is sometimes used as a condiment.

Other Uses

Carrot essential oil is used in perfumery and anti-wrinkle lotions.

Constituents

Seed: essential oil (asarone, carotol, limonene, pinene)
Root: carotene, pectin, alkaloids (daucine, asparagine), vitamin C, potassium
Leaf: flavonoids (kaempferol, quercitin), potassium, porphyrins

Energetic Correspondences

- Flavor: sweet
- Temperature: warm
- Moisture: moist
- Polarity: yang
- Planet: Mars
- Element: fire

Contraindications

Avoid the seeds during pregnancy. Carrots and their leaves can increase photosensitivity in some people.

Range and Appearance

Native to Eurasia but widely naturalized, wild carrot is a biennial that can grow to 4 feet in height. The roots of ancient wild carrots were bitter tasting and purple and black in color, but today they are usually white on the inside and brown on the outside, and sweet to the taste. The plant features ribbed stems and aromatic, hermaphroditic, white flowers that grow in flat-topped umbels, often with a central flower that is maroon to purple in color. The plant prefers moist, well-drained soil and full sun.

WILD CHERRY

Botanical Name

Prunus avium, P. serotina (black cherry), *P. virens, P. virginiana* (chokecherry)

Family

Rosaceae (Rose Family)

Etymology

The genus name *Prunus* derives from the Latin name for plum, *prunum*. The common name *cherry* traces back to the ancient Greek name for the fruit, *kerasos*.

Also Known As

English: black cherry, chokecherry
Finnish: kiitotuomi, virginiahägg
French: cerisier
German: kirsche, spätblühende traubenkirsche, trauben-kirsche
Italian: ciliegio, pruno
Spanish: cerezo
Swedish: glanshägg
Turkish: kiraz ag

Parts Used

Inner bark (collected in fall and dried)

Physiological Effects

Antitussive, astringent, bitter, carminative, diuretic, expectorant, sedative, tonic

Medicinal Uses

Wild cherry contains the substances amygdalin and prunasin, which in the body break down into hyrocyanic acid, which, though toxic in large amounts, in small amounts can increase respiration, improve digestion, inhibit the development of cancer cells, and improve mood. Wild cherry also improves circulation, relaxes the nerves, reduces inflammation, and dries up mucus. It relieves the urge to cough, probably thanks to its prunasin content.

The inner bark is used in the treatment of asthma, bronchitis, colds, cough, fever, diarrhea, dysentery, dyspepsia (due to nerves), measles, and whooping cough. Some Native American tribes used the bark to relax women in childbirth.

To prepare a tea from the bark, simply steep it in hot water, rather than boiling it, to avoid diminishing its essential oil content.

Topically, the bark can be prepared as an eyewash to reduce inflammation in the eyes.

Edible Uses

The bark is not generally considered edible, aside from as tea. The berry can be eaten raw or cooked and have varying flavors; *Prunus avium* is the ancestor of many modern cherry varieties. The berry encourages the release of uric acid from the body, thus relieving joint pain and inflammation.

Other Uses

The leaves yield a green dye, while the fruit yield a green to dark gray dye. A dried resin made from the tree bark or the dried blossoms can be burned as an incense. The wood is used in woodworking. In Japanese folklore, tying one strand of one's own hair to a blossoming cherry tree is said to help one find love.

Constituents

Cyanogenic glycosides (prunasin), benzaldhyde, essential oil, coumarins, gallitannins, amygdalin, scopoletin, tannin, resin

Energetic Correspondences

- Flavor: bitter, sweet
- Temperature: warm
- Moisture: dry
- Polarity: yang
- Planet: Venus/Mars
- Element: fire

Contraindications

Wild cherry bark is toxic in large doses, so use only in small doses. It may cause drowsiness. Though it helps soothe coughs, it does not address any infection that may be causing the cough. Do not use in cases of severe infection.

The seeds (pits) of the fruit should not be consumed unless they have been dried or cooked, as they contain high concentrations of toxic compounds.

Range and Appearance

Wild cherry is a deciduous tree, native to North America and Eurasia, that grows up to 10 feet tall. It prefers full sun to partial shade and moist, well-drained soil. The leaves are sharply serrated and range from ovate to obovate. The tree bears white or pinkish hermaphroditic flowers and red to dark purple fruits. Each fruit contains a single large seed (pit).

WILD LETTUCE

Botanical Name

Lactuca canadensis, L. serriola (prickly wild lettuce), *L. virosa* (bitter wild lettuce)

Family

Asteraceae (Daisy Family)

Etymology

The genus name, *Lactuca*, derives from the Latin *lac*, "milk," alluding to the plant's milky white sap.

Also Known As

English: acrid lettuce, bitter lettuce, lettuce opium, poor man's opium, prickly lettuce, strong-scented lettuce

Finnish: rohtosalaati

French: laitue sauvage

German: wilder lattich

Italian: lattuga

Swedish: giftsallet

Parts Used

Leaf, latex

Physiological Effects

Analgesic, anaphrodisiac, anodyne, antispasmodic, antitussive, digestive, diuretic, expectorant, febrifuge, galactagogue, hypnotic, hypoglycemic, narcotic, sedative

Medicinal Uses

Wild lettuce calms the nervous system, aids sleep, and relieves pain. It is used in the treatment of anxiety, bronchitis, coughs, hyperactivity, insomnia, nausea, neuroses, pain, restlessness, and whooping cough. The dried leaves can be smoked to ease pain.

Topically, wild lettuce can be prepared as a wash or included in lotions to get rid of acne. The latex can be applied topically to get rid of warts or calm the itch of poison ivy.

Edible Uses

This plant is the wild ancestor of some of our cultivated lettuces. The young leaves (under 10 inches tall) can be eaten raw or cooked. The leaves get bitter as they mature. Soaking or cooking the leaves in two changes of water decreases some of the bitterness. An edible oil can be made from the seeds.

Other Uses

Wild lettuce contains a milky white latex that when dried has euphoric properties similar to those of opium, though it is not addictive or distressing to the digestive system. The seeds yield an oil that is used in making paints, varnishes, and soaps.

Constituents

Lactucarium, sesquiterpene alkaloids (lactucine, lactucopicrin, lactucic acid), mannitol, caoutchouc, flavonoids (quercetin), coumarins, phenethylamine

Energetic Correspondences

- Flavor: bitter
- Temperature: cool
- Moisture: moist
- Polarity: yin
- Planet: moon
- Element: water

Contraindications

Wild lettuce is best used only under the guidance of a qualified health-care professional. Moderate doses can cause drowsiness, while large doses can give rise to excessive sexual urges or insomnia. Very large doses can be fatal.

The latex from the plant can cause eye irritation or contact dermatitis in some individuals.

Range and Appearance

Wild lettuce is native to North America and Eurasia. It grows as an annual or biennial, often in colonies, and can reach a height of 6 feet. It features basal leaves that are obovate, shallowly lobed, and sharply toothed, with bases that firmly grasp the stem. The hermaphroditic flowers are small and numerous. The plant grows best in moist soil with plenty of sunshine.

WILD YAM

Botanical Name

Dioscorea polystachya (syn. *D. batatas*), *D. bulbifera*, *D. japonica*, *D. villosa*

Family

Dioscoreaceae (Yam Family)

Etymology

The genus name *Dioscorea* was given in honor of Dioscorides, a renowned first-century Greek herbalist and physician. The common name *yam* derives from the Spanish name for the plant, *ñame,* a term of unknown African origin.

Also Known As

Afrikaans: wildejam
Aztec: chipahuacxituitl ("graceful plant")
Cantonese: wai san
English: colic root, devil's bones, rheumatism root
French: igname
German: yamswurzel
Hindi: gendhi, zamin-kand
Japanese: sanyaku
Korean: sanyak
Mandarin: shan yao ("mountain medicine")
Sanskrit: varahikand
Zulu: isidakwa

Parts Used

Root, rhizome

Physiological Effects

Analgesic, anti-inflammatory, antirheumatic, antispasmodic, aphrodisiac, chi tonic, cholagogue, demulcent, diaphoretic (mild), diuretic, expectorant, nutritive, rejuvenative, reproductive tonic, restorative, vasodilator

Medicinal Uses

Wild yam contains discin, a compound the body converts to diosgenin, which is a precursor to progesterone, was once used to make birth control pills, and is also made into steroidal compounds. Wild yam also promotes the normalization of progesterone and estrogen levels, moves stagnant chi, calms the liver, relaxes the nerves, tonifies the stomach and spleen, and stimulates interferon production. In Zulu tradition it is used as a remedy for convulsions, epilepsy, and hysteria.

Wild yam is used in the treatment of colic, cough (dry), depression, diarrhea, diabetes, diverticulitis, dysmenorrhea, emotional weakness, enteritis, enuresis, erectile dysfunction, exhaustion, fatigue, flatulence, hemorrhoids, immune-system weakness, infertility, irritable bowel syndrome, labor pain, leg cramps, low sperm count, lung weakness, menopause symptoms, morning sickness, muscle spasms, neuralgia, night sweats, ovarian pain, polyruria, premenstrual syndrome, rheumatoid arthritis, rheumatism, senility, and spermatorrhea. It can also be of use in cases of threatened miscarriage.

Topically, wild yam can be made into a salve to treat eczema or a poultice to treat bruises and scabies. In recent times wild yam has been incorporated into a number of salves designed to enhance hormone production and balance in women.

Edible Uses

The roots of wild yam species with opposite leaves are edible. However, the roots of species with alternate leaves are poisonous. Of the edible species, some roots are more starchy-tasting than sweet; *D. betata* and *D. villosa* are among the best of the edible wild yams, once their tough outer skin has been removed.

Other Uses

None reported

Constituents

Vitamin C, choline, calcium, chromium, copper, iron, amino acids (arginine, glutamine, leucine, tyrosine), steroidal saponins (dioscin), starch, mucilage, tannins, amylase

Energetic Correspondences

- Flavor: sweet, bitter
- Temperature: warm
- Moisture: moist
- Polarity: yin
- Planet: Venus/Jupiter
- Element: water

Contraindications

Avoid large doses during pregnancy, except under the guidance of a qualified health-care practitioner. Avoid large doses in cases of constipation or high blood pressure.

Many species in the genus have poisonous tubers, so eat only those that are known to be edible.

Range and Appearance

This perennial is rather beanlike, with meandering, twisting, climbing vines. *Dioscorea japonica* and *D. polystachya* are native to eastern Asia, while *D. bulbifera* is native to Africa and Asia and *D. villosa* is native to North America. The flowers are yellow, green, or lavender, the roots long and tuberous, and the leaves simple or palmately lobed.

WILLOW

Botanical Name

Salix spp., including *S. alba* (white willow), *S. bonplandiana* (red willow), *S. cinerea* (gray willow), *S. daphnoides* (violet willow), *S. discolor* (pussy willow), *S. fragilis* (crack willow), *S. melanopsis* (dusky willow), *S. nigra* (black willow), *S. purpurea* (purple osier), *S. sitchensis* (Sitka willow)

Family

Salicaceae (Willow Family)

Etymology

The genus name, *Salix,* derives from the Celtic *sal lis,* "near water." The common name *willow* derives from the Old English name for this tree, *welig.*

Also Known As

Danish: hvidpil
English: with, withy
Finnish: valkopaju
French: saule, osier
German: felbinger, weide, wilgenbaum
Italian: salice, salcio
Norwegian: kvitpil
Spanish: jarita, sauz
Swedish: vitpil
Turkish: ak sogut, soynd

Part Used

Inner bark

Physiological Effects

Alterative, anaphrodisiac, analgesic, anodyne, anti-bacterial, antifungal, anti-inflammatory, antirheumatic, antiseptic, astringent, bitter, diaphoretic, digestive, diuretic, febrifuge, hypnotic, sedative, tonic, vermifuge

Medicinal Uses

Willow was used in ancient Greece for the treatment of fevers. The bark contains a chemical called salicin, also known as methyl salicylate, that is also found in birch, meadowsweet, and wintergreen. Salicin relieves pain and reduces fever and inflammation. A chemist at the Bayer Corporation discovered that combining salicin with acetyl acid made it work more efficiently. The new compound, called aspirin, was launched into the marketplace in 1899.

Willow helps clear heat, deter infection, and reduce inflammation, in part by inhibiting prostaglandin production. It has an action similar to quinine in reducing fever. It is used in the treatment of angina, arthritic pain, back pain, colds, colic, diarrhea, dysentery, dyspepsia, fever, flu, gonorrhea, gout, hangover, hay fever, headache, heartburn, hot flashes, insomnia, irritability, malaria, migraine, neuralgia, night sweats, nymphomania, pain, rheumatic pain, urinary tract infection, and worms. It is also used in the prevention of cancer, stroke, and heart attack, in part because of its ability to thin the blood, prevent blood clots, and deter stagnation and the resulting toxic buildup in the body.

Topically, willow can be used as a mouthwash to relieve gum soreness, as a gargle to relieve sore throat and tonsillitis, as a hair rinse to get rid of dandruff, or as a poultice to treat arthritic pain, bunions, burns, corns, eczema, gangrene, poison ivy or oak, toothache, warts, and wounds.

As a flower essence, willow helps users to take personal responsibility for their actions and to have increased optimism. It is useful for those feeling bitterness or resentment or tending to blame others.

Edible Uses

Young willow shoots and leaves and the inner bark can be gathered in spring as edibles, they are rich in vitamin C. The inner bark can be eaten raw but is best if dried and made into flour.

Other Uses

Willow wood is an excellent pliable material for making baskets, wicker furniture, and dowsing rods. Willow is also used to make artist's charcoal. White willow is used commercially for making paper. Willow branches have long been used to douse for water. The leaves can be used as livestock fodder.

Constituents

Phosphorous, flavonoids (catechin), glycosides (salicin, populin, salicoside), salicortine, tannin; female willow buds contain phytoestrogens

Energetic Correspondences

- Flavor: bitter
- Temperature: cold
- Moisture: dry
- Polarity: yin
- Planet: Neptune/Moon/Saturn
- Element: water

Contraindications

Willow is not recommended during pregnancy. Avoid in cases of hemophilia or other risk of hemorrhage, and do not use in conjunction with blood-thinning medications or iodine supplements. Avoid giving willow bark to children with a viral infection accompanied by headache to avoid the risk of Reye's syndrome. Those who suffer from tinnitus or who are allergic to aspirin should use willow with caution.

Range and Appearance

Willows are fast-growing, deciduous trees that can grow to 70 feet tall. The leaves are long, narrow, and lance shaped, with a silvery color that appears on both sides but is more pronounced on the back. Small glands can be found on the edges of the leaves. The trees are dioecious, meaning that male and female flowers (catkins) appear on separate trees.

Willow likes to have wet feet and is often found in damp woods and along streams or bodies of water. It is native to northern Africa, Asia, Europe, and North America but is widely naturalized and cultivated.

WINTERGREEN

Botanical Name

Gaultheria procumbens

Family

Ericaceae (Heath Family)

Etymology

The genus name, *Gaultheria,* was given in honor of Jean François Gaultier, a mid-1700s physician from Quebec. The species name, *procumbens,* is Latin for "face down," in reference to the manner in which the stems trail along the ground. The common name *wintergreen* refers to the fact that the plant stays green throughout the winter.

Also Known As

Cantonese: lok ham chou, lok heun chou
English: boxberry, Canada tea, checkerberry, creeping wintergreen, deer berry, ground berry, hillberry, mountain tea, teaberry, wax cluster berry
Finnish: lamosalali
French: gaulthérie, pirole à feuilles rondes, pyrole
German: wintergrün
Mandarin: lu han cao, lu ti cao, lu xian cao
Sanskrit: gandapura

Parts Used

Leaf, flowering top

Physiological Effects

Analgesic, anodyne, antibacterial, antirheumatic, antiseptic, antispasmodic, aromatic, astringent, carminative, decongestant, diuretic, emmenagogue, expectorant, hemostatic, hypotensive, rubefacient, stimulant, tonic, vulnerary

Medicinal Uses

Native Americans have used wintergreen to treat rheumatism and chewed the leaves to increase their respiratory capacity, such as when running long distances or performing difficult labor. Settlers in Early America had their children chew the leaves for several weeks each spring to prevent tooth decay. The leaf was an official remedy in the United States Pharmacopoeia from 1820 to 1984, and essential oil of wintergreen is still listed there as an astringent, diuretic, and stimulant.

Wintergreen clears toxins from the body, promotes tissue repair, relieves pain, combats infection, and reduces inflammation. It is used in the treatment of amenorrhea, angina, arthritis, asthma, colds, colic, cystitis, diarrhea, fever, flatulence, flu, gout, headache, hookworm, hypertension, pain, prostatitis, rheumatism, spermatorrhea, tuberculosis, and urinary tract infection.

Topically, wintergreen can be used as an ingredient in massage oil, salve, or liniment or as a bath herb to treat cellulite, gout, headache, joint pain, lumbago, muscle soreness, paralysis, rheumatism, and sciatica.

The essential oil of wintergreen can be used, in diluted form, as a gargle to relieve sore throat.

Edible Uses

Wintergreen tea is a longtime favorite; it was used as a substitute for black tea during the American Revolution. The leaves can be used to make traditional root beers and as a flavoring for candy. Wintergreen berries are edible; they can be blended with honey or made into pies or jam. The berries are an important winter food for deer, bear, turkeys, grouse, partridges, and other wild creatures.

Other Uses

Native Americans smoked the leaves. The essential oil of wintergreen is sometimes included in toothpastes and mouthwashes for its breath-freshening properties. In folkloric tradition, placing the berries in children's pillows is said to protect them from harm and grant them a good life.

Constituents

Calcium, magnesium, phosphorous, potassium, zinc, glycoside, arbutin, ericolin, phenols (gaultherin), salicin, tannin, mucilage, gallic acid, ursolic acid, methylhydroquinone

Energetic Correspondences

- Flavor: bitter, sweet, pungent
- Temperature: cold
- Moisture: dry
- Polarity: yin
- Planet: Venus/Saturn/Moon
- Element: water

Contraindications

The methyl salicylate found in wintergreen is closely related to the acetylsalicylic acid found in aspirin; those allergic to aspirin or taking blood-thinning medications should use wintergreen cautiously. Do not use the essential oil undiluted, as it can irritate the skin. Do not ingest the essential oil, except under the guidance of a qualified health-care practitioner.

Nowadays most oil marketed as wintergreen essential oil is actually derived from birch or is totally synthetic. Make sure you're getting the real thing!

Range and Appearance

Wintergreen is a native American evergreen perennial found most often in coniferous forests. The plant reaches a height of about 6 inches. The leaves are oval, leathery, and glossy; they grow in a basal rosette and then alternately. The reddish stem produces an inflorescence of hermaphroditic white flowers with an open cup shape. The berries are red. The plant grows in full sun to partial shade in moist soil. It is excellent as a ground cover or in a rock garden.

WITCH HAZEL

Botanical Name

Hamamelis virginiana

Family

Hamamelidaceae (Witch Hazel Family)

Etymology

The genus name, *Hamamelis,* is thought to be a Greek term meaning the medlar tree or any fruit tree.

One reason the plant was given the common name *witch hazel* is that its forked branches were made into divining rods for dowsing. This technique was known in ancient Britain as *witching,* a term taken from *wice,* the Old English name for a tree with pliable branches.

Also Known As

Danish: hamamelia, troldnoed
Dutch: toverhazelaar, virginische hamamelis
English: American witch hazel, pistachio tree, snapping hazelnut, spotted alder, Virginia witch hazel, winterbloom
Finnish: amerikantaiapähkinä
French: hamamelida, hamamélis, noisetier des sorcieres
German: mamelide, zauberstrauch, zaubernuss
Italian: amamelide, hamamelis, trilopo
Portuguese: hamamélis
Spanish: hamamelis
Swedish: amerikansk trollhassel
Turkish: guvercin ag

Parts Used

Bark, twig, leaf

Physiological Effects

Antibacterial, anti-inflammatory, antioxidant, astringent, hemostatic, sedative, styptic, tonic

Medicinal Uses

Native Americans introduced European settlers to witch hazel, which quickly became popular among them. Witch hazel was listed in the United States Pharmacopoeia from 1862 through 1916 and in the National Formulary from 1916 to 1955. Its flavonoid content helps heal damaged blood vessels and contributes to the plant's astringent properties. Witch hazel has long been used in the treatment of colitis, diarrhea, dysentery, hemorrhage, hemorrhoids, leukorrhea, menorrhagia, organ prolapse, threat of miscarriage, and varicose veins.

For the preparation of topical applications, only the twigs are used, not the leaves or bark. The tannins found in the twigs precipitate the protein in wounds, thus helping to form a healing protective coating. Witch hazel can be used as a compress or salve to treat bruises, hemorrhoids, insect bites, muscle soreness, phlebitis, poison ivy, sunburn, swellings, and varicose veins. It also can be prepared as a sitz bath to treat hemorrhoids, as a douche to treat vaginitis, or as a wash to treat eye soreness. It is excellent as a gargle to relieve sore throat and tonsillitis and as a mouthwash to relieve gum inflammation. The Potawatomi Indians burned the twigs in sweat lodges to relieve sore muscles.

Distilled witch hazel is still a popular over-the-counter preparation, available in any drugstore. It can be applied directly to the skin to treat bedsores, blemishes, bruises, eczema, insect bites, pimples, poison ivy or oak, and sunburn. It is also used as an aftershave and to shrink enlarged pores. Athletes are known to rub witch hazel on their limbs prior to workouts to prevent muscle strain. Witch hazel can be frozen in ice-cube form (clearly labeled) and applied for cool, soothing relief in cases of bruises or swellings.

As a flower essence, witch hazel is helpful for those who allow themselves to be sacrificed while trying to live up to others' expectations.

Edible Uses

The barks, leaves, and twigs are not generally considered edible, aside from as tea. Witch hazel has edible black seeds that taste like pistachios. They ripen the summer following the fall flowering. They can be eaten raw or cooked.

Other Uses

Witch hazel is sometimes included in lotions, toners, and deodorants for its astringent properties.

Constituents

Choline, tannins (gallic acid), flavonoids (catechins, kaempferol, proanthocyanins, quercitin), saponins, essential oils (carvacol, eugenol, hexaenol)

Energetic Correspondences

- Flavor: bitter, pungent
- Temperature: cool
- Moisture: dry
- Polarity: yang
- Planet: Sun/Venus/Saturn
- Element: fire

Contraindications

Because of its high tannin content, witch hazel is very astringent. Topical applications of witch hazel should use only products made from the twigs, as those made from the bark or leaves may be disfiguring. Tincture of witch hazel can be too astringent for topical skin use. Use witch hazel internally only for short periods of time, as the high tannin content can be too astringent for the liver and constipating.

Although distilled witch hazel does not contain tannins, it often does contain rubbing alcohol, and it should not be used internally or applied close to mucous membranes, on broken skin, or in the eyes.

Range and Appearance

Witch hazel is a deciduous shrub native to North America. It most often grows in damp woods with acidic soil. Several trunks branch up from a single root, and they can reach a height of 8 to 12 feet. The leaves are alternate and elliptical, with hairy undersides; they turn yellow in autumn. The ribbonlike, hermaphroditic, sweet-scented, yellow flowers bloom in late autumn, after the leaves have fallen.

WOOD BETONY

Botanical Name

Stachys hyssopifolia, S. officinalis (formerly
   Betonica officinalis; syn. *S. betonica*),
   S. palustris (marsh betony), *S. sylvatica*

Family

Lamiaceae (Mint Family)

Etymology

The genus name *Stachys* is an ancient Greek term meaning "spike," in reference to the way the flowers grow. The name *betony* is thought to derive from the Latin *vettonica*, a reference to the Vettones, a people who inhabited a part of the Iberian Peninsula in ancient times. *Betony* could also derive from the Celtic *bew*, "head," and *ton*, "good," in reference to the herb's use for ailments of the head.

Also Known As

Danish: betonie
English: betony, bidney, bishop's wort, hedge nettle,
   wild hop
Finnish: rohtopähkämö
French: bétoine, epiare à feuilles minces
German: betonie, heil-ziest, ziest, ziestkraut
Italian: betonica
Norwegian: betonie
Spanish: betónica
Swedish: humlesuga, läkebetonika

Part Used

Aboveground plant

Physiological Effects

Alterative, analgesic, antispasmodic, astringent, aromatic, bitter, carminative, cerebral tonic, circulatory stimulant, diuretic, hepatotonic, hypoglycemic, hypotensive, nervine, sedative (mild), styptic, vulnerary

Medicinal Uses

Wood betony has long been held in high regard, as evidenced by the Spanish compliment, "He has as many virtues as betony," and the Italian saying, "It is better to sell your coat than be without betony." The ancient Anglo-Saxons wore wood betony as a protective charm.

Wood betony breaks up chi stagnation, relaxes the nerves, and relieves pain. One of its constituents, the alkaloid trigonelline, has been shown to help lower blood sugar levels. Wood betony is used in the treatment of alcoholism, allergies, anxiety, asthma, catarrh, colic, diarrhea, dyspepsia, drunkenness, edema, exhaustion, fear, flatulence, gout, headache, head cold, hearing loss, heartburn, hyperactivity, hypertension, hysteria, indigestion, insomnia, kidney dysfunction, migraine, neuralgia, nightmares, rheumatism, sore throat, stress, varicose veins, vertigo, worms, and worry.

Topically, wood betony can be applied to wounds to stop bleeding and prevent scarring. It also can be used as a poultice to draw out splinters and boils and to treat varicose veins. As a mouthwash and gargle it can be used to treat sores, sore gums, and sore throat. It was once used as a snuff and smoke to treat headache; because the snuff was apt to cause sneezing it dispelled congestion in the head.

As a flower essence, wood betony enhances pineal gland function, thus improving the user's sense of well-being. It fosters a desire for higher principles and inner calm and can be useful for those who are dealing with excessive sexual energy.

Edible Uses

The young shoots and leaves of all *Stachys* species can be eaten raw or cooked.

Other Uses

The fresh plant can be made into a hair rinse yielding golden highlights. It also can be used to make a yellow dye for wool. The dried plant has been burned as a purifying incense.

Constituents

Calcium, magnesium, manganese, phosphorous, potassium, choline, tannins, saponins, glucosides, alkaloids (betonicine, stachydrine, trigonelline), betaine, coffeic acid

Energetic Correspondences

- Flavor: bitter
- Temperature: cool
- Moisture: dry
- Polarity: yang
- Planet: Jupiter/Venus
- Element: fire

Contraindications

Wood betony is generally regarded as safe. However, large doses may cause vomiting. Pregnant women should avoid large doses, except during labor, and then only under the guidance of a qualified healthcare practitioner.

Do not confuse *Stachys* species with *Pedicularis* species, which are also known as *betony,* as their uses are not interchangeable.

Range and Appearance

A perennial native to Europe, Asia, and northern Africa, wood betony grows in shady woods where lime is present in the soil. It has a tall, hairy stem and rough, fringed leaves. The two-lipped flowers range in color from pink to purple and bloom in whorls from short spikes. The spikes have the unique quality of having a break in the flower rings, so that the spike is interrupted.

WOODRUFF

Botanical Name

Galium odoratum (syn. *Asperula odorata*)

Family

Rubiaceae (Madder Family)

Etymology

The genus name *Galium* derives from the Greek *gala,* "milk." The species name *odoratum* is Latin for "fragrant." The common name *woodruff* derives from the Old English *wudurofe,* from *wudu,* "wood," and *rofe,* most likely from the French *rouvelle,* "wheel," in reference to the whorl of leaves surrounding the stem.

Also Known As

Dutch: walstroo
English: hay plant, master of the woods, musk of the woods, Our Lady's bedstraw, sweet woodruff, wood root, wood-rova, woodward, wuderove
French: aspérule odorante, belle-etoile, muge-des-bois, petit muguet, reine des bois
German: ackermeir, waldmeie, waldmeister ("master of the woods")
Italian: asperula dei campi, piccolo mughetto, raspello, regina dei boschi, stellina odorosa
Spanish: cuaja leche

Part Used

Aboveground plant

Physiological Effects

Alterative, anti-inflammatory, antispasmodic, astringent, cardiotonic, carminative, cholagogue, diuretic, digestive, liver tonic, sedative (mild), tonic

Medicinal Uses

Woodruff clears obstructions in the body, which aids in the elimination of toxins. It is used in the treatment of depression, digestive weakness, dropsy, dysmenorrhea, epilepsy, hepatitis, insomnia, jaundice, menopause symptoms, phlebitis, and varicose veins.

Topically, woodruff can be used as a poultice to treat boils, headaches, and wounds. Such a poultice would also function as an anticoagulant on wounds, should that be the desired effect. Woodruff can also be prepared as a soothing footbath for tired feet.

Edible Uses

The leaves are edible raw or cooked. They should be picked just a few hours prior to use to allow the flavor to develop. Woodruff leaf is often used to improve the flavor of teas and sweet wines such as German May wine. The flowers are also edible.

Other Uses

When dried, woodruff becomes delightfully scented, smelling something like new-cut grass, vanilla, and honey. Woodruff is used to make perfume, insect repellent, potpourri, and snuffs. It was once used to stuff mattresses and was a popular strewing herb during the Middle Ages. When mixed with animal fodder, it gives cow's milk a delicious aroma. Woodruff rhizome, like all those in the *Galium* genus, yields a red dye. In magical traditions, woodruff is carried to attract prosperity, bring victory, and give protection from harm.

Constituents

Coumarinic compounds (which release coumarin as the plant breaks down), iridoids (asperuloside, monotropein), anthraquinones, flavonoids, organic acids (citric acid, rubichloric acid), tannin

Energetic Correspondences

- Flavor: sweet
- Temperature: warm
- Moisture: dry
- Polarity: yang
- Planet: Venus/Mars/Moon
- Element: water/fire

Contraindications

Large doses may cause dizziness and possibly internal bleeding. Avoid using in conjunction with blood-thinning medications. Avoid during pregnancy.

Range and Appearance

Native to Europe and Asia but naturalized elsewhere, woodruff is a perennial most often found in deciduous forests, especially among beech trees. It reaches a height of 8 to 12 inches. The leaves are lanceolate and grow in whorls of six to eight. The flowers are small, tubular, white, four-petaled, six to nine in number, and arranged in a terminal corymb.

WORMWOOD

Botanical Name

Artemisia absinthium, A. maritima, A. pontica

Family

Asteraceae (Daisy Family)

Etymology

The species name *Artemisia* derives from that of the Greek goddess Artemis, who is said to have given this herb to the centaur Chiron. The common name *wormwood* derives from the Old English *wermode*, "mind preserver."

Also Known As

Cantonese: ta-feng ai
Croatian: gorski pelin
Danish: malurt
Dutch: absint, alsem
English: absinthe, green ginger, madderwort, old woman, southernwood

Finnish: koiruoho, mali
French: absinthe, absinthium, armoise amère
German: absinth, wermut
Italian: assenzio
Japanese: niga yomogi
Norwegian: malurt
Polish: piolun
Portuguese: absinto, losna
Russian: polin
Sanskrit: indhana
Spanish: absintio, ajenjo
Swedish: malört
Vietnamese: cây nga'i dang

Part Used

Aboveground plant

Physiological Effects

Alterative, anthelmintic, antibiotic, antidepressant, anti-inflammatory, antiparasitic, antiseptic, antispasmodic, aromatic, bitter, carminative, cholagogue, choleretic, digestive, emmenagogue, febrifuge, hypnotic, stimulant, stomachic, vermifuge

Medicinal Uses

Wormwood's bitter flavor stimulates digestive secretions, the liver, and the gallbladder's production of bile. Wormwood also improves the body's absorption of nutrients. One of its constituents, thujone, works as a brain stimulant. Wormwood has been used in the treatment of anemia, anorexia, arthritis, bloating, childbirth (pain and placenta retention), colds, depression, fever, flatulence, gallstones, gastritis, hepatitis, jaundice, lead poisoning, rheumatism, and worms (roundworms, threadworms).

Topically, wormwood can be used in liniments, poultices, and compresses to treat bruises, insect bites and stings, and pain. It also can be made into a wash to get rid of lice or scabies and to soothe itchy skin.

Edible Uses

Wormwood is sometimes used in stuffings for geese. Its most renowned edible use was as an ingredient in absinthe, a green alcoholic liqueur that functioned as a narcotic analgesic, affecting the medullary portion of the brain concerned with pain and anxiety. Absinthe induces a dreamy, altered state of mind. It was especially popular in the late 1800s and early 1900s with artists such as Baudlaire, Degas, Gauguin, Manet, Toulouse Lautrec, and Van Gogh and was also used by writers such as Jack London, Edgar Allan Poe, and Oscar Wilde. Because of its addictive qualities, and the at times deranged states of mind that it caused (possibly resulting from the copper stills and salts used to give the drink color), absinthe has been banned in many countries.

Other Uses

The leaves are sometimes dried and burned as a purifying incense or added to smoking mixtures. Wormwood is sometimes used as a strewing herb, and as a beneficial side effect it repels insects and mice (though it can attract dogs). The plant is sometimes made into a spray to deter pests in the garden, and it can be added to sachets to keep moths away from clothes. In folkloric tradition, wormwood is said to give protection from the "evil eye."

Constituents

Essential oils (absinthol, azulenes, camphene, cineol, isovaleric acid, pinene, thujone), sesquiterpene lactones (absinthin), bitters (absinthium), flavonoids (quercetin), polyacetylenes

Energetic Correspondences

- Flavor: bitter
- Temperature: cold
- Moisture: dry
- Polarity: yin
- Planet: Moon/Mars/Pluto
- Element: air

Contraindications

Avoid during pregnancy. Do not give to children. Large doses are toxic and can cause nausea, vomiting, vertigo, restlessness, and delirium; small doses, however, are generally safe to use.

Range and Appearance

Native to western Asia, Europe and northern Africa but naturalized in North America, wormwood is a perennial reaching 2 to 4 feet in height. It features alternate, silvery green leaves and small, yellow, hermaphroditic flowers. It requires full sun but will tolerate varying soil and moisture conditions, including drought.

YARROW

Botanical Name

Achillea millefolium (syn. *A. lanulosa*)

Family

Asteraceae (Daisy Family)

Etymology

The genus name *Achillea* derives from that of Achilles, the hero Greek legend, who was taught herbology by the centaur Chiron. Achilles is said to have used yarrow to staunch his wounds during the Trojan War. The species name *millefolium* is Latin for "a thousand leaves." The common name yarrow derives from the Old English name for the plant, *gearwe*.

Also Known As

English: carpenter's weed, herba militaris, life
   medicine, milfoil, soldier's woundwort,
   staunchweed
French: millefoille
German: schargarbe
Italian: achillea
Sanskrit: rojmari
Spanish: plumajillo

Part Used

Flowering top

Physiological Effects

Analgesic, anodyne, antifungal, anti-inflammatory, antiseptic, antispasmodic, aromatic, astringent, carminative, cholagogue, circulatory stimulant, diaphoretic, digestive, diuretic, emmenagogue, expectorant, febrifuge, hemostatic, hypotensive, nerve relaxant, odontalgic, parturient, stimulant, stomachic, styptic, sudorific, tonic, urinary antiseptic, uterine decongestant, uterine stimulant, vasodilator, vulnerary

Medicinal Uses

Yarrow opens the pores, purifies the blood, soothes inflammation, circulates chi, regulates liver function, relaxes spasms, strengthens the venous system, and calms the nerves. It also helps relax peripheral blood vessels, thereby improving circulation. Drinking yarrow as a hot tea increases body temperature and produces sweating; drinking it cold has more of a diuretic effect. A classic tea to relieve the symptoms of colds and flus is prepared from yarrow, peppermint, and ginger.

Yarrow is used in the treatment of amenorrhea, anorexia, Bright's disease, catarrh (due to allergies), chicken pox, colds, coronary thrombosis, cystitis, diarrhea, dysentery, dysmenorrhea, dyspepsia, eczema, fever, flatulence, flu, hay fever, headache, hemorrhage, hyperacidity, incontinence, indigestion, irregular menses, jaundice, leukorrhea, measles, menorrhagia, nephritis, pneumonia, postpartum hemorrhage, rheumatism, stomachache, typhoid, tuberculosis, ulcers, urethritis, and varicose veins.

Topically, yarrow is an excellent herb to promote tissue repair. A poultice of fresh leaves helps stop the bleeding of wounds, and fresh leaves placed in the nose will stop a nosebleed. Yarrow also can be prepared as a compress to treat blood blisters, hemorrhoids, migraine, toothache, and varicose veins. A steam inhalation of yarrow treats asthma and hay fever and is useful for clearing up oily or blemished skin. Yarrow can be used as a wash for acne, blemishes, oily skin, and eczema; as a hair rinse for hair loss; as a bath herb for skin complaints; as a douche or sitz bath for female complaints; and as a mouthwash for inflamed gums.

As a flower essence, yarrow gives protection against negative environmental influences. It is of benefit for those who work under fluorescent lights or in front of computers, helping them to be less stressed from the effects of modern living.

Edible Uses

The bitter young leaves and flowers are edible, raw or cooked. Yarrow is sometimes used in making liqueurs, and it is used in making Swedish beer to increase the intoxicating effects and preserve the beer. The essential oil of yarrow is used as a soda flavoring agent.

Other Uses

Dried yarrow stalks were once used to throw the I Ching, an ancient Chinese system for guidance and wisdom. Druids used yarrow stems to foretell the weather. In medieval times it was used as a strewing herb. The herb is sometimes used to flavor tobacco and as a snuff. A yellow and green dye can be made from the flowers. The blue essential oil distilled from yarrow is used in cosmetics as an anti-inflammatory agent.

In folkloric tradition, holding yarrow over one's eyes is said to enhance clairvoyance. Putting some under one's pillow is said to bring dreams of one's true love. And hanging yarrow over the bed of a married couple is said to ensure their love for at least seven years.

Constituents

Beta-carotene, B-complex vitamins, vitamin C, vitamin E, choline, inositol, calcium, copper, magnesium, phosphorous, potassium, silicon, essential oils (proazulene, azulene, borneol, camphor, cineole, eugenol, linalool, pinene, sabinene, thujone), isovalerianic acid, achillein, formic acid, salicylic acid, polyacetylenes, asparagin, sterols, glycoalkaloid (achilleine), flavonoids (apigenin, luteolin, quercitin), coumarins, tannins

Energetic Correspondences

- Flavor: bitter, sweet, pungent
- Temperature: cool
- Moisture: dry
- Polarity: yin
- Planet: Venus
- Element: water

Contraindications

Overuse may cause skin photosensitivity, dizziness, and headache in some people. Rare individuals may be sensitive to yarrow and experience dermatitis after use. Avoid yarrow during pregnancy.

Range and Appearance

Yarrow, a perennial native to the northern hemisphere, thrives in partial shade to full sun with well-drained soil. It does best with low to moderate watering, but it can tolerate drought better than most plants. It grows from 1 to 3 feet tall on an angular stem. The alternate leaves have a feathery appearance, are 3 to 4 inches long, and clasp the stem at the base. The aromatic, hermaphroditic flowers are five-petaled rays that can be white to pink to pale purple, look like miniature daisies, and grow in flattened terminal loose heads.

Added to a compost pile, yarrow will accelerate its breakdown. When grown in the garden, it helps other plants nearby be more disease resistant.

YELLOW DOCK

Botanical Name

Rumex crispus

Family

Polygonaceae (Buckwheat Family)

Etymology

Rumex is an ancient Latin word for "lance," referring to the shape of the leaves. *Crispus* is Latin for "curly," in reference to the edges of the leaf. The common name *dock* derives from the Old English name for this plant, *docce*.

Also Known As

English: curly dock, garden patience, narrow dock, sour dock, spurdock
Finnish: poimuhierakka
French: churelle, herbe britannique, oreille de vache, parielle, patience, rhubarbe sauvage

German: gelber ampfer, grindampfer, krauser ampfer, mengelwurz, wilder mangolt, zitterwurz

Italian: erba britannica, romice

Sanskrit: amlavetasa

Spanish: acedera, bandana, canagria, lengua de vaca

Swedish: krusskräppa, krussyra

Part Used

Root

Physiological Effects

Alterative, anti-inflammatory, antiscorbutic, aperient, antiseptic, astringent, blood tonic, cholagogue, depurative, diuretic, laxative, tonic

Medicinal Uses

Though introduced from Europe, yellow dock root was widely used by the Native Americans. This herb was included in the United States Pharmacopoeia from 1863 to 1905. It clears toxins, moves stagnation, promotes bowel cleansing and bile flow, reduces inflammation, and inhibits the growth of *E. coli* and staph. Yellow dock helps to free up iron stored in the liver, thus making it more available to the rest of the body. As a tea, it aids in the digestion of fatty foods.

Yellow dock is used in the treatment of acne, anemia, appetite loss, arsenic poisoning, arthritis, boils, cancer, catarrh, constipation, dermatitis, eczema, glandular tumors, indigestion, jaundice, leprosy, liver congestion, lumbago, lymph node enlargement, malabsorbtion, psoriasis, rheumatism, scrofula, sore throat, and syphilis. It also is used to encourage convalescence.

Topically, yellow dock can be used as a poultice to soothe stings from nettle plants and as a poultice or salve to treat athlete's foot, boils, eczema, hives, itchy skin, ringworm, scabies, skin infection, swellings, ulcers, and wounds. It can be prepared as a tooth powder to treat gingivitis or a gargle to treat laryngitis. It also can be made into a douche or bolus to treat vaginitis.

Edible Uses

The leaves and peeled stems are nutritive. Eat them in spring and late fall (after the first hard frost). The young greens can be eaten raw or cooked as a potherb. Older leaves need to be soaked or cooked in two changes of water to remove bitterness. The leaves have a flavor similar to that of rhubarb and can be used in pie. The seeds are used as a grain; they are usually dried, threshed, and ground into flour. They can also be roasted and used as a coffee substitute.

Other Uses

Yellow dock is useful for animals as well as humans; it can be prepared as a poultice to treat saddle sores on horses, mules, and donkeys and mange on dogs. The roots yield a brown to dark gray dye.

In folkloric tradition, a woman will wear yellow dock seeds on her left arm to increase her chances of conceiving a child. The seeds are also used in prosperity rituals and are sprinkled about a place of business to attract customers.

Constituents

Calcium, iron, magnesium, sulfur, anthraquinones, glycosides (nepodin, emodin, chryysophanol), quercitrin, mucilage, tannins, resins, oxalates

Energetic Correspondences

- Flavor: bitter
- Temperature: cool
- Moisture: dry
- Polarity: yang
- Planet: Mars/Jupiter/Saturn
- Element: air

Contraindications

Yellow dock leaves are high in oxalate, which can impair calcium absorption and potentially aggravate kidney stones, arthritis, gout, and hyperacidity. Large amounts of the root or leaves may cause nausea, vomiting, or diarrhea. In rare cases handling the plant may result in contact dermatitis.

Range and Appearance

Native to northern Africa, Asia, and Europe, yellow dock is a perennial that can reach a height of 1 to 5 feet. It has large, curly basal leaves. The hermaphroditic flowers are greenish. The seeds are three-sided winged capsules that turn rusty red when mature. The roots are russet on the outside and a deep yellow or orange within.

YERBA MANSA

Botanical Name

Anemopsis californica (syn. *Houttuynia californica*)

Family

Saururaceae (Lizard Tail Family)

Etymology

The genus name, *Anemopsis,* derives from the Greek *anemos,* "wind," and *opsis,* "likeness" or "similarity." The species name *californica* alludes to the plant's native range in California. *Yerba mansa* is Spanish for "gentle herb." The Spanish common name *yerba del manso* means "herb of the *manso,*" a reference to the Indians who worked at Spanish missions in California, who were known as *mansos.* The common name *lizard's tail* refers to the long, pinkish runners the plant sends out in spring.

Also Known As

English: lizard's tail, swamp root
Spanish: bavisa, raiz del manso, yerba del manso

Parts Used

Root, leaf

Physiological Effects

Alterative, analgesic, antibacterial, antiemetic, antifungal, anti-inflammatory, antiseptic, aromatic, astringent, carminative, diuretic, immune stimulant, stomachic, tonic, vulnerary

Medicinal Uses

Yerba mansa improves the body's fluid transport, helps remove matter that interferes with tissue repair, and tonifies the structure of the mucous membranes. It is a traditional panacea of Native Americans of the Southwest, used to treat colds, cramps, diabetes, pain, and tuberculosis. It is often recommended for treating infections that are not healing properly. It is also used to treat asthma, bronchitis, catarrh, colds, cough, diarrhea, digestive weakness, dysentery, flu, gonorrhea, herpes, indigestion, laryngitis, lung infection, malaria, pleurisy, ulcers, urinary tract infection, and vaginitis.

Topically, yerba mansa can be prepared as a wash to treat wounds; a salve or compress to help heal fungal infections and sores; a mouthwash or gargle to soothe and treat receding and inflamed gums as well as sore throat; a nasal spray to remedy hay fever; a snuff to treat nasal polyps; a powder to treat athlete's foot; a bath herb to relieve arthritis and sore muscles; a sitz bath to treat Bartholin gland cysts and anal fissures; and a douche to treat yeast infection.

Edible Uses

The root is edible raw or cooked. The seeds can be dried, ground, and used in place of grain to make cereal.

Other Uses

The roots are sometimes made into decorative beads.

Constituents

Methyleugenol, esdragole, thymol, linalool, asarinin, tannin

Energetic Correspondences

- Flavor: bitter, pungent
- Temperature: warm
- Moisture: dry
- Polarity: yang
- Planet: Mars
- Element: fire

Contraindications

Generally considered safe.

Range and Appearance

Yerba mansa is an evergreen shrub native to the American West and northern Mexico. It grows in stands in moist, swampy areas. Its stem reaches about 1 to 2 feet in height. The large, flat basal leaves are 3 to 6 inches long, have toothless margins, and often are fuzzy around the edges. The plant bears clusters of conelike, hermaphroditic, fragrant white flowers, encircled by white bracts that are often tinged with red. The entire plant turns rust red in the fall.

YERBA MATÉ

Botanical Name

Ilex paraguariensis (syn. *I. domestica, I. mate, I. sorbilis*)

Family

Aquifoliaceae (Holly Family)

Etymology

The term *ilex* is taken from the botanical name of the holly oak, *Quercus ilex,* whose foliage resembles that of holly; as a genus name, it indicates that this plant is in the Holly Family. The species name is a Latin term meaning "a native of Paraguay." The common name *maté* derives from the Quechua *mati,* the name of the hollowed-out gourd (*Lagenaria vulgaris*) used as a cup for drinking maté.

Also Known As

English: Brazil tea, green gold of the Indios, hervea, Jesuit's tea, maté, Paraguay tea, St. Bartholomew's tea, South American holly, yaupon holly
Finnish: matee
French: arbre à maté, houx, thé du Paraguay
German: matebaum, matéstrauch, stechpalme
Italian: aquifoglio, maté, paragua
Mandarin: mao dong qing
Portuguese: erve mate
Quechua: ka'a
Spanish: aceba, yerva de palos

Part Used

Leaf

Physiological Effects

Alterative, antibacterial, antioxidant, antiscorbutic, antispasmodic, aperient, aphrodisiac, astringent, cardiotonic, depurative, diaphoretic, digestive, diuretic, immune stimulant, nervous system stimulant, purgative (in large amounts), rejuvenative, stimulant, stomachic, sudorific, thermogenic, tonic

Medicinal Uses

Yerba maté cleanses the blood, decreases the appetite, and stimulates the mind, the respiratory system, and the nervous system. It is said to help users better tolerate hot, humid weather. Because maté helps cleanse the body of wastes without harming beneficial intestinal flora, some people drink it when they are on a cleanse, diet, or fast. It is often used to improve memory and concentration. It also delays the buildup of uric acid after a workout, thereby improving motor response.

Yerba maté is used in the treatment of allergies, arthritis, colds, constipation, depression, diabetes, fatigue, hay fever, headache, heavy metal toxicity, hemorrhoids, hypotension, migraines, neuralgia, obesity, rheumatic pain, scurvy, sinusits, and stress.

The tea's saponin and tannin content make it useful as a wash in cleansing wounds and as a compress to speed the healing process.

Edible Uses

Yerba maté is not generally considered edible, aside from as tea. As a tea, however, it has achieved widespread renown. In some places in South America it is consumed more frequently than coffee or black tea. It is often served with burnt sugar and lemon juice, and it is traditionally sipped through the metal straw called a *bombilla* (which strains out the herbs).

Maté tea comes in green (unfermented) and black (fermented) varieties. In general, the leaves are collected when the berries are ripe, then heated briefly to preserve their color. However, maté grows in a wide variety of conditions and, like green and black tea, has many different methods of cultivation and processing, each contributing to the tea's flavor.

Other Uses

In South American folkloric tradiation, maté tea is

used in love potions: a couple that wants to stay together drinks it together, while someone wanting to break off a relationship sprinkles some on the floor.

Constituents

Beta-carotene, vitamin B, vitamin C, calcium, iron, magnesium, manganese, potassium, quercitin, silicon, sulfur, xanthine derivatives (caffeine citronate, theobromine, theophylline), neocholerogenic acid, chlorogenic acid, essential oils (eugenol, gerniol), tannins

Energetic Correspondences

- Flavor: slightly bitter
- Temperature: cool
- Moisture: dry
- Polarity: yang
- Planet: Mars/Saturn
- Element: fire

Contraindications

Maté contains caffeine; however, its tannins tend to bind with the caffeine, thereby reducing both compounds' effects. Most people who find that caffeine impairs their sleep will not experience this effect with maté. But those suffering from anxiety, heart palpitations, or insomnia should use maté cautiously.

It is best to avoid consuming maté with meals, as the high tannin content can impair nutrient assimilation.

Range and Appearance

This South American shrub grows from 4 to 20 feet in height. It has four-petaled, greenish white flowers with alternate, oval or lanceolate, broadly toothed, hollylike leaves. It bears a red, yellow, or black fruit the size of a peppercorn. The plant can grow in full sun or shade in climates with hot, wet summers and cold, dry winters. It prefers iron-rich soils.

YERBA SANTA

Botanical Name

Eriodictyon californicum

Family

Hydrophyllaceae (Waterleaf Family)

Etymology

The genus name *Eriodictyon* derives from the Greek *erodios,* "heron," in reference to the long beak on the fruit. The genus name, *californicum,* indicates that the plant is native to California. *Yerba santa* is Spanish for "holy herb"; the name was given to this herb by early Spanish settlers in the American Southwest.

Also Known As

English: bear's weed, consumptive weed, eriodictyon, gum bush, holy herb, mountain balm, tarweed, sacred herb, wild balsam
German: santakraut
Spanish: hierba santa

Part Used

Leaf

Physiological Effects

Alterative, antiasthmatic, antiseptic, antispasmodic, aromatic, astringent, bronchial dilator, carminative, decongestant, expectorant, pectoral, siliagogue, stimulant, tonic

Medicinal Uses

Yerba santa was one of the most widely used herbs of the Native Americans of Mendocino County in northern California at the time when European explorers first began to venture through. It was an official herb in the United States Pharmacopoeia from 1894 to 1905, and again from 1916 to 1947. It is effective for decreasing mucus in the lungs and normalizing the mucus-secreting cells in the respiratory, urinary, and digestive tract. It also strengthens capillaries and helps stimulate the cilia of the lungs.

Yerba santa is used in the treatment of asthma, bronchitis, catarrh, colds, cough, cystitis, dysentery, fever, flu, hay fever, hemorrhoids, laryngitis, pneumonia, rheumatism, sinus congestion, sore throat, and urinary tract infection.

Topically, yerba santa can be used as a wash or poultice to treat broken bones, bruises, fever, insect bites, poison oak and ivy, rash, sprains, and sores. The herb is also used in saunas and steam baths for its pleasant, decongesting odor and its ability to soothe the pain of rheumatism. The leaves were once smoked to treat asthma and bronchial spasms.

As a flower essence, yerba santa gladdens the emotional heart and enables emotions to flow freely, helping to relieve repressed grief. It can be beneficial for those who are wasting away and especially susceptible to lung disorders.

Edible Uses

The leaves can be chewed like gum and help quench thirst. They were at one time mixed with alcohol to make an intoxicating beverage. They were also used to disguise the flavor of quinine. They yield a flavoring that can be used to flavor confections and beverages. They make an aromatic tea.

Other Uses

The leaves have been woven to make clothing. They are sometimes burned as incense. In folkloric tradition yerba santa is used to enhance beauty and increase psychic ability.

Constituents

Flavonoids (eriodictyol), hemoeriodictyl, chrysocriol, zanthoeridol, eridonel, phytosterol, pentatriacontane acid, cerotonic acid, glucose, resin (eriodonol)

Energetic Correspondences

- Flavor: pungent, sweet
- Temperature: warm
- Moisture: dry
- Polarity: yin
- Planet: Mercury
- Element: air

Contraindications

Avoid during pregnancy. Large doses may cause excessively dry sinuses, nausea, vomiting, or diarrhea.

Range and Appearance

Yerba santa is native to the mountains and deserts of the American West and northwestern Mexico. It is a resinous evergreen bush that can form thickets and grow up to 10 feet tall. The stems are sticky and hairless. The leaves are alternate, leathery, and hairy, with coarsely toothed margins. The trumpet-shaped, purplish to white flowers grow in flat clusters. The plant requires full sun and sandy, well-drained soil.

YOHIMBE

Botanical Name

Pausinystalia yohimbe (formerly *Corynanthe yohimbe*)

Family

Rubiaceae (Madder Family)

Etymology

The name *yohimbe* is thought to have been borrowed from a Bantu language of southern Cameroon.

Also Known As

Danish: johimbe
English: johimbe, quebrachin
German: yohimbe

Part Used

Bark

Physiological Effects

Analgesic, antidiuretic, aphrodisiac, cardiac stimulant, cerebral stimulant, hallucinogen (mild), hypertensive, kidney yang tonic, serotonin inhibitor, stimulant, vasodilator

Medicinal Uses

Yohimbe has been used medicinally in Africa for hundreds of years, especially by the Bantu people. It increases blood flow to the genitals, compresses the veins, and prevents the blood from flowing back out of the genital area, while also stimulating the ganglian nerve center at the base of the spine and thus stimulating erection. It has been found to restore erectile function in many cases of psychogenic (psychological) impotence. It is also sometimes recommended as an herb for weight loss (though there are safer herbs one could choose for this purpose), and it increases adrenaline production. It is used in the treatment of angina, depression, dysmenorrhea, erectile dysfunction, low libido, and narcolepsy.

Topically, yohimbe can be used as a poultice for pain relief, to treat skin infection and itchiness, and as an analgesic. The powdered bark is sometimes smoked, used as snuff, or rubbed on the body as an aphrodisiac.

Edible Uses

Not generally considered edible, aside from as tea.

Other Uses

None known

Constituents

Indole alkaloids (yohimbine, yohimbiline, ajmaline, pseudoyohimbine, corynantheine), tannins

Energetic Correspondences

- Flavor: pungent, bitter
- Temperature: warm
- Moisture: dry
- Polarity: yang
- Planet: Mars
- Element: fire

Contraindications

Yohimbe is best used under the guidance of a qualified health-care practitioner. It should be ingested no more than twice a week and used only in small doses, as large doses can cause depression and reduced sex drive. Yohimbe can elevate blood pressure and cause insomnia, mania, tremors, nausea, and vomiting. Avoid using in conjunction with pharmaceuticals, particularly MAO inhibitors and medications for treating diabetes, high blood pressure, and

heart problems. Avoid in cases of diabetes, heart disease, hypertension, kidney disease, liver disease, prostate inflammation, bipolar conditions, and schizophrenia. It's also best to avoid tyramine-rich foods (bananas, cheese, chocolate, sauerkraut, red wine) for twelve hours before using yohimbe, as the combination can elevate blood pressure.

Range and Appearance

Native to tropical West Africa, yohimbe is a fast-growing evergreen tree that can reach a height of 90 feet. It has sessile, obovate leaves that grow in whorls of three. Its reddish brown bark has many furrows. The flowers are white at first and later turn yellow and red. A tree must be at least ten years old before its bark is ready to be harvested, and harvesting the bark can kill the tree. Overharvesting of this plant is contributing to its decreased populations, so use this herb with care and only when needed.

YUCCA

Botanical Name

Yucca spp., including *Yucca baccata* (banana yucca, Our Lord's candle), *Y. brevifolia* (Joshua tree), *Y. filamentosa* (Adam's needle), *Y. glauca* (soapweed), *Y. schidigera* (Mojave yucca)

More than two dozen yuccas grow in North America, and they are used almost interchangeably.

Family

Agavaceae (Agave Family)

Etymology

The word *yucca* is a Caribbean name (probably Taino, a native language of Haiti) for cassava, a plant that was once believed to be in the same genus.

Also Known As

English: datil, guardian of the desert, needle palm, Spanish bayonet, Spanish dagger, Our Lord's candle

Finnish: hapsijukka
German: palmlilie
Spanish: amole, yuca
Swedish: palmlilja

Part Used

Root (dried)

Physiological Effects

Alterative, anti-inflammatory, antirheumatic, antispasmodic, astringent, laxative, oxytocic

Medicinal Uses

The saponins in yucca root are believed to accelerate the breakdown of organic wastes. Yucca can be used in the treatment of arthritis, constipation, diarrhea, gout, indigestion, rheumatism, prostatitis, and urethritis.

Topically, yucca root can be prepared as a poultice to treat inflammation, sprains, and skin diseases. Chopping the root and mixing it with water causes it to lather, making an excellent biodegradable soap that can also be used as shampoo to prevent hair loss, get rid of dandruff, and deter lice and other parasites.

Although traditionally the root of yucca is used medicinally, the fresh, undried flowers are being investigated for their antitumor activity.

Edible Uses

Yucca has long served as a wild food. The flower stalks can be harvested before the flowers open and consumed raw or cooked as a vegetable. The flowers can be eaten raw; they also are sometimes made into tempura or added to stir-fry dishes. Some yucca varieties have fruits that dry up at maturity, while fruits of other species remain fleshy. Those that dry at maturity can be eaten unripe, but they must be peeled and are often more edible if boiled. The fleshy varieties can be consumed raw. Yucca seed pods can be eaten as a vegetable or ground into flour. Some species of yucca are made into the intoxicating beverages tequila and mescal.

Other Uses

Fibers can be peeled from the leaves after they have been soaked; the fiber is used to make shoes, rope, mats, fishing line, brooms, paintbrushes, baskets, and sewing needles. The core of the plant's center stalk can be used as tinder.

The roots of *Y. filamentosa* were once pounded by native peoples and added to corralled fish to stupefy them. The juice from the leaf was used to make poison arrows.

Steroidal saponins extracted from yucca have been found to improve the growth rate of alfalfa, citrus trees, onions, potatoes, strawberries, and tomatoes.

Constituents

Galactose, arabinose, glucose, saponins (sapogenins, tigogenin)

Energetic Correspondences

- Flavor: sweet
- Temperature: cool
- Moisture: moist
- Polarity: yang
- Planet: Mars/Pluto
- Element: fire

Contraindications

Use only dried yucca root, as the fresh root can irritate the digestive system. Avoid during pregnancy. The fresh leaves have been reported to be toxic to livestock and should not be consumed.

Range and Appearance

Yuccas are perennials native to the arid desert regions of North America. Their long, sword-shaped leaves grow in a rosette and are stiff with a sharp tip. The flowers are whitish, six-petaled bells that partially close during the day and open at night. They are more fragrant at night.

Y. baccata's leaves extend up to 3 feet in length and are spine tipped, with margins that shred into coarse fibers; its flowers are somewhat reddish brown on the outside and cream colored inside. *Y. filamentosa* has fraying, twisting threads on its leaf margins and whitish green flowers on smooth, branched stalks. *Y. brevifolia* can reach a height of 30 feet and has stiff green-blue leaves that are clustered at the ends of the branches. *Y. glauca's* flowers are more whitish, and its leaves are rounded on the back, with their edges curving in.

A pronuba moth lives in the flowers and also pollinates them. Before eating freshly collected yucca flowers, spread them out for a few hours so that any resident moths can escape.

ZEDOARY

Botanical Name

Curcuma zedoaria

Family

Zingiberaceae (Ginger Family)

Etymology

The genus name *Curcuma* derives from the Arabic *kurkum,* "yellow dye." The species name, *zedoaria,* from which the common name *zedoary* derives, derives from the Arabic name for this plant, *jadwaar.*

Also Known As

Cantonese: ngoh seuht
Croatian: bijeli isiot, sekvar
Czech: zedoár
Dutch: zedoarwortl
English: white turmeric
Estonian: tsitverijuur
French: zédoaire
German: zitwer
Hindi: kachura, kachur sugandhi
Hungarian: fehér kurkuma, zedoária-gyökér
Indonesian: kunir putih
Italian: zedoaria
Japanese: gajutsu
Korean: ach'ul
Mandarin: é zhú
Portuguese: zedoária
Russian: zedoari
Sanskrit: shati

Spanish: cedoaria
Swedish: zittverrot
Thai: kha min khao
Turkish: cedvar
Ukrainian: kurkuma zedoarskaya
Vietnamese: nga truât
Yiddish: tsitver-kurkume

Part Used

Rhizome

Physiological Effects

Antiemetic, antitumor, aromatic, astringent, bitter, carminative, circulatory stimulant, febrifuge

Medicinal Uses

Zedoary breaks up blood and chi congestion and helps alleviate pain. It is being investigated for its potential in the treatment of cervical cancer and to increase the effectiveness of chemotherapy and radiotherapy. In India it is given to babies and invalids, mixed with cinnamon, pepper, and honey, in the treatment of colds. It is also an ingredient in some bitter digestive tonics.

Zedoary is used in the treatment of bloating, cancer, flatulence, indigestion, sore throat, and spleen enlargement.

Topically, zedoary can be prepared as a poultice to draw out infection from wounds or as a gargle to relieve sore throat.

Edible Uses

The rhizome and leaves are edible. The root has a smell like a cross between turmeric and mango and is used similarly to ginger, though it is more bitter. The root is sometimes used in making cordials and wines.

Other Uses

The essential oil is sometimes used in some perfumery. The root yields a yellow dye.

Constituents

Carbohydrates, essential oil, sesquiterpenes (curcumenone, curcumanolide A and B, zederone, germacrone), mucilage

Energetic Correspondences

- Flavor: pungent
- Temperature: warm
- Moisture: dry
- Polarity: yang
- Planet: Mars/Saturn
- Element: fire

Contraindications

Avoid therapeutic dosages during pregnancy. In cases of menorrhagia, use under the guidance of a qualified health-care practitioner.

Range and Appearance

Native to the subtropical forests of India, zedoary prefers partial shade and moderate moisture. It grows to about 3 feet in height and features yellow and pink flowers with red and green bracts. The large, tuberous, yellow roots take two years to mature.

Glossary of Physiological Effects

Abortifacient. Can stimulate miscarriage.

Adaptogen. Increases the body's resistance to stress and normalizes immune system.

Adrenal tonic. Strengthens and nourishes the adrenal glands.

Alterative. Alters one's condition. Usually increases blood flow to tissues, normalizes body functions, aids digestive assimilation, stimulates metabolism, and promotes waste excretion.

Anabolic. Builds the muscles and tissues of the body.

Analgesic. Relieves pain.

Anaphrodisiac. Curbs sex drive.

Androgenic. Increases levels of the hormone androgen.

Anesthetic. Deadens sensation.

Anodyne. Relieves pain by lessening nerve excitability at nerve centers.

Antacid. Brings an overacidic condition back to neutral.

Anthelmintic. Destroys or expels intestinal worms.

Antiabortifacient. Works to prevent threatened miscarriage.

Antiallergenic. Relieves the symptoms of allergies.

Antiandrogenic. Decreases levels of the hormone androgen.

Antiarthritic. Relieves the inflammation of arthritis and protects the joints from further degeneration.

Antiasthmatic. Relieves the symptoms associated with asthma, such as wheezing.

Antibacterial. Suppresses or combats the growth of bacteria.

Antibiotic. Destroys or suppresses the growth of microbes.

Anticarcinogenic. Reduces the number or activity of cancer cells.

Anticatarrhal. Reduces mucus levels in the body as well as inflammation of the mucous membranes.

Anticoagulant. Prevents blood coagulation.

Anticonvulsant. Reduces the frequency and severity of seizures.

Antidepressant. Supports the nervous system and alleviates depression.

Antidiarrheal. Remedies diarrhea.

Antidiuretic. Causes water retention.

Antiemetic. Counteracts nausea and vomiting.

Antiestrogenic. Decreases levels of estrogen.

Antifungal. Inhibits the overgrowth of fungal organisms.

Antigalactagogue. Decreases lactation in a nursing mother.

Antihistamine. Reduces the body's production of anti-inflammatory histamines.

Anti-inflammatory. Reduces inflammation.

Antimicrobial. Inhibits the activity of microbes.

Antimucoid. Decreases the amount of mucus in the body.

Antimutagenic. Works to prevent cell mutation.

Antineoplastic. Decreases growths such as tumors.

Antioxidant. Prevents free-radical damage.

Antiparasitic. Destroys parasites and worms.

Antiphlogistic. Reduces fever and/or inflammation.

Antirheumatic. Relieves rheumatic pain and stiffness in joints and muscles.

Antiscorbutic. Prevents scurvy by providing the body with vitamin C.

Antiseptic. Prevents bacterial growth, inhibits pathogens, and counters sepsis.

Antispasmodic. Eases muscle cramps and psychological stress.

Antisudorific. Decreases perspiration.

Antithrombotic. Prevents the formation of blood clots.

Antitumor. Reduces tumors.

Antitussive. Relieves coughing.

Antivenomous. Reduces the harm from venom, such as that of a snake or insect.

Antiviral. Inhibits viral replication.

Anxiolytic. Lessens anxiety.

Aperient. Is mildly laxative and stool softening. Typically used in cases of sluggish bowels.

Aphrodisiac. Increases sexual desire and potency.

Aromatic. Is fragrant, often pungent, and often stimulating to the digestive tract. Often improves the flavor of bitter herbs.

Astringent. Tightens and tones tissues and dries secretions. Often contains tannins.

Biogenic stimulator. Stimulates new cellular growth.

Bitter. Stimulates the flow of digestive secretions, as well as pituitary, liver, and duodenum secretions. Clears heat and aids digestion. Can be tonic, aromatic, or pungent and usually has a contractive force. Often considered cooling and drying.

Bladder tonic. Strengthens and nourishes the bladder.

Blood tonic. Strengthens and nourishes the blood.

Bone tonic. Strengthens and nourishes the bones.

Brain tonic. Strengthens and nourishes the brain.

Bronchial dilator. Relaxes the bronchial muscles, thus facilitating breathing.

Calmative. Gently relaxes the nerves.

Cardiac sedative. Calms heart activity.

Cardiac stimulant. Stimulates heart activity.

Cardioprotective. Protects heart function.

Cardiotonic. Strengthens and protects the heart.

Cardiovascular stimulant. Stimulates the heart and circulatory system.

Carminative. Relieves gas and nausea and relaxes griping in the bowel. Often used in cases of indigestion and appetite loss.

Cataleptic. Lessens response to external stimuli.

Cathartic. Stimulates intense bowel evacuation.

Central nervous system depressant. Decreases nervous system activity.

Central nervous system stimulant. Increases nervous system activity.

Cephalic. Has an effect upon the head, such as relieving headache or improving memory.

Cerebral sedative. Lessens brain activity.

Cerebral stimulant. Increases brain activity.

Cerebral tonic. Strengthens and nourishes brain function.

Cerebral vasodilator. Increases circulation and dilates blood vessels in the brain.

Cerebral vasorelaxant. Relaxes blood vessels in the brain.

Chi regulator. Promotes the smooth movement of chi (life-force energy) throughout the body.

Chi tonic. Nourishes and strengthens chi (life-force energy) in the body.

Cholagogue. Promotes bile flow from the liver.

Choleretic. Stimulates the production of bile in the liver.

Circulatory stimulant. Increases circulation throughout the body.

Circulatory tonic. Nourishes and strengthens the circulation system.

Cordial. Invigorates and stimulates body activities.

Counterirritant. Counteracts irritation.

Decongestant. Decreases swelling and congestion.

Demulcent. Soothes irritated tissues, especially of the mucous membranes (such as are found in the throat), ulcers, and the bladder. Usually contains mucilage.

Deobstruent. Works to remove obstructions.

Depurative. Cleanses body systems, especially the blood.

Detergent. Promotes cleansing of the body structure and systems.

Diaphoretic. Promotes perspiration by relaxing the pores and increasing elimination through the skin.

Digestive. Nourishes and strengthens the digestive system.

Discutient. Dissolves tumors and abnormal growths. Used internally in moderation and also topically.

Disinfectant. Lessens the activity of microbes.

Diuretic. Increases the secretion and expulsion of urine by promoting the activity of the kidneys and bladder.

Emetic. Stimulates vomiting.

Emmenagogue. Stimulates menstruation.

Emollient. Soothes, softens, and protects the skin; used externally.

Endocrine tonic. Nourishes and strengthens the endocrine system.

Entheogenic. Psychoactive, promoting a spiritual or mystical experience.

Escharotic. Has a caustic action.

Estrogenic. Increases the production of estrogen.

Euphoric. Causes emotional upliftment.

Expectorant. Promotes the discharge of mucus from respiratory passages.

Febrifuge. Reduces or eliminates fever.

Female tonic. Strengthens and nourishes the female reproductive system.

Fiber laxative. Increases bowel action due to its high fiber content.

Galactagogue. Increases milk secretions in nursing mothers.

Genitourinary antiseptic. Curbs infection in the bladder, kidneys, and urinary system.

Hallucinogen. Causes hallucinations.

Hemostatic. Arrests bleeding or hemorrhaging. Can be used internally and externally.

Hepatic. Strengthens, stimulates, and tones the liver.

Hepatoprotective. Has a protective effect upon the liver.

Hepatotonic. Strengthens and nourishes the liver and gallbladder.

Hormone regulator. Promotes the normalization of hormone production.

Hormone tonic. Supports and nourishes the organs that produce hormones.

Hyperglycemic. Elevates blood sugar levels.

Hypertensive. Elevates blood pressure.

Hypnotic. Induces deep nerve relaxation and a healing sleep state.

Hypoglycemic. Lowers blood sugar levels.

Hypotensive. Lowers blood pressure.

Immune stimulant. Enhances the body's ability to defend itself against illness or disease.

Immune tonic. Nourishes and strengthens the immune system.

Insecticide. Kills or deters insects.

Interferon stimulant. Stimulates the body's production of interferon.

Intoxicant. Causes a state of intoxication or inebriation.

Kidney cleanser. Aids in cleansing the kidneys.

Kidney stimulant. Increases the activity of the kidneys.

Kidney tonic. Strengthens and nourishes the kidneys.

Kidney yang tonic. Supports the activity of the kidneys.

Kidney yin tonic. Supports the fluid balance of the kidneys.

Laxative. Stimulates bowel action.

Lithotriptic. Reduces, suppresses, or dissolves calculi (stones in the body).

Liver cleanser. Aids in cleansing and detoxifying the liver.

Liver decongestant. Promotes the clearing of obstructions and stagnation from the liver.

Liver stimulant. Increases circulation to and activity in the liver.

Liver tonic. Strengthens and nourishes the liver.

Lung tonic. Strengthens and nourishes the lungs.

Lymphatic cleanser. Promotes cleansing of the lymph system.

Lymphatic decongestant. Promotes the clearing of obstructions and stagnation from the lymph system.

Metabolic stimulant. Increases metabolism.

Molluscidal. Kills or deters mollusks.

Mucilaginous. Has a slippery, soothing consistency.

Mucous membrane tonic. Strengthens and nourishes the mucous membranes.

Muscle relaxant. Relaxes the muscles.

Mucolytic. Reduces the stickiness of mucus.

Narcotic. Relieves pain or induces anesthesia.

Nerve relaxant. Relaxes the nerves.

Nerve restorative. Restores nerves that have been stressed or damaged.

Nervous system stimulant. Stimulates activity of the nervous system.

Nervous system tonic. Strengthens and nourishes the nervous system.

Nervine. Calms and nourishes the nerves.

Neuromuscular stimulant. Stimulates activity of the nerves and muscles.

Neuroprotective. Protects the nervous system.

Nootropic. Increases the activity and supply of nutrients in the brain.

Nutritive. Supplies a multitude of nutrients that build and tone the body.

Odontalgic. Gives temporary relief from dental pain.

Ophthalmic. Treats and prevents ocular (eye) disorders and improves vision.

Oxytocic. Stimulates uterine contractions by increasing the production of the hormone oxytocin.

Parasitacide. Kills or deters parasites.

Parturient. Assists in labor and delivery.

Pectoral. Relieves lung disorders and diseases.

Pediculocide. Kills lice.

Peripheral vasoconstrictor. Causes constriction of blood vessels at the periphery of the body.

Phytoandrogenic. Provides the raw material the body needs to produce the hormone androgen.

Phytoestrogenic. Contains the raw material to help the body produce its own estrogen.

Phytoprogesteronic. Contains the raw material to help the body produce its own progesterone.

Postpartum tonic. Helps a woman regain strength after birthing.

Prostate tonic. Nourishes and strengthens the prostate gland.

Psychoactive. Causes an altered state of perception.

Purgative. Increases bile secretions, causing intestinal peristalsis. Often used in conjunction with carminatives to prevent gripe.

Refrigerant. Lowers body temperature and relieves thirst.

Rejuvenative. Renews the body, mind, and spirit. May also slow the aging process, counteract stress, and increase endurance.

Reproductive tonic. Strengthens and nourishes the reproductive system.

Resolvent. Reduces inflammation and swelling.

Respiratory stimulant. Increases respiratory activity.

Restorative. Works to rebuild a depleted condition and normalize body functions.

Rubefacient. Increases blood flow to the surface of the skin and draws out deep impurities. Generally used topically.

Sedative. Slows body actions and strongly quiets the nerves.

Sialagogue. Stimulates the flow of saliva, thus aiding digestion.

Soporific. Causes sleepiness and drowsiness.

Spermicide. Kills or inactivates sperm.

Spinal cord tonic. Strengthens and nourishes the spinal column.

Spleen chi tonic. Supports the flow of chi (life-force energy) in the spleen.

Spleen tonic. Strengthens and nourishes the spleen.

Stimulant. Quickens various body actions, improves circulation, and warms the body.

Stomachic. Strengthens and tones the stomach, improves digestion, and reduces gas.

Stomach tonic. Strengthens and nourishes the stomach.

Styptic. Stops bleeding by constricting blood vessels. Generally is astringent and can be used externally and internally.

Sudorific. Increases perspiration, like a diaphoretic, but with a stronger action.

Thermogenic. Increases metabolism and body temperature, thus aiding in weight loss.

Thyroid stimulant. Increases thyroid activity.

Thyroid tonic. Strengthens and nourishes the thyroid gland.

Tonic. Promotes general health and well-being, sometimes for a particular organ system.

Urinary antiseptic. Deters infection and pathogens in the urinary tract.

Urinary stimulant. Increases circulation and activity in the urinary system.

Uterine decongestant. Promotes the clearing of ob-structions and stagnation from the uterus, such as cysts and fibroids.

Uterine relaxant. Relaxes the uterus.

Uterine stimulant. Increases activity in the uterus.

Uterine tonic. Nourishes and strengthens the uterus.

Uterine vasodilator. Increases circulation to and expands blood vessels in the uterus.

Vasoconstrictor. Causes constriction of the blood vessels.

Vasodilator. Expands blood vessels, thus lowering blood pressure.

Vasorelaxant. Relaxes blood vessels.

Vermifuge. Expels intestinal worms.

Vulnerary. Encourages wound healing by promoting cellular growth and repair. Usually used topically in the treatment of minor wounds.

Yang tonic. Nourishes and strengthens the activity of the body's functions.

Yin tonic. Nourishes and strengthens the fluids of the body.

Resources

Herbal Products

Asia Natural Products
590 Townsend Street
San Francisco, CA 94103
415-522-1668
www.drkangformulas.com
Quality Oriental herbs.

Blessed Herbs
109 Barre Plains Road
Oakham, MA 01068
508-882-3839
www.blessedherbs.com
Fresh and dried organic herbs.

Frontier Herbs
P.O. Box 299
Norway, IA 52318
800-669-3275
www.frontiercoop.com
Mail-order herbs and herbal products.

Guayaki Yerba Maté
P.O. Box 14730
San Luis Obispo, CA 93406
888-482-9254
www.guayaki.com
*Quality organic yerba maté environmentally
cultivated and harvested.*

Herb Pharm
P.O. Box 116
Williams, OR 97544

541-846-6262 or 800-545-739
www.herb-pharm.com
Makers of excellent-quality herbal tinctures.

Horizon Herbs
P.O. Box 69
Williams, OR 97544-0069
541-846-6704
www.horizonherbs.com
Excellent selection of herb seeds and seedlings.

Mountain Rose Herbs
25472 Dilley Lane
Eugene, OR 97405
800-879-3337
www.mountainrose.com
*Herbs and herbal products such as strainers,
empty tea bags, tincture bottles, et cetera.*

Primal Essence
1351 Maulhardt Avenue
Oxnard, CA 93030
805-981-2409
www.primalessence.com
*Makes excellent tea additions such as cinnamon,
chai, ginger, and peppermint essences.*

StarWest Botanicals
11253 Trade Center Drive
Rancho Cordova, CA 95742
916-853-9354 or 800-800-4372
www.starwest-botanicals.com
Mail-order herbs and herbal products.

Sunburst Bottle Company
5710 Auburn Boulevard, #7
Sacramento, CA 95841
916-348-3803
www.sunburstbottle.com
Glass and plastic bottles and containers for herbal preparations.

Education

American Botanical Council
P.O. Box 14445
Austin, TX 78714-4345
800-373-7105
www.herbalgram.org
Publishes Herbalgram; *sells herbal books.*

American Herbalists Guild
141 Nob Hill Road
Cheshire, CT 06410
203-272-6731
www.americanherbalist.com
Offers a member directory of peer-reviewed herbal practitioners.

American Herb Association
P.O. Box 1673
Nevada, CA 95959
530-265-9552
www.jps.net/ahaherb
Provides listing of herb schools throughout country and an excellent newsletter.

California School of Herbal Studies
P.O. Box 39
Forestville, CA 95436

707-887-7457
www.cshs.com
Provides in-depth, on-site herbal education with many fine teachers.

Herb Research Foundation
4140 15th Street
Boulder, CO 80304
303-449-2265
www.herbs.org
Clearinghouse for herbal information.

The Science and Art of Herbalism
   Correspondence Course
P.O. Box 420
East Barre, VT 05649
An excellent home-study program designed by beloved herbalist Rosemary Gladstar.

Tai Sophia Institute
7750 Montpelier Road
Laurel, MD 20723
410-888-9048
www.tai.edu
Provides in-depth herbal education and degree program.

United Plant Savers
P.O. Box 98
East Barre, VT 05649
802-479-9825
www.plantsavers.org
Group that promotes awareness about rare and endangered species. Great newsletter.

Bibliography

Bensky, Dan, and Andrew Gamble. *Chinese Herbal Medicine*. Seattle: Eastland, 1986.

Berger, Judith. *Herbal Rituals*. New York: St. Martin's, 1998.

Castleman, Michael. *The Healing Herbs*. Emmaus, PA: Rodale, 1991.

Cech, Richo. *Making Plant Medicine*. Williams, OR: Horizon Herbs, 2000.

Chevallier, Andrew. *The Encyclopedia of Medicinal Plants*. London: Dorling Kindersley, 1996.

Cunningham, Scott. *Cunninghams's Encyclopedia of Magical Herbs*. St. Paul, MN: Llewellyn, 1994.

Davies, Jill. *A Garden of Miracles: Herbal Drinks*. New York: Beaufort Books, 1985.

Duke, James A. *The Green Pharmacy*. Emmaus, PA: Rodale, 1997.

Dwyer, James, and David Rattray. *Reader's Digest Magic and Medicine of Plants*. Pleasantville, NY: Reader's Digest Association, 1986.

Edwards, Gail Faith. *Opening Our Wild Hearts to the Healing Herbs*. Woodstock, NY: Ash Tree, 2000.

Frawley, David. *Ayurvedic Healing*. Salt Lake City: Morson, 1992.

French, Jackie. *Book of Mint*. New York: Harper Collins, 1993.

Gladstar, Rosemary. *Rosemary Gladstar's Family Herbal: A Guide to Living Life with Energy, Health, and Vitality*. North Adams, MA: Storey Books, 2001.

Gladstar, Rosemary. *The Science and Art of Herbology*, Lesson 2. East Barre, VT: Sage Mountain.

Gordon, Lesley. *A Country Herbal*. Exeter, England: Webb and Bower, 1980.

Green, James. *Herbal Medicine Maker's Handbook: The Art and Science of Herbal Medicine Making as Taught at the California School of Herbal Studies*. Forestville, CA: Crossing Press, 1987.

Grieve, Maude. *A Modern Herbal*, vol. 1 and 2. London: Dover, 1971.

Hallowell, Michael. *Herbal Healing*. Bath, England: Ashgrove, 1990.

Hartung, Tammi. *Growing 101 Herbs That Heal: Gardening Techniques, Recipes, and Remedies*. North Adams, MA: Storey Books, 2000.

Heinerman, John. *The Complete Book of Spices*. New Canaan, CT: Keats, 1983.

Heinerman, John. *Heinerman's Encyclopedia of Healing Herbs and Spices*. Englewod Cliffs, NJ: Parker, 1996.

Heinerman, John. *Science of Herbal Medicine*. Orem, UT: Bi-World, 1979.

Hobbs, Christopher. *Handmade Medicines: Simple Recipes for Health*. Loveland, CO: Interweave, 1998.

Hoffmann, David. *The Herb User's Guide: The Basic Skills of Medical Herbalism*. Rochester, VT: Thorson's, 1987.

Hoffman, David. *The Holisistic Herbal*. Moray, Scotland: Findhorn, 1983.

Holmes, Peter. *The Energetics of Western Herbs*, vol. 1 and 2. Boulder, CO: Artemis, 1989.

Hyam, Roger, and Richard Pankhurst. *Plants and Their Names*. Oxford, England: Oxford University Press, 1995.

Keville, Kathi. *Herbs for Health and Healing: A Drug-Free Guide to Prevention and Cure*. Emmaus, PA: Rodale, 1996.

Keville, Kathi. *The Illustrated Herb Encyclopedia.* New York: Mallard, 1991.

Lehane, Brendan. *The Power of Plants.* New York: McGraw-Hill, 1977.

Levetin, Estelle, and Karen McMahon. *Plants and Society.* Chicago, IL: William C. Brown, 1996.

Lewis, Walter, and Memory Elvin-Lewis. *Medical Botany.* New York: John Wiley and Sons, 1977.

Lust, John. *The Herb Book.* New York: Bantam Books, 1974.

Mars, Brigitte. *The Herbal Pharmacy CD-ROM.* Boulder, CO: Hale Software, 1998.

McGuffin, Michael, Christopher Hobbs, Roy Upton, and Alicia Goldberg. *Botanical Safety Handbook.* Boca Raton, FL: CRC, 1997.

McIntyre, Anne. *Flower Power.* New York: Henry Holt, 1996.

Moore, Michael. *Medicinal Plants of the Desert and Canyon West.* Santa Fe: Museum of New Mexico Press, 1989.

Murray, Michael, and Joseph Pizzorno. *Encyclopedia of Natural Medicine.* Rocklin, CA: Prima, 1991.

Ody, Penelope. *The Complete Medicinal Herbal.* New York: Dorling Kindersley, 1993.

Onstad, Dianne. *Whole Foods Companion.* White River Junction, VT: Chelsea Green, 1996.

Ortiz, Elisabeth Lambert. *The Encyclopedia of Herbs, Spices and Flavorings: A Cook's Compendium.* New York: Dorling Kindersley, 1992.

Pedersen, Mark. *Nutritional Herbology.* Warsaw, IN: Wendell W. Whitman, 1994.

Phillips, Nancy and Michael. *The Village Herbalist: Sharing Plant Medicines with Family and Community.* White River Junction, VT: Chelsea Green, 2001.

Pollak, Jeanine. *Healing Tonics: 101 Herbal Concoctions.* North Adams, MA: Storey Books, 2000.

Rose, Jeanne. *Herbs and Things.* New York: Grosset and Dunlap, 1976.

Rosengarten, Frederic Jr. *The Book of Spices.* New York: Pyramid Books, 1973.

Saint Claire, Debra. *The Herbal Medicine Cabinet: Preparing Natural Remedies at Home.* Berkeley, CA: Celestial Arts, 1997.

Santillo, Humbart. *Natural Healing with Herbs.* Prescott Valley, AZ: Hohm, 1984.

Scalzo, Richard. *Naturopathic Handbook of Herbal Formulas.* Durango, CO: Kivaki, 1994.

Schivelbusch, Wolfgang. *Tastes of Paradise: A Social History of Spices, Stimulants, and Intoxicants.* New York: Pantheon, 1992.

Smith, Ed. *Therapeutic Herb Manual.* Williams, OR: Herb Pharm, 1993.

Stuart, Malcolm. *The Encyclopedia of Herbs and Herbalism.* New York: Crescent Books, 1989.

Svoboda, Robert E. *Ayurveda: Life, Health and Longevity.* New York: Penguin, 1993.

Svoboda, Robert E. *Prakuti: Your Ayurvedic Constitution.* Albuquerque, NM: Geocom, 1988.

Theiss, Barbara and Peter. *The Herbal Family.* Rochester, VT: Healing Arts, 1989.

Thomson, Robert. *The Grosset Encyclopedia of Natural Medicine.* New York: Grosset & Dunlap, 1980.

Tierra, Michael. *Planetary Herbology.* Santa Fe: Lotus Press, 1988.

Tierra, Michael. *The Way of Herbs.* New York: Washington Square, 1983.

Trattler, Ross. *Better Health through Natural Healing.* New York: McGraw Hill, 1988.

Tyler, Varro E. *The Honest Herbal.* New York: Pharmaceutical Products, 1993.

Weiner, Michael A. and Janet. *Herbs That Heal.* Mill Valley, CA: Quantum, 1994.

Weiss, Rudolf Fritz. *Herbal Medicine.* Beaconsfield, England: Beaconsfield, 1988.

Willard, Terry. *The Wild Rose Scientific Herbal.* Calgary, Canada: Wild Rose College of Natural Healing, 1991.

Wren, R. C. *Potter's New Encyclopedia of Botanical Drugs and Preparations.* Essex, England: Saffron Walden, 1994.

Zak, Victoria, *Twenty Thousand Secrets of Tea.* New York: Dell, 1999.

Zevin, Igor Vilevich. *A Russian Herbal.* Rochester, VT: Healing Arts, 1997.

Index of Alternative English Common Names

beechdrops *see* blue cohosh *or* cistanches

bee's nest *see* wild carrot

beggar's blanket *see* mullein

beggar's buttons *see* burdock

Belgian endive *see* chicory

bellflower *see* codonopsis

benefit mother plant *see* motherwort

betony *see* wood betony

bhringaraj *see* eclipta

bidney *see* wood betony

big sting nettle *see* nettle

big taper *see* mullein

big tobacco *see* mullein

birdlime mistletoe *see* mistletoe

bird pepper *see* cayenne

bird's foot *see* fenugreek

bird's nest *see* wild carrot

bishop's hat *see* epimedium

bishop's wort *see* wood betony

bitterbark *see* cascara sagrada

bitter bloom *see* centaury

bitter buttons *see* tansy

bitter clover *see* centaury

bitter herb *see* centaury

bitter lettuce *see* wild lettuce

bitter orange *see* orange

bitter root *see* gentian

bitter wintergreen *see* pipsissewa

bitterworm *see* buckbean

bitterwort *see* dandelion

black bush *see* chaparral

blackberry *see* blackberry

black cherry *see* wild cherry

black cottonwood *see* balm of Gilead

black forest mushroom *see* shiitake

black larch *see* larch

black pepper *see* pepper

black Sampson *see* echinacea

black snakeroot *see* black cohosh

black sugar *see* licorice

black tany *see* bladder wrack

blackwort *see* comfrey

bladderpod *see* lobelia

blatter dock *see* butterbur

blessed cardus *see* blessed thistle

blessed thistle *see* blessed thistle

blind buff *see* poppy

blind weed *see* shepherd's purse

blonde ispaghula *see* psyllium

blond psyllium *see* psyllium

blood elder *see* elder

blowball *see* chicory *or* dandelion

blueberry root *see* blue cohosh

blue curls *see* self-heal

blue daisy *see* chicory

blue dandelion *see* chicory

blue ginseng *see* blue cohosh

blue malee *see* eucalyptus

blue mountain tea *see* goldenrod

blue pimpernel *see* skullcap

blue sailors *see* chicory

bobea *see* redroot

bogbean *see* buckbean

bog-hop *see* buckbean

bog myrtle *see* bayberry

bog nut *see* buckbean

bog rhubarb *see* butterbur

bogshorn *see* butterbur

boldina *see* boldo

boldu *see* boldo

boneset *see* boneset

bookoo *see* buchu

bottlebrush *see* horsetail

bour tree *see* elder

bow wood *see* p'au d'arco

boxberry *see* wintergreen

boxthorn *see* goji

brain plant *see* bacopa

bramble *see* blackberry *or* raspberry

brandy mint *see* mint

Brazilian cocoa *see* guarana

Brazil tea *see* yerba maté

bread and cheese tree *see* hawthorn

bridewort *see* meadowsweet

brindal berry *see* garcinia

British tobacco   *see* coltsfoot
broomrape   *see* cistanches
bruisewort   *see* comfrey
brunella   *see* self-heal
brushes and combs   *see* teasel
bucco   *see* buchu
buchu   *see* buchu
buckbean   *see* buckbean
buckeye   *see* horse chestnut
buckthorn   *see* cascara sagrada
bucku   *see* buchu
Buddha's fingernails   *see* ginkgo
buffalo grass   *see* alfalfa
bugbane   *see* black cohosh
bugloss   *see* borage
Bulgarian saffron   *see* saffron
bull pipes   *see* horsetail
bull's blood   *see* horehound
bull's eye   *see* calendula
bull's foot   *see* coltsfoot
bumble bees   *see* self-heal
burrage   *see* borage
burr marigold   *see* agrimony
butterbur   *see* coltsfoot
butterdock   *see* butterbur
butterfly milkweed   *see* pleurisy
butterfly weed   *see* pleurisy
butternut   *see* walnut
buttons   *see* peyote
cacaotier   *see* cacao
cactus pudding   *see* peyote
caltrop   *see* tribulus
Canada root   *see* pleurisy
Canada tea   *see* wintergreen
Canby's licorice root   *see* osha
cancer root   *see* cistanches *or* poke
candleberry   *see* bayberry
candlewick   *see* mullein
candy leaf   *see* stevia
canker root   *see* coptis
cankerwort   *see* dandelion
cannabis   *see* marijuana
capdockin   *see* butterbur
capon's tail   *see* valerian

cardin   *see* blessed thistle
cardinal flower   *see* lobelia
carnation clove   *see* clove
carpenter's herb   *see* self-heal
carpenter's weed   *see* yarrow
carrageenan   *see* Irish moss
carragheen   *see* Irish moss
carvies   *see* caraway
case wort   *see* shepherd's purse
cassia   *see* cinnamon
catchweed   *see* cleavers
catmint   *see* catnip
catnep   *see* catnip
catswort   *see* catnip
catwort   *see* valerian
chaparro   *see* chaparral
charas resin   *see* marijuana
chaste tree   *see* vitex
chastity tree   *see* hawthorn
checkerberry   *see* wintergreen
cheeses   *see* marshmallow
chewing John   *see* galangal
chichira   *see* maca
chicoria   *see* dandelion
chiggerflower   *see* pleurisy
chile   *see* cayenne
Chilean clover   *see* alfalfa
chili   *see* cayenne
chinaberry tree   *see* neem
China root   *see* galangal *or* poria
Chinese anise   *see* star anise
Chinese cornbind   *see* ho shou wu
Chinese date   *see* jujube
Chinese foxglove   *see* rehmannia
Chinese parsley   *see* coriander
Chinese senega root   *see* polygala
chinghai rhubarb   *see* rhubarb
chipmunk's apples   *see* uva-ursi
chittambark   *see* cascara sagrada
chocolate   *see* cacao
chokecherry   *see* wild cherry
Christ's ladder   *see* centaury
chrondus   *see* Irish moss
church brooms   *see* teasel

elixir of life	*see* gotu kola
ellanwood	*see* elder
ellhorn	*see* elder
emblic myrobalan	*see* amla
emetic weed	*see* lobelia
empress of the dark forest	*see* osha
enchanter's plant	*see* vervain
endive	*see* chicory
Englishman's foot	*see* plantain
epifagus	*see* cistanches
eriodictyon	*see* yerba santa
essence of man	*see* ginseng
ettle	*see* nettle
euphrasia	*see* eyebright
euphrosyne	*see* eyebright
European mistletoe	*see* mistletoe
everlasting friendship	*see* cleavers
eye balm root	*see* goldenseal
eyebright	*see* lobelia
eye of the star	*see* horehound
fairy clock	*see* dandelion
false daisy	*see* eclipta
false indigo	*see* baptisia
false saffron	*see* safflower
false wintergreen	*see* pipsissewa
fan palm	*see* saw palmetto
fastening herb	*see* goldenrod
featherfew	*see* feverfew
featherfoil	*see* feverfew
featherfowl	*see* feverfew
feather-full pyrethrum	*see* feverfew
felon herb	*see* mugwort
female ginseng	*see* dong quai
fennel wood	*see* sassafras
fever grass	*see* lemongrass
fever tree	*see* elder *or* eucalyptus
feverweed	*see* gravel root
feverwort	*see* boneset *or* centaury
field balm	*see* catnip
field poppy	*see* poppy
field sorrel	*see* sheep's sorrel
filius ante patrem	*see* coltsfoot
filwort	*see* centaury
five fingers	*see* ginseng

five-flavor fruit	*see* schizandra
five-taste berry	*see* schizandra
flame flower	*see* California poppy
Flanders poppy	*see* poppy
flapper dog	*see* butterbur
flea seeds	*see* psyllium
flirtwort	*see* feverfew
flower of the five wounds	*see* passionflower
flower velure	*see* coltsfoot
flowery knotweed	*see* ho shou wu
flux root	*see* pleurisy
foal's foot	*see* coltsfoot
food of the gods	*see* cacao
fortune-teller	*see* dandelion
fossil tree	*see* ginkgo
fo-ti	*see* ho shou wu
French tarragon	*see* tarragon
gagan-gagan	*see* gotu kola
gag weed	*see* lobelia
galibanum	*see* frankincense
galingale	*see* galangal
garabato	*see* cat's claw
garbato casha	*see* cat's claw
garclive	*see* agrimony
garden heliotrope	*see* valerian
garden marigold	*see* calendula
garden mint	*see* mint
garden patience	*see* yellow dock
garden poppy	*see* poppy
garden rue	*see* rue
garden sage	*see* sage
ghost plant	*see* cistanches
gladdon	*see* calamus
glossagyne	*see* shiitake
glossy ganoderma	*see* reishi
goat's beard	*see* meadowsweet
goat's head	*see* tribulus
goat's thorn	*see* astragalus
goat's tit bellflower	*see* codonopsis
goatweed	*see* Saint John's wort
gold and silver flower	*see* honeysuckle
gold buttons	*see* tansy
golden apple	*see* orange
golden bough	*see* mistletoe

herb of grace	*see* bacopa, rue, *or* vervain	human root	*see* ginseng
herb of Paraguay	*see* stevia	hundred-rooted vine	*see* asparagus
herb of repentance	*see* rue	hurr burr	*see* burdock
herb of the cross	*see* vervain	hylder	*see* elder
herby grass	*see* rue	immortal	*see* pleurisy
Hercules's club	*see* prickly ash	Indian anise	*see* star anise
Hercules's woundwort	*see* self-heal	Indian bedellium	*see* guggulu
herpestris monniera	*see* bacopa	Indian bread	*see* poria
hervea	*see* yerba maté	Indian cedar	*see* neem
he shou wu	*see* ho shou wu	Indian corn	*see* cornsilk
hidgy-pidgy	*see* nettle	Indian dreamer	*see* marijuana
hikuli	*see* peyote	Indian dye	*see* goldenseal
hillberry	*see* wintergreen	Indian echinacea	*see* andrographis
hindberry	*see* raspberry	Indian elm	*see* slippery elm
hoama	*see* Syrian rue	Indian ginseng	*see* ashwagandha
hoarhound	*see* horehound	Indian gooseberry	*see* amla
hock herb	*see* marshmallow	Indian hyssop	*see* vervain
hoelen	*see* poria	Indian lilac	*see* neem
hog cranberry	*see* uva-ursi	Indian paint	*see* bloodroot *or* goldenseal
hoky-poky	*see* nettle	Indian plantain	*see* psyllium
holigold	*see* calendula	Indian root	*see* osha
holly grape	*see* Oregon grape	Indian saffron	*see* turmeric
holly mahonia	*see* Oregon grape	Indian sage	*see* boneset
holy herb	*see* vervain *or* yerba santa	Indian spice	*see* vitex
holy thistle	*see* blessed thistle	Indian spikenard	*see* spikenard
holy wood	*see* mistletoe	Indian spinach	*see* nettle
holy wort	*see* vervain	Indian tobacco	*see* lobelia
honeygrass	*see* licorice	Indian toilet paper	*see* mullein
honey leaf	*see* stevia	indigo broom	*see* baptisia
honeystalks	*see* red clover	indigo weed	*see* baptisia
honey vine	*see* honeysuckle	inebriating pepper	*see* kava kava
honeywort	*see* dong quai	intoxicating long pepper	*see* kava kava
hooded willow herb	*see* skullcap	Irish daisy	*see* dandelion
hoodwort	*see* skullcap	iron bark	*see* eucalyptus
hook heal	*see* self-heal	ispaghul plantain	*see* psyllium
hop bine	*see* hops	istan	*see* isatis
horny goat weed	*see* epimedium	Jacob's staff	*see* mullein
horse elder	*see* elecampane	Jamaica feverplant	*see* tribulus
horsefly weed	*see* baptisia	Jamaican pepper	*see* allspice
horseheal	*see* elecampane	Jamaica sorrel	*see* hibiscus
horsehoof	*see* coltsfoot	jaundice root	*see* goldenseal
houndsbane	*see* horehound	Java pepper	*see* cubeb
		jelly moss	*see* Irish moss

manroot	*see* spikenard
many-heired vine	*see* asparagus
manzanita	*see* uva-ursi
maracoc	*see* passionflower
marapama	*see* muira puama
marapuama	*see* muira puama
margosa	*see* neem
María pastora	*see* divining sage
Marian thistle	*see* milk thistle
marl grass	*see* red clover
marsh clover	*see* buckbean
marsh drain	*see* alisma
marsh milkweed	*see* gravel root
marsh parsley	*see* celery
marsh pennywort	*see* gotu kola
Mary bud	*see* calendula
Mary Jane	*see* marijuana
Mary thistle	*see* milk thistle
master of the woods	*see* woodruff
masterwort	*see* angelica
maté	*see* yerba maté
matrimony vine	*see* goji
May blossom	*see* hawthorn
May bush	*see* hawthorn
May Day flower	*see* hawthorn
maypop	*see* passionflower
mayweed	*see* chamomile *or* feverfew
meadow honeysuckle	*see* red clover
meadow sorrow	*see* sheep's sorrel
meadow trefoil	*see* red clover
meadwort	*see* meadowsweet
mealberry	*see* uva-ursi
Mecca balsam	*see* balm of Gilead
medicine plant	*see* aloe
Mediterranean thistle	*see* milk thistle
melissa	*see* lemon balm
menthol mint	*see* mint
mescal button	*see* peyote
Mexican parsley	*see* coriander
midsummer daisy	*see* feverfew
milfoil	*see* yarrow
milk gowan	*see* dandelion
milk sweet	*see* cleavers
milk vetch	*see* astragalus
milkweed	*see* pleurisy
milk witch	*see* dandelion
milkwort	*see* polygala
miracle fruit	*see* gymnema
mishmi bitter	*see* coptis
mock pennyroyal	*see* pennyroyal
monk's head	*see* dandelion
monk's pepper	*see* vitex
moonflower	*see* buckbean
moonwort	*see* valerian
moose elm	*see* slippery elm
mortification plant	*see* marshmallow
mosquito plant	*see* pennyroyal
mother herb	*see* feverfew
mother of herbs	*see* rue
mother of plants	*see* mugwort
mothers' hearts	*see* shepherd's purse
mountain balm	*see* yerba santa
mountain box	*see* uva-ursi
mountain carrot	*see* osha
mountain celery	*see* dong quai
mountain cranberry	*see* cascara sagrada *or* uva-ursi
mountain flax	*see* polygala
mountain ginseng	*see* osha
mountain grape	*see* Oregon grape
mountainsweet	*see* redroot
mountain tea	*see* wintergreen
moutan	*see* peony
mouthroot	*see* coptis
moxa	*see* mugwort
mukul tree	*see* guggulu
mushroom of immortality	*see* reishi *or* shiitake
musk of the woods	*see* woodruff
myrtle flag	*see* calamus
myrtle pepper	*see* allspice
naald tea	*see* rooibos
nard	*see* lavender
narrow dock	*see* yellow dock
naughty man	*see* mugwort
needle palm	*see* yucca
nep	*see* catnip
New Jersey tea	*see* redroot

newspice	*see* allspice	Paraguay cress	*see* spilanthes
nine hooks	*see* lady's mantle	paraguayo	*see* cat's claw
nipbone	*see* comfrey	Paraguay tea	*see* yerba maté
nipo	*see* osha	parrot plant	*see* safflower
nosebleed	*see* feverfew	passiflora	*see* passionflower
oak mushroom	*see* shiitake	passionaria	*see* passionflower
ocularia	*see* eyebright	patchouli	*see* anise hyssop
odostemon	*see* Oregon grape	Paul's betony	*see* bugleweed
Ohio curcuma	*see* goldenseal	pearl moss	*see* Irish moss
oilnut	*see* butternut	peasant's cloak	*see* dandelion
old man	*see* rosemary	pellitory	*see* prickly ash
old man's beard	*see* usnea	pellote	*see* peyote
old man's friend	*see* saw palmetto	pennywort	*see* gotu kola
old man's pharmacetly	*see* shepherd's purse	pepper and salt	*see* shepherd's purse
old man's root	*see* spikenard	peppermint	*see* mint
old woman	*see* wormwood	pepperweed	*see* maca
olibanum	*see* frankincense	perceley	*see* parsley
oliva	*see* olive	periploca of the woods	*see* gymnema
opium poppy	*see* poppy	persiana	*see* cascara sagrada
orange root	*see* goldenseal	Persian walnut	*see* walnut
orange swallow wort	*see* pleurisy	persil	*see* parsley
organ tea	*see* pennyroyal	Peruvian ginseng	*see* maca
Oriental black mushroom	*see* shiitake	pestilence wort	*see* butterbur
origanum	*see* oregano	petty morel	*see* spikenard
ortiga	*see* nettle	pewterwort	*see* horsetail
oshá	*see* osha	peyotl	*see* peyote
oshala	*see* osha	philantropos	*see* agrimony
Our Lady's bedstraw	*see* woodruff	philtron	*see* wild carrot
Our Lady's flannel	*see* mullein	phu	*see* valerian
Our Lady's mantle	*see* lady's mantle	picklooker	*see* shepherd's purse
Our Lady's rose	*see* rosemary	pickpocket	*see* shepherd's purse
Our Lady's thistle	*see* milk thistle	pick purse	*see* shepherd's purse
Our Lord's candle	*see* yucca	piddly bed	*see* dandelion
owl's blanket	*see* coltsfoot	pigeon berry	*see* poke
oxalis	*see* sheep's sorrel	pigeon grass	*see* vervain
ox balm	*see* collinsonia	pikake	*see* jasmine
Pacific ginseng	*see* devil's club	pimento	*see* allspice
paddock pipes	*see* horsetail	pimpernel	*see* self-heal
paddy tang	*see* bladder wrack	pipe tree	*see* elder
pagan wound herb	*see* goldenrod	pistachio tree	*see* witch hazel
pannag	*see* ginseng	plague flower	*see* butterbur
pan pipes	*see* elder	plant's physician	*see* chamomile
papoose root	*see* blue cohosh	pokeweed	*see* poke
Para cress	*see* spilanthes	poor man's ginseng	*see* codonopsis

poor man's opium   *see* wild lettuce
poor Robin   *see* cleavers
popping wrack   *see* bladder wrack
Porter's licorice root   *see* osha
Porter's lovage   *see* osha
pot   *see* marijuana
potency wood   *see* muira puama
pot marigold   *see* calendula
prairie indigo   *see* baptisia
pretty mugget   *see* cleavers
prickly lettuce   *see* wild lettuce
prickly porcupine ginseng *see* devil's club
pride of the meadow   *see* meadowsweet
priest's crown   *see* dandelion
Prince of Wale's feathers *see* tansy
prince's pine   *see* pipsissewa
pudding grass   *see* pennyroyal
puffball   *see* dandelion
pukeweed   *see* lobelia
puncture vine   *see* tribulus
purple boneset   *see* gravel root
purple clover   *see* red clover
purple medic   *see* alfalfa
purple osier   *see* willow
purslet   *see* shepherd's purse
pussy willow   *see* willow
quack grass   *see* couch grass
Quaker's hat   *see* skullcap
Quebec oak   *see* white oak
quebrachin   *see* yohimbe
quechua   *see* maca
Queen Anne's lace   *see* wild carrot
queen of flowers   *see* rose
queen of the meadow   *see* gravel root *or*
                          meadowsweet
queen of the night   *see* jasmine
quickens   *see* couch grass
quick grass   *see* couch grass
quitch grass   *see* couch grass
ragged sailors   *see* chicory
ram's horn   *see* gymnema
rangaya   *see* cat's claw
rattle brush   *see* baptisia
rattle pouches   *see* shepherd's purse

rattle root   *see* black cohosh
rattlesnake root   *see* polygala
red berry   *see* ginseng
red bush tea   *see* rooibos
red date   *see* jujube
red elm   *see* slippery elm
red fucus   *see* bladder wrack
red ink plant   *see* poke
red ornamental rhubrab   *see* rhubarb
red pepper   *see* cayenne
red pucoon   *see* bloodroot
red root   *see* bloodroot *or*
                          redroot
red sage   *see* sage
red sorrel   *see* sheep's sorrel
red-top sorrel   *see* sheep's sorrel
red weed   *see* sheep's sorrel
relative root   *see* codonopsis
rheumatism root   *see* wild yam
rheumatism weed   *see* pipsissewa
ribwort   *see* plantain
rich weed   *see* collinsonia
ripplegrass   *see* plantain
rock elm   *see* slippery elm
rock parsley   *see* parsley
rockwrack   *see* bladder wrack
Roman cumin   *see* caraway
rooibosch   *see* rooibos
rooitea   *see* rooibos
rooitee   *see* rooibos
root of the Holy Ghost   *see* angelica
rosella   *see* hibiscus
rosemallow   *see* hibiscus
rose of Sharon   *see* hibiscus
rose pink   *see* centaury
roseroot   *see* rhodiola
rosin rose   *see* Saint John's wort
rosin weed   *see* grindelia
royal protector   *see* white oak
rub-by-the-ground   *see* pennyroyal
rudbeckia   *see* echinacea
ruddles   *see* calendula
Russian rhubarb   *see* rhubarb
sabal   *see* saw palmetto

southernwood	*see* wormwood	swamp daisy	*see* eclipta
Spanish bayonet	*see* yucca	swamp root	*see* yerba mansa
Spanish chestnut	*see* horse chestnut	sweating plant	*see* boneset
Spanish dagger	*see* yucca	sweet briar	*see* rose
Spanish hay	*see* alfalfa	sweet bugle	*see* bugleweed
Spanish juice	*see* licorice	sweet coltsfoot	*see* butterbur
Spanish saffron	*see* saffron	sweet cumin	*see* fennel
sparrowgrass	*see* asparagus	sweet elm	*see* slippery elm
spearmint	*see* mint	sweet flag	*see* calamus
speld tea	*see* rooibos	sweet gale	*see* bayberry
spiceberry	*see* spikenard	sweet hay	*see* meadowsweet
spice ginger	*see* galangal	sweet herb	*see* stevia
spignet	*see* spikenard	sweet jujube	*see* jujube
spike	*see* lavender	sweet laurel	*see* bay
spirit herb	*see* ginseng	sweet leaf	*see* stevia
spogel	*see* psyllium	sweet plantain	*see* plantain
spotted alder	*see* witch hazel	sweet root	*see* licorice
spotted thistle	*see* blessed thistle	sweet slumber	*see* bloodroot
spurdock	*see* yellow dock	sweet violet	*see* violet
squaw root	*see* black cohosh *or* blue cohosh	sweet weed	*see* marshmallow
		sweet wood	*see* cinnamon
squinant	*see* lemongrass	sweet woodruff	*see* woodruff
squirrel corn	*see* corydalis	swine's snout	*see* dandelion
star flower	*see* borage	tacamahac	*see* balm of Gilead
starweed	*see* chickweed	tad broom	*see* horsetail
starwort	*see* chickweed	taheebo	*see* p'au d'arco
staunchweed	*see* yarrow	tahuari	*see* p'au d'arco
sticklewort	*see* agrimony	tailed pepper	*see* cubeb
sticky willie	*see* cleavers	tajibo	*see* p'au d'arco
stinging nettle	*see* nettle	tajylapacho	*see* p'au d'arco
stinking balm	*see* pennyroyal	tall boneset	*see* gravel root
stinking rose	*see* garlic	tallow shrub	*see* bayberry
stinking willie	*see* tansy	tamarack	*see* larch
stitchwort	*see* chickweed	tambor huasca	*see* cat's claw
stoneroot	*see* collinsonia	tang kuei	*see* dong quai
stringy bark tree	*see* eucalyptus	tang kwei	*see* dong quai
strong-scented lettuce	*see* wild lettuce	tangerine	*see* orange
succory	*see* chicory	tanging nettle	*see* nettle
sugar leaf	*see* stevia	tangled vine	*see* ho shou wu
summer dry herb	*see* self-heal	tanner's bark	*see* white oak
sun apple	*see* orange	tartar root	*see* ginseng
sun-in-the-grass	*see* dandelion	tarweed	*see* grindelia *or* yerba santa
sun medicine	*see* goldenrod		
suterberry	*see* prickly ash	tazzel	*see* teasel

teaberry	*see* wintergreen	triticum	*see* couch grass
tedral	*see* boneset	true nettle	*see* nettle
tell time	*see* dandelion	true saffron	*see* saffron
terrestrial sun	*see* Saint John's wort	true tarragon	*see* tarragon
terror of the earth	*see* tribulus	trumpet bush	*see* p'au d'arco
tetterwort	*see* bloodroot	trumpetweed	*see* gravel root
theobroma	*see* cacao	tuckahoe	*see* poria
theriak herb	*see* valerian	turkey corn	*see* cornsilk *or* corydalis
thickweed	*see* pennyroyal		
thin-leaf milkwort	*see* polygala	turmeric root	*see* goldenseal
thorough-stem	*see* boneset	turnera	*see* damiana
thoroughwax	*see* bupleurum	turragi	*see* ashwagandha
thoroughwort	*see* boneset *or* gravel root	twitchgrass	*see* couch grass
thorow wax	*see* bupleurum	umbellate wintergreen	*see* pipsissewa
thousand guilder herb	*see* centaury	umbrella plant	*see* butterbur
thread-the-heart lotus	*see* andrographis	una de gavilan	*see* cat's claw
three-leaves grass	*see* red clover	ungangui	*see* cat's claw
throw-wort	*see* motherwort	upland cranberry	*see* uva-ursi
thunderbesam	*see* mistletoe	vandal root	*see* valerian
thyme-leaved gratiola	*see* bacopa	variegated thistle	*see* milk thistle
tickweed	*see* pennyroyal	varnished conk	*see* reishi
tin weed	*see* horsetail	vegetable antimony	*see* boneset
tipton weed	*see* Saint John's wort	vegetable gold	*see* coptis
toad pipes	*see* horsetail	vegetable silica	*see* horsetail
tobacco root	*see* valerian	vegetable tallow	*see* bayberry
toothache plant	*see* spilanthes	velvet dock	*see* elecampane *or* mullein
toothache tree	*see* prickly ash		
torches	*see* mullein	Venus basin	*see* teasel
toron	*see* cat's claw	Venus bath	*see* teasel
touch-and-heal	*see* Saint John's wort	Venus thistle	*see* milk thistle
toywort	*see* shepherd's purse	verbena	*see* vervain
tramp with the golden head	*see* dandelion	vetter-voo	*see* feverfew
treacle	*see* valerian	Viking elder	*see* elder
treefold	*see* buckbean	village pharmacy	*see* neem
tree hydrangea	*see* hydrangea	violon	*see* larch
tree moss	*see* usnea	Virginia witch hazel	*see* witch hazel
tree of life	*see* olive	vomit weed	*see* lobelia
tree of medicine	*see* elder	vomitwort	*see* lobelia
tree of music	*see* elder	vraic	*see* bladder wrack
tree peony	*see* peony	walewort	*see* elder
trefoil	*see* red clover	walnoot	*see* walnut
trifoil	*see* red clover	Walpole tea	*see* redroot
		walwort	*see* comfrey
		ward seed	*see* shepherd's purse

watcher of the road	*see* chicory
water bugle	*see* bugleweed
water horehound	*see* bugleweed
water hyssop	*see* bacopa
water plantain	*see* alisma
water shamrock	*see* buckbean
water thistle	*see* teasel
water trefoil	*see* buckbean
wati	*see* kava kava
waxberry	*see* bayberry
wax cluster berry	*see* wintergreen
wax myrtle	*see* bayberry
waybread	*see* plantain
welcome winter flower	*see* coltsfoot
wet-a-bed	*see* dandelion
wheatgrass	*see* couch grass
white horehound	*see* horehound
white hyssop	*see* bacopa
white mallow	*see* marshmallow
white man's footsteps	*see* plantain
white mule	*see* peyote
white root	*see* gotu kola *or* pleurisy
white sage	*see* mugwort
whitethorn	*see* hawthorn
white turmeric	*see* zedoary
white walnut	*see* butternut
whitewort	*see* feverfew
wild artichoke	*see* milk thistle
wild balsam	*see* yerba santa
wild celery	*see* angelica
wild chamomile	*see* feverfew
wild curcuma	*see* goldenseal
wild endive	*see* dandelion
wild hop	*see* wood betony
wild indigo	*see* baptisia
wild Isaac	*see* boneset
wild lovage	*see* osha
wild marjoram	*see* oregano
wild sarsaparilla	*see* spikenard
wild snowball	*see* redroot
wild succory	*see* centaury

wild sunflower	*see* elecampane
wind root	*see* pleurisy
winterbloom	*see* witch hazel
winter cherry	*see* ashwagandha
wintersweet	*see* oregano
winterweed	*see* chickweed
witches' pouches	*see* shepherd's purse
witch grass	*see* couch grass
witch's broom	*see* mistletoe *or* usnea
witch's candle	*see* mullein
with	*see* willow
withania	*see* ashwagandha
withy	*see* willow
witloof	*see* chicory
woad	*see* isatis
wolfberry	*see* goji
wolverine's foot	*see* coltsfoot
wombwort	*see* mugwort
woodbine	*see* honeysuckle
wood boneset	*see* boneset
wood cotton	*see* eucommia
woodland bonnet	*see* codonopsis
wood of the cross	*see* mistletoe
wood root	*see* woodruff
wood-rova	*see* woodruff
wood spider	*see* devil's claw
woodward	*see* woodruff
wound weed	*see* goldenrod
woundwort	*see* comfrey *or* self-heal
wuderove	*see* woodruff
wymote	*see* marshmallow
yaupon holly	*see* yerba maté
yellow broom	*see* baptisia
yellow ginger	*see* turmeric
yellow ginseng	*see* blue cohosh
yellow gowan	*see* dandelion
yellow puccoon	*see* goldenseal
yellow root	*see* coptis *or* goldenseal
yellow vetch	*see* astragalus
yellow weed	*see* goldenrod
yellow wood	*see* prickly ash
yoqona	*see* kava kava

Index of Botanical Names

Astragalus membranaceus	*see* astragalus	*Centella asiatica*	*see* gotu kola
Astragalus mongolicus	*see* astragalus	*Chamaemelum nobile*	*see* chamomile
Atractylodes alba	*see* atractylodes	*Chamomilla recutita*	*see* chamomile
Atractylodes japonica	*see* atractylodes	*Chimaphila menziesii*	*see* pipsissewa
Atractylodes macrocephala	*see* atractylodes	*Chimaphila umbellata*	*see* pipsissewa
Avena fatua	*see* oat	*Chondrus crispus*	*see* Irish moss
Avena sativa	*see* oat	*Chrysanthemum partheniem*	*see* feverfew
Azadirachta indica	*see* neem	*Chrysanthemum vulgare*	*see* tansy
Bacopa monnieri	*see* bacopa	*Cichorium intybus*	*see* chicory
Baptisia alba	*see* baptisia	*Cimicifuga racemosa*	*see* black cohosh
Baptisia tinctoria	*see* baptisia	*Cinnamomum aromaticum*	*see* cinnamon
Barosma betulina	*see* buchu	*Cinnamomum cassia*	*see* cinnamon
Berberis aquifolium	*see* Oregon grape	*Cinnamomum verum*	*see* cinnamon
Berberis nervosa	*see* Oregon grape	*Cinnamomum zeylanicum*	*see* cinnamon
Berberis pinnata	*see* Oregon grape	*Cistanche deserticola*	*see* cistanches
Betonica officinalis	*see* wood betony	*Cistanche salsa*	*see* cistanches
Betula spp.	*see* birch	*Citrus reticulata*	*see* orange
Blainvillea acmella	*see* spilanthes	*Citrus* x *sinensis*	*see* orange
Borago officinalis	*see* borage	*Citrus* x *aurantium*	*see* orange
Boswellia carteri	*see* frankincense	*Cnicus benedictus*	*see* blessed thistle
Boswellia sacra	*see* frankincense	*Codonopsis lanceolata*	*see* codonopsis
Boswellia thurifera	*see* frankincense	*Codonopsis pilosula*	*see* codonopsis
Bupleurum chinense	*see* bupleurum	*Collinsonia canadensis*	*see* collinsonia
Bupleurum falcatum	*see* bupleurum	*Commiphora africana*	*see* guggulu
Bupleurum fruticosum	*see* bupleurum	*Commiphora molmol*	*see* myrrh
Bupleurum rotundifolium	*see* bupleurum	*Commiphora mukul*	*see* guggulu
Bupleurum scorzoneraefolium	*see* bupleurum	*Commiphora myrrha*	*see* myrrh
Calendula officinalis	*see* calendula	*Commiphora wightii*	*see* guggulu
Camellia sinensis	*see* tea	*Coptis* spp.	*see* coptis
Cannabis sativa	*see* marijuana	*Coriandrum sativum*	*see* coriander
Capsella bursa-pastoris	*see* shepherd's purse	*Corydalis ambigua*	*see* corydalis
Capsicum spp.	*see* cayenne	*Corydalis aurea*	*see* corydalis
Carbenia benedicta	*see* blessed thistle	*Corydalis bulbosa*	*see* corydalis
Carduus benedictus	*see* blessed thistle	*Corydalis cava*	*see* corydalis
Carduus marianus	*see* milk thistle	*Corydalis formosa*	*see* corydalis
Carthamus tinctorius	*see* safflower	*Corydalis solida*	*see* corydalis
Carum carvi	*see* caraway	*Corydalis turtschaninovii*	*see* corydalis
Cassia senna	*see* senna	*Corydalis yanhusuo*	*see* corydalis
Caulophyllum thalictroides	*see* blue cohosh	*Corynanthe yohimbe*	*see* yohimbe
Ceanothus americanus	*see* redroot	*Crataegus* spp.	*see* hawthorn
Centaurium erythraea	*see* centaury	*Crocus sativus*	*see* saffron
Centaurium exaltatum	*see* centaury	*Cuminum cyminum*	*see* cumin
Centaurium umbellatum	*see* centaury	*Cupania americana*	*see* guarana

Curcuma longa	*see* turmeric	*Euphrasia canadensis*	*see* eyebright
Curcuma zedoaria	*see* zedoary	*Euphrasia nemorosa*	*see* eyebright
Cymbopogon citratus	*see* lemongrass	*Euphrasia officinalis*	*see* eyebright
Daucus carota	*see* wild carrot	*Euphrasia rostkoviana*	*see* eyebright
Dioscorea batatas	*see* wild yam	*Filipendula ulmaria*	*see* meadowsweet
Dioscorea bulbifera	*see* wild yam	*Foeniculum officinale*	*see* fennel
Dioscorea japonica	*see* wild yam	*Foeniculum vulgare*	*see* fennel
Dioscorea polystachya	*see* wild yam	*Fucus vesiculosus*	*see* bladder wrack
Dioscorea villosa	*see* wild yam	*Galium aparine*	*see* cleavers
Diosma betulina	*see* buchu	*Galium odoratum*	*see* woodruff
Dipsacus spp.	*see* teasel	*Galium trifida*	*see* cleavers
Echinacea angustifolia	*see* echinacea	*Galium triflorum*	*see* cleavers
Echinacea pallida	*see* echinacea	*Galium verum*	*see* cleavers
Echinacea purpurea	*see* echinacea	*Ganoderma lucidum*	*see* reishi
Echinopanax horridus	*see* devil's club	*Garcinia atroviridis*	*see* garcinia
Eclipta alba	*see* eclipta	*Garcinia cambogia*	*see* garcinia
Eclipta prostrata	*see* eclipta	*Garcinia gummi-gutta*	*see* garcinia
Elettaria cardamomum	*see* cardamom	*Garcinia indica*	*see* garcinia
Elytrigia repens	*see* couch grass	*Gaultheria procumbens*	*see* wintergreen
Emblica officinalis	*see* amla	*Gentiana andrewsii*	*see* gentian
Ephedra distachya	*see* ephedra	*Gentiana lutea*	*see* gentian
Ephedra equisetina	*see* ephedra	*Gentiana macrophylla*	*see* gentian
Ephedra sinica	*see* ephedra	*Gentiana officinalis*	*see* gentian
Ephedra vulgaris	*see* ephedra	*Gentiana scabra*	*see* gentian
Epimedium spp.	*see* epimedium	*Gentiana villosa*	*see* gentian
Equisetum spp.	*see* horsetail	*Ginkgo biloba*	*see* ginkgo
Eriodictyon californicum	*see* yerba santa	*Glycyrrhiza glabra*	*see* licorice
Erythraea centaurium	*see* centaury	*Glycyrrhiza inflata*	*see* licorice
Erythroxylum catuaba	*see* catuaba	*Glycyrrhiza lepidota*	*see* licorice
Eschscholtzia californica	*see* California poppy	*Glycyrrhiza uralensis*	*see* licorice
Eschscholtzia mexicana	*see* California poppy	*Grindelia camporum*	*see* grindelia
		Grindelia rigida	*see* grindelia
Eucalyptus spp.	*see* eucalyptus	*Grindelia robusta*	*see* grindelia
Eucommia ulmoides	*see* eucommia	*Grindelia squarrosa*	*see* grindelia
Eugenia aromatica	*see* clove	*Gymnema sylvestre*	*see* gymnema
Eupatorium maculatum	*see* gravel root	*Hamamelis virginiana*	*see* witch hazel
Eupatorium perfoliatum	*see* boneset	*Harpagophytum procumbens*	*see* devil's claw
Eupatorium purpureum	*see* gravel root	*Hedeoma pulegioides*	*see* pennyroyal
Eupatorium rebaudianum	*see* stevia	*Hibiscus* spp.	*see* hibiscus
Eupatorium ternifolium	*see* gravel root	*Hippophae rhamnoides*	*see* sea buckthorn
Eupatorium verticullatum	*see* gravel root	*Houttuynia californica*	*see* yerba mansa
Euphrasia americana	*see* eyebright	*Humulus americanus*	*see* hops
		Humulus lupulus	*see* hops

Hydrangea arborescens	*see* hydrangea
Hydrastis canadensis	*see* goldenseal
Hydrocotyle asiatica	*see* gotu kola
Hypericum spp.	*see* Saint John's wort
Hyssopus officinalis	*see* hyssop
Ilex domestica	*see* yerba maté
Ilex mate	*see* yerba maté
Ilex paraguariensis	*see* yerba maté
Ilex sorbilis	*see* yerba maté
Illicium verum	*see* star anise
Inula conyzae	*see* elecampane
Inula helenium	*see* elecampane
Isatis indigotica	*see* isatis
Isatis tinctoria	*see* isatis
Jasminum grandiflorum	*see* jasmine
Jasminum officinale	*see* jasmine
Jasminum sambac	*see* jasmine
Juglans cinerea	*see* butternut
Juglans nigra	*see* walnut
Juglans regia	*see* walnut
Kadsura chinensis	*see* schizandra
Lactuca canadensis	*see* wild lettuce
Lactuca serriola	*see* wild lettuce
Lactuca virosa	*see* wild lettuce
Larix spp.	*see* larch
Larrea divaricata	*see* chaparral
Larrea glutinosa	*see* chaparral
Larrea mexicana	*see* chaparral
Larrea tridentata	*see* chaparral
Laurus nobilis	*see* bay
Laurus sassafras	*see* sassafras
Lavandula spp.	*see* lavender
Lentinula edodes	*see* shiitake
Lentinus edodes	*see* shiitake
Leonurus cardiaca	*see* motherwort
Lepidium meyenii	*see* maca
Lepidium peruvianum	*see* maca
Ligusticum canbyi	*see* osha
Ligusticum filicinum	*see* osha
Ligusticum grayi	*see* osha
Ligusticum porteri	*see* osha
Ligusticum scoticum	*see* osha

Ligusticum tenuifolium	*see* osha
Linum lewisii	*see* flax
Linum perenne	*see* flax
Linum usitatissimum	*see* flax
Lobelia cardinalis	*see* lobelia
Lobelia inflata	*see* lobelia
Lobelia siphilitica	*see* lobelia
Lonicera japonica	*see* honeysuckle
Lophanthus anisatus	*see* anise hyssop
Lophophora diffusa	*see* peyote
Lophophora williamsii	*see* peyote
Lycium barbarum	*see* goji
Lycium chinense	*see* goji
Lycopus americanus	*see* bugleweed
Lycopus europaeus	*see* bugleweed
Lycopus virginicus	*see* bugleweed
Mahonia aquifolium	*see* Oregon grape
Mahonia nervosa	*see* Oregon grape
Mahonia pinnata	*see* Oregon grape
Mahonia repens	*see* Oregon grape
Marrubium vulgare	*see* horehound
Matricaria chamomilla	*see* chamomile
Matricaria recutita	*see* chamomile
Medicago sativa	*see* alfalfa
Melia azadirachta	*see* neem
Melissa officinalis	*see* lemon balm
Mentha pulegium	*see* pennyroyal
Mentha spp.	*see* mint
Menyanthes trifoliata	*see* buckbean
Myrica cerifera	*see* bayberry
Myristica fragrans	*see* nutmeg
Nepeta cataria	*see* catnip
Ocimum spp.	*see* basil
Olea europaea	*see* olive
Oplopanax horridus	*see* devil's club
Origanum spp.	*see* oregano
Orobanche spp.	*see* cistanches
Paeonia albiflora	*see* peony
Paeonia lactiflora	*see* peony
Paeonia officinalis	*see* peony
Paeonia rubra	*see* peony
Paeonia suffruticosa	*see* peony
Panax ginseng	*see* ginseng

Senna italica	*see* senna	*Tilia* spp.	*see* linden
Senna marilandica	*see* senna	*Tribulus cistoides*	*see* tribulus
Senna alexandrina	*see* senna	*Tribulus terrestris*	*see* tribulus
Serenoa repens	*see* saw palmetto	*Trifolium pratense*	*see* red clover
Serenoa serrulata	*see* saw palmetto	*Trigonella foenum-graecum*	*see* fenugreek
Silybum marianum	*see* milk thistle	*Triticum repens*	*see* couch grass
Smilax aristolochiifolia	*see* sarsaparilla	*Turnera aphrodisiaca*	*see* damiana
Smilax aspera	*see* sarsaparilla	*Turnera diffusa*	*see* damiana
Smilax medica	*see* sarsaparilla	*Turnera microphylla*	*see* damiana
Smilax officinalis	*see* sarsaparilla	*Tussilago farfara*	*see* coltsfoot
Smilax ornata	*see* sarsaparilla	*Tussilago hybrida*	*see* butterbur
Smilax papyracea	*see* sarsaparilla	*Ulmus fulva*	*see* slippery elm
Smilax regelii	*see* sarsaparilla	*Ulmus rubra*	*see* slippery elm
Solidago spp.	*see* goldenrod	*Uncaria guianensis*	*see* cat's claw
Spilanthes acmella	*see* spilanthes	*Uncaria tomentosa*	*see* cat's claw
Spilanthes oleracea	*see* spilanthes	*Urtica dioica*	*see* nettle
Spiraea betulifolia	*see* meadowsweet	*Urtica urens*	*see* nettle
Spiraea lucida	*see* meadowsweet	*Usnea* spp.	*see* usnea
Spiraea ulmaria	*see* meadowsweet	*Valeriana* spp.	*see* valerian
Stachys betonica	*see* wood betony	*Vanilla planifolia*	*see* vanilla
Stachys hyssopifolia	*see* wood betony	*Vanilla pompona*	*see* vanilla
Stachys officinalis	*see* wood betony	*Verbascum densiflorum*	*see* mullein
Stachys palustris	*see* wood betony	*Verbascum phlomoides*	*see* mullein
Stachys sylvatica	*see* wood betony	*Verbascum thapsus*	*see* mullein
Stellaria alsine	*see* chickweed	*Verbena citriodora*	*see* lemon verbena
Stellaria graminea	*see* chickweed	*Verbena* spp.	*see* vervain
Stellaria media	*see* chickweed	*Verbena triphylla*	*see* lemon verbena
Stevia rebaudiana	*see* stevia	*Verbesina alba*	*see* eclipta
Stigmata maidis	*see* cornsilk	*Verbesina prostrata*	*see* eclipta
Symphytum caucasicum	*see* comfrey	*Viola odorata*	*see* violet
Symphytum officinale	*see* comfrey	*Viscum album*	*see* mistletoe
Symphytum peregrinum	*see* comfrey	*Vitex agnus-castus*	*see* vitex
Symphytum uplandicum	*see* comfrey	*Withania somnifera*	*see* ashwagandha
Syzygium aromaticum	*see* clove	*Yucca* spp.	*see* yucca
Tabebuia spp.	*see* p'au d'arco	*Zanthoxylum americanum*	*see* prickly ash
Tabeuia spp.	*see* p'au d'arco	*Zanthoxylum clava-herculis*	*see* prickly ash
Tanacetum parthenium	*see* feverfew	*Zea mays*	*see* cornsilk
Tanacetum vulgare	*see* tansy	*Zingiber officinale*	*see* ginger
Taraxacum officinale	*see* dandelion	*Ziziphus jujuba*	*see* jujube
Thea sinensis	*see* tea	*Ziziphus sativa*	*see* jujube
Theobroma cacao	*see* cacao	*Ziziphus vulgaris*	*see* jujube
Thymus spp.	*see* thyme	*Ziziphus zizyphus*	*see* jujube

General Index

Other Works by Brigitte Mars

BOOKS

Addiction Free Naturally: Liberating Yourself from Sugar, Caffeine, Food Addiction, Tobacco, Alcohol and Prescription Drugs. Rochester, VT: Healing Arts, 2001.

Dandelion Medicine: Remedies and Recipes to Detoxify, Nourish and Stimulate. North Adams, MA: Storey Books, 1999.

Beauty by Nature: Complete Body Care. Summertown, TN: Healthy Living, 2006

Elder: The Amazing Healing Benefits of Elder, the Premier Herbal Remedy for Colds and Flu. New Canaan, CT: Keats, 1997.

Healing Herbal Teas: A Complete Guide to Making Delicious, Healthful Beverages. North Bergen, NJ: Basic Health, 2006.

The HempNut Cookbook: Tasty, Omega-Rich Meals from Hempseed. Coauthored with Richard Rose and Christina Pirello. Summertown, TN: The Farm, 2004.

Herbs for Healthy Skin, Hair and Nails: Banish Eczema, Acne and Psoriasis with Healing Herbs That Cleanse the Body Inside and Out. New Canaan, CT: Keats, 1998.

Natural First Aid: Herbal Treatments for Ailments and Injuries, Emergency Preparedness, and Wilderness Safety. North Adams, MA: Storey Books, 1999.

Rawsome! Maximizing Health, Energy, and Culinary Delight with the Raw Foods Diet. North Bergen, NJ: Basic Health, 2004.

Sex, Love & Health: A Self-Help Guide to Love and Sex. North Bergen, NJ: Basic Health, 2002.

AUDIO TAPES

The Herbal Renaissance: How to Heal with Common Plants and Herbs. Louisville, CO: Sounds True, 1990.

Natural Remedies for a Healthy Immune System. Louisville, CO: Sounds True, 1990.

For information on lectures, herb walks, raw food workshops, formulations, and health consultations by the author, e-mail brigitte@indra.com, call 303-442-4967, or visit www.brigittemars.com.

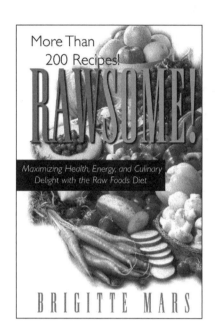

RAWSOME!

Maximizing Health, Energy, and Culinary Delight with the Raw Foods Diet

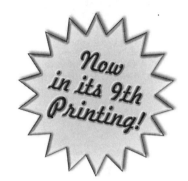

Now in its 9th Printing!

A raw foods diet advocates exactly that: raw foods. No cooking, no grilling, no steaming, no application of heat of any kind. Why? Because eating food closest to its natural state engenders a tremendous exchange of energy between food and body. The result, over time, is a feeling of buoyant, radiant health.

Tackling head-on the skepticism likely to greet proponents of what the world sees as a "fad" diet, renowned nutritionist and long-time raw-foods adherent Brigitte Mars presents historical data, case studies, and scientific evidence confirming the efficacy of raw foods diets in increasing energy levels, boosting immune system function, improving digestive function, dispelling depression, supporting emotional stability, clearing the skin, and sustaining overall good health.

In addition, Mars points out the environmental benefits of the raw foods diet, making a case for eating raw foods as a means of reducing waste, making the most of agricultural practice, and reducing the human footprint on the earth. Whether the reader wants to jump right into an all-raw diet or just wants to introduce more raw foods into the diet, Mars offers gentle encouragement and practical instruction. Readers will find advice on planning a balanced diet to meet their nutritional needs, combining foods for best effect, preserving raw foods, equipping the raw kitchen, sprouting, juicing, and every other technique that makes the raw foods diet simple, delicious, and healthful. In-depth profiles describe the nutritional and health benefits of hundreds of fruits, vegetables, nuts, and seasonings.

Perhaps most important, Mars provides more than 200 kitchen-tested, real-people-approved raw foods recipes. Under Mars's instruction, readers will enjoy making everything from juices and shakes to salads, soups, dressings, yogurts, crackers, spreads, dips, vegetable burgers, curries, vegetable pastas, wraps, and more. And let's not forget dessert: brownies, ice cream, lemon bars, fruit leathers, pies, cakes, puddings, and other delectable treats. For people who want the vibrant energy and health that raw foods offer but don't want to give up the taste of good cooking, *Rawsome!* provides the answer.

$18.95 • Trade Paperback • 368 Pages • ISBN: 978-1-59120-060-4

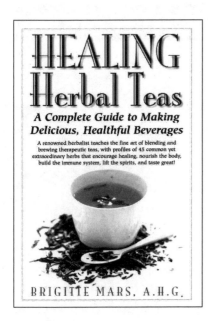

HEALING Herbal Teas

A Complete Guide to Making Delicious, Healthful Beverages

Tea infuses the precious commodity of water with plants that have transmuted the elements of sunshine and earth into nourishing constituents. It is quickly absorbed into the body, inexpensive, and easy to prepare, and its physiological interaction with the body has been proven time and again in scientific studies. In an age when people are becoming ever more aware of the importance of taking responsibility for their own health, herbal tea is an essential ally in the prevention and treatment of illness and the nourishment and support of the body, mind, and spirit.

In quick-study format, this book profiles forty-five common herbs with extraordinary healing potential. Each profile outlines the herb's major constituents, physiological effects, traditional applications, contraindications, and flavor, as well as its growth habits both in the wild and in the garden.

Mars's years of experience and talent for bringing together the wisdom of disparate cultures shine through in the author's discussion of guidelines and theories for preparing herbal formulas and maintaining good health.

$17.95 • Trade Paperback • 176 Pages • ISBN: 978-1-59120-110-6

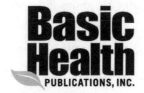

Basic Health PUBLICATIONS, INC.